POCKET BOOK

OF

Hospital care for children

GUIDELINES FOR THE MANAGEMENT OF COMMON ILLNESSES WITH LIMITED RESOURCES

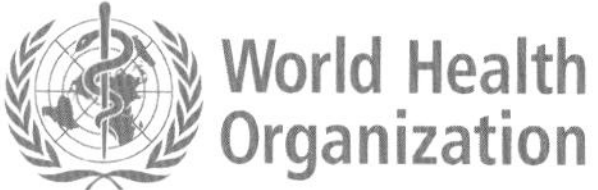

WHO Library Cataloguing-in-Publication Data

Pocket book of hospital care for children: guidelines for the management of common illnesses with limited resources.

1.Pediatrics 2.Child care 3.Hospitals 4.Child, Hospitalized 5.Developing countries 6.Practice guidelines 7.Manuals I.World Health Organization.

ISBN 92 4 154670 0 (NLM classification: WS 29)

Designed by minimum graphics
Printed in China

Contents

CHARTS

TABLES

Acknowledgements

This pocket book is the result of an international effort coordinated by the World Health Organization's Department of Child and Adolescent Health and Development.

A special debt of gratitude is owed to Dr Harry Campbell, University of Edinburgh, Scotland for the overall coordination of the preparation of the chapters of the document and significant contributions to individual chapters.

WHO would like to thank the following for their preparation of and contributions to the chapters:

Dr Ann Ashworth (UK); Dr. Stephen Bickler (USA); Dr Jacqueline Deen (Philippines), Dr Trevor Duke (PNG/Australia); Dr Greg Hussey (South Africa); Dr Michael English (Kenya); Dr Stephen Graham (Malawi); Dr Elizabeth Molyneux (Malawi); Dr Nathaniel Pierce (USA); Dr Haroon Saloojee (South Africa); Dr Barbara Stoll (USA); Dr Giorgio Tamburlini (Italy); Dr Bridget Wills (Vietnam); and Fabienne Jäger (Switzerland) for assistance in the review and revision process.

WHO is grateful to the following for reviewing the manuscript at different stages:

L. Adonis-Koffy, Côte d'Ivoire; E. Agyei-Yobo, Ghana; M. Agyemang, Ghana; R. Ahmed, Maldives; E. Akrofi-Mantey, Ghana; H., Almaraz Monzon; A. Amanor, Ghana; E. Aranda, Bolivia; W. , Asamoah, Ghana; C. Assamoi Bodjo, Côte d'Ivoire; A. Bartos, Bolivia; Z. Bhutta, Pakistan; U. Bodhankar, India; L. Bramante, Italy; L. Bravo, Philippines; D. Brewster, Vanuatu; J. Bunn, UK; K. Bylsma, Ghana; C. Casanovas, Bolivia; N. Chintu, Zambia; B. Coulter, UK; S. Cywes, South Africa; A. da Cunha, Brazil; S.-C. Daka, Cambodia; A. Deorari, India; G.F. Ding, China; V. Doku, Ghana; P. Enarson, France; J. Erskine, Gambia; F.A. Eshgh, Iran; A. Falade, Nigeria; J. Farrar, Vietnam, C. Frago, Philippines; M. Funk, Ghana; S. C. Galina, Russia; E. Gallardo, Philippines; R. Gie, South Africa; A. Grange, Nigeria; A. Hansmann, Germany; H. Hartmann, Germany; S. Heinrich, Cambodia; E.M. Hubo, Philippines; R. Ismail, Indonesia; P. Jeena, South Africa; A. Jhukral, India; S. Junge, Switzerland; V. Kapoor, India; M. Kazemian, Iran; N. Kesaree, India; E. Keshishian, Russia; H. T. Kim, Vietnam; E. Kissi Owusu, Ghana; A. Klufio, Ghana; J. Kouawo, Côte d'Ivoire; M. Krawinkel, Germany; B. Kretschmer, Germany; C. Krueger, Germany; A. Krug, South Africa; M. Langaroodi; J. Lawn, UK; J. Lim, Philippines; W. Loening, South Africa;

M.P. Loscertales, Spain; C. Maclennan, Australia; A. Madkour, Egypt; I. Mahama, Ghana; D. Malchinkhuu, Mongolia; N. Manjavidze, Georgia; P. Mazmanyan, Armenia; D. Mei, China; A. Mekasha, Ethiopia; C.A. Melean Gumiel, Bolivia; C. Meng, Cambodia; W. Min, China; H. Mozafari, Iran; K. Mulholland, Australia; A. Narang, India; S. Nariman, Iran; K.J. Nathoo, Zimbabwe; K. Nel, South Africa; S. K. Newton, Ghana; K. Olness, USA; K. Pagava, Georgia; V. Paul, India; I. Rahman, Sudan; M. Rakha, Egypt; S.E. Razmikovna, Russia; R. Rios, Chile; H. Rode, South Africa; E. Rodgers, Fiji; I. Ryumina, Russia; I. Sagoe-Moses, Ghana; G. Sall, Senegal; L. C. Sambath, Cambodia; W. Sangu, Tanzania; J. Schmitz, France; F. Shann, Australia; P. Sharma, Nepal; M. Shebbe, Kenya; L. Sher, South Africa; N. Singhal, Canada; D. Southall, UK; J.-W. Sun, China; G. Swingler, South Africa; T.T. Tam, Vietnam; E. Tanoh; M. Taylor, Ghana; E. Teye Adjase, Ghana; I. Thawe, Malawi; M. Timite-Konan, Côte d'Ivoire; P. Torzillo, Australia; R. Turki, Tunisia; F. Uxa, Italy; D.-H. Wang, China; D. Woods, South Africa; B.J. Wudil, Nigeria; A.J. Yao, Côte d'Ivoire.

Valuable inputs were provided by the WHO Clusters of Communicable Diseases and of Non Communicable Diseases, and WHO Departments of Disability/Injury Prevention and Rehabilitation, Essential Drugs and Medicines Policy, Essential Health Technology, HIV/AIDS, Nutrition for Health and Development, Protection of the Human Environment, Reproductive Health and Research, Roll Back Malaria, Stop Tuberculosis, and Vaccines and Biologicals and by WHO Regional Offices.

WHO wishes to thank the following organizations who contributed to the production of the pocket book:

Australian Agency for International Development (AusAID); Institute for Child Health IRCCS "Burlo Garofolo", Trieste, Italy; and the International Paediatric Association.

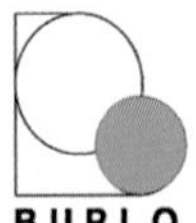

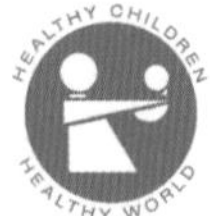

international pediatric association
association internationale de pédiatrie
asociación internacional de pediatría

Foreword

This pocket book is for use by doctors, senior nurses and other senior health workers who are responsible for the care of young children at the first referral level in developing countries. It presents up-to-date clinical guidelines which are based on a review of the available published evidence by subject experts, for both inpatient and outpatient care in small hospitals where basic laboratory facilities and essential drugs and inexpensive medicines are available. In some settings, these guidelines can be used in the larger health centres where a small number of sick children can be admitted for inpatient care.

The guidelines require the hospital to have (1) the capacity to carry out certain essential investigations—such as blood smear examinations for malaria parasites, estimations of haemoglobin or packed cell volume, blood glucose, blood grouping and cross-matching, basic microscopy of CSF and urine, bilirubin determination for neonates, chest radiography and pulse oximetry—and (2) essential drugs available for the care of seriously ill children. Expensive treatment options, such as new antibiotics or mechanical ventilation, are not described.

These guidelines focus on the inpatient management of the major causes of childhood mortality, such as pneumonia, diarrhoea, severe malnutrition, malaria, meningitis, measles, and related conditions. They contain guidance on the management of children with HIV infection, neonates with problems, and of the surgical management of children. Details of the principles underlying the guidelines can be found in technical review papers published by WHO. A companion background book has also been published by WHO which gives details of burden of disease, pathophysiology and technical basis underlying the guidelines for use by medical/nursing students or as part of inservice training of health workers. The evidence-base underlying these recommendations is published on the WHO website as well. (See Further Reading, page 301.)

This pocket book is part of a series of documents and tools that support the Integrated Management of Childhood Illness (IMCI) and is consistent with the IMCI guidelines for outpatient management of sick children. It is presented in a format that could be carried by doctors, nurses and other health workers during their daily work and so be available to help guide the management of sick children. Standard textbooks of paediatrics should be consulted for rarer conditions not covered in the pocketbook. These guidelines are applicable in most areas of the world and may be adapted by countries to suit their specific circumstances. Blank pages have been left at the end of each chapter to allow individual readers to include their own notes—for example, on locally important conditions not covered in this pocket book.

WHO believes that their widespread adoption would improve the care of children in hospital and lead to lower case fatality rates.

Abbreviations

AIDS	acquired immunodeficiency syndrome
AVPU	simple consciousness scale (**a**lert, responding to **v**oice, responding to **p**ain, **u**nconscious)
BP	blood pressure
CMV	cytomegalovirus
CSF	cerebrospinal fluid
DHF	dengue haemorrhagic fever
DPT	diphtheria, pertussis, tetanus
DSS	dengue shock syndrome
EPI	expanded programme of immunization
FG	French gauge
G6PD	glucose 6-phosphate dehydrogenase
HIV	human immunodeficiency virus
HUS	haemolytic uraemic syndrome
IM	intramuscular injection
IMCI	Integrated Management of Childhood Illness
IV	intravenous injection
JVP	jugular venous pressure
LIP	lymphoid interstitial pneumonitis
LP	lumbar puncture
NG	nasogastric
OPV	oral polio vaccine
ORS	oral rehydration salts
ORT	oral rehydration therapy
PCP	*Pneumocystis carinii* pneumonia
PCV	packed cell volume
PPD	purified protein derivative (used in a test for tuberculosis)
ReSoMal	rehydration solution for malnutrition
RDA	recommended daily allowance
SD	standard deviation
SP	sulfadoxine-pyrimethamine
STI	sexually transmitted infection
TB	tuberculosis
TMP	trimethoprim
TPHA	treponema pallidum haemogglutination
SMX	sulfamethoxazole
UTI	urinary tract infection
VDRL	veneral disease research laboratories
WBC	white blood cell count
WHO	World Health Organization
°C	degrees Celsius
°F	degrees Fahrenheit

■ diagnostic sign or symptom

➤ treatment recommendation

CHART 1. Stages in the management of the sick child admitted to hospital: summary of key elements

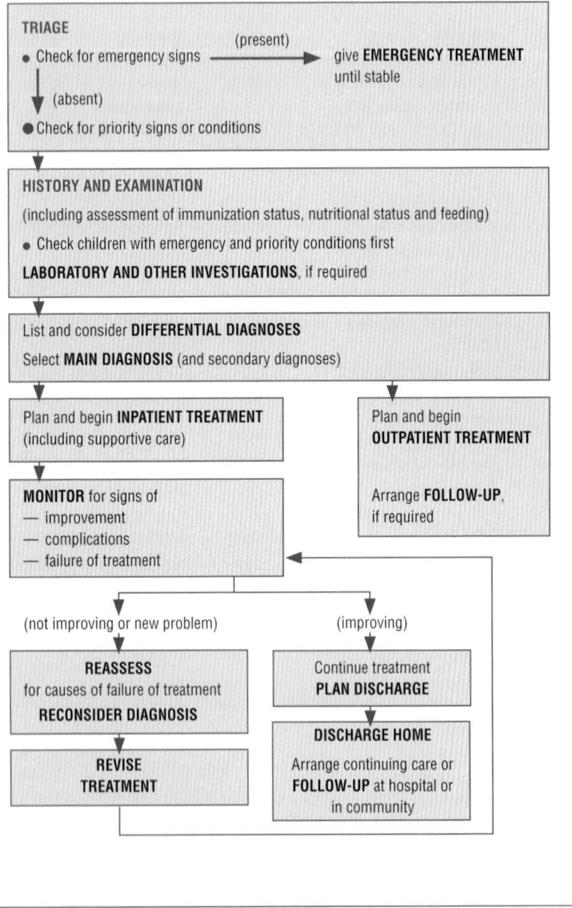

CHAPTER 1

Triage and emergency conditions

Triage is the process of rapidly screening sick children soon after their arrival in hospital in order to identify:

- — those with ***emergency signs***, who require immediate emergency treatment;
- — those with ***priority signs***, who should be given priority while waiting in the queue so that they can be assessed and treated without delay;
- — ***non-urgent*** cases, who have neither emergency nor priority signs.

Emergency signs include:

- obstructed breathing
- severe respiratory distress
- central cyanosis
- signs of shock (cold hands; capillary refill longer than 3 seconds; weak, fast pulse)
- coma
- convulsions
- signs of severe dehydration in a child with diarrhoea (lethargy, sunken eyes, very slow return after pinching the skin—any two of these).

Children with emergency signs require ***immediate*** treatment to avert death.

The priority signs (see below, page 5) identify children who are at higher risk of dying. These children should be ***assessed without unnecessary delay***.

1.1 Summary of steps in emergency triage assessment and treatment

The process of emergency triage assessment and treatment is summarized in the Charts on pages 4–16.

First, check for ***emergency signs****.*

Check for emergency signs in two steps:

- **Step 1**. If there is any airway or breathing problem, start immediate treatment to restore breathing.
- **Step 2**. Quickly determine if the child is in shock or unconscious or convulsing, or has diarrhoea with severe dehydration.

If emergency signs are found:

- Call an experienced health professional to help if available, but do not delay starting the treatment. Stay calm and work with other health workers who may be required to give the treatment, because a very sick child may need several treatments at once. The most experienced health professional should continue assessing the child (see Chapter 2, page 37), to identify all underlying problems and develop a treatment plan.

- Carry out emergency investigations (blood glucose, blood smear, haemoglobin). Send blood for typing and cross-matching if the child is in shock, or appears to be severely anaemic, or is bleeding significantly.
- After giving emergency treatment, proceed immediately to assessing, diagnosing and treating the underlying problem.

Tables of common differential diagnoses for emergency signs are provided from page 20 onwards.

If no emergency signs are found, check for priority signs:

- **T**iny baby: any sick child aged under 2 months
- **T**emperature: child is very hot
- **T**rauma or other urgent surgical condition
- **P**allor (severe)
- **P**oisoning
- **P**ain (severe)
- **R**espiratory distress
- **R**estless, continuously irritable, or lethargic
- **R**eferral (urgent)
- **M**alnutrition: visible severe wasting
- **O**edema of both feet
- **B**urns (major)

The above can be remembered with the help of "3TPR MOB".

These children need prompt assessment (no waiting in the queue) to determine what further treatment is needed. Move the child with any priority sign to the front of the queue to be assessed next. If a child has trauma or other surgical problems, get surgical help where available.

CHART 2. Triage of all sick children

EMERGENCY SIGNS

If any sign positive: give treatment(s), call for help, draw blood for emergency laboratory investigations (glucose, malaria smear, Hb)

ASSESS		TREAT *Do not move neck if cervical spine injury possible*
Airway and breathing ■ Obstructed breathing, *or* ■ Central cyanosis, *or* ■ Severe respiratory distress	***ANY SIGN POSITIVE***	**If foreign body aspiration** ➤ Manage airway in choking child (Chart 3) **If no foreign body aspiration** ➤ Manage airway (Chart 4) ➤ Give oxygen (Chart 5) ➤ Make sure child is warm
Circulation Cold hands with: ■ Capillary refill longer than 3 seconds, *and* ■ Weak and fast pulse	***ANY SIGN POSITIVE*** *Check for severe malnutrition*	➤ Stop any bleeding ➤ Give oxygen (Chart 5) ➤ Make sure child is warm **If no severe malnutrition:** ➤ Insert IV and begin giving fluids rapidly (Chart 7) If not able to insert peripheral IV, insert an intraosseous or external jugular line (see pages 310, 312) **If severe malnutrition:** *If lethargic or unconscious:* ➤ Give IV glucose (Chart 10) ➤ Insert IV line and give fluids (Chart 8) *If not lethargic or unconscious:* ➤ Give glucose orally or by NG tube ➤ Proceed immediately to full assessment and treatment

CHART 2. Triage of all sick children (*continued*)

EMERGENCY SIGNS

If any sign positive: give treatment(s), call for help, draw blood for emergency laboratory investigations (glucose, malaria smear, Hb)

ASSESS		TREAT *Do not move neck if cervical spine injury possible*
Coma/convulsing ■ Coma *or* ■ Convulsing (now)	***IF COMA OR CONVULSING***	➤ Manage airway (Chart 3) ➤ If convulsing, give diazepam or paraldehyde rectally (Chart 9) ➤ Position the unconscious child (if head or neck trauma is suspected, stabilize the neck first) (Chart 6) ➤ Give IV glucose (Chart 10)
Severe dehydration *(only in child with diarrhoea)* Diarrhoea plus any two of these: ■ Lethargy ■ Sunken eyes ■ Very slow skin pinch	***DIARRHOEA plus*** ***TWO SIGNS POSITIVE*** *Check for severe malnutrition*	➤ Make sure child is warm. **If no severe malnutrition:** ➤ Insert IV line and begin giving fluids rapidly following Chart 11 and Diarrhoea Treatment Plan C in hospital (Chart 13, page 114) **If severe malnutrition:** ➤ Do **not** insert IV ➤ Proceed immediately to full assessment and treatment (see section 1.3, page 18)

PRIORITY SIGNS

These children need prompt assessment and treatment

- Tiny baby (<2 months)
- Temperature very high
- Trauma or other urgent surgical condition
- Pallor (severe)
- Poisoning (history of)
- Pain (severe)
- Respiratory distress
- Restless, continuously irritable, or lethargic
- Referral (urgent)
- Malnutrition: visible severe wasting
- Oedema of both feet
- Burns (major)

Note: If a child has trauma or other surgical problems, get surgical help or follow surgical guidelines

NON-URGENT

Proceed with assessment and further treatment according to the child's priority

CHART 3. How to manage the choking infant

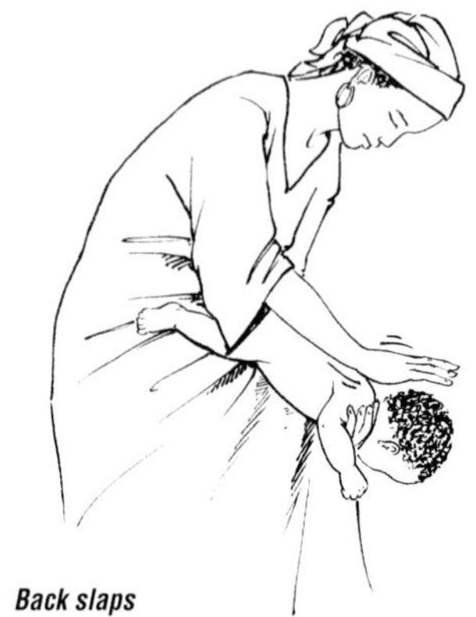

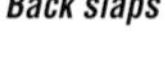

Back slaps

- ➤ Lay the infant on your arm or thigh in a head down position
- ➤ Give 5 blows to the infant's back with heel of hand
- ➤ If obstruction persists, turn infant over and give 5 chest thrusts with 2 fingers, one finger breadth below nipple level in midline (see diagram)
- ➤ If obstruction persists, check infant's mouth for any obstruction which can be removed
- ➤ If necessary, repeat sequence with back slaps again

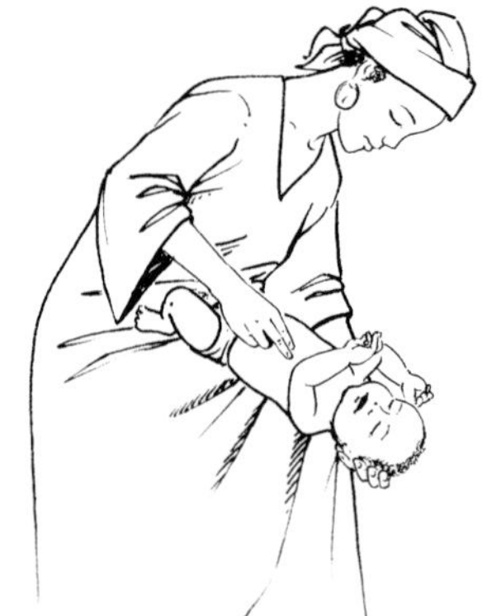

Chest thrusts

CHART 3. How to manage the choking child (over 1 year of age)

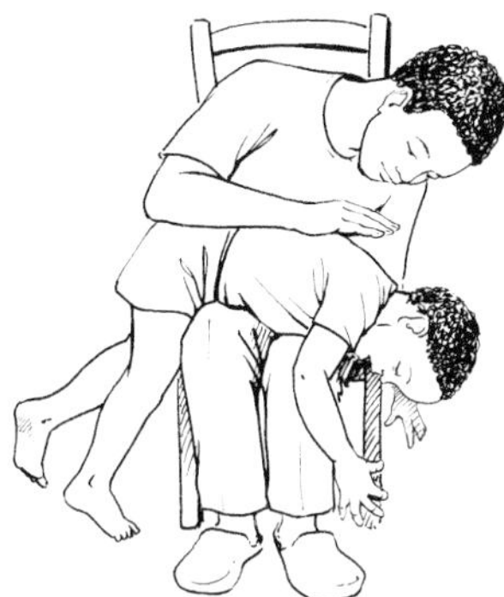

Slapping the back to clear airway obstruction in a choking child

- Give 5 blows to the child's back with heel of hand with child sitting, kneeling or lying
- If the obstruction persists, go behind the child and pass your arms around the child's body; form a fist with one hand immediately below the child's sternum; place the other hand over the fist and pull upwards into the abdomen (see diagram); repeat this Heimlich manoeuvre 5 times
- If the obstruction persists, check the child's mouth for any obstruction which can be removed
- If necessary, repeat this sequence with back slaps again

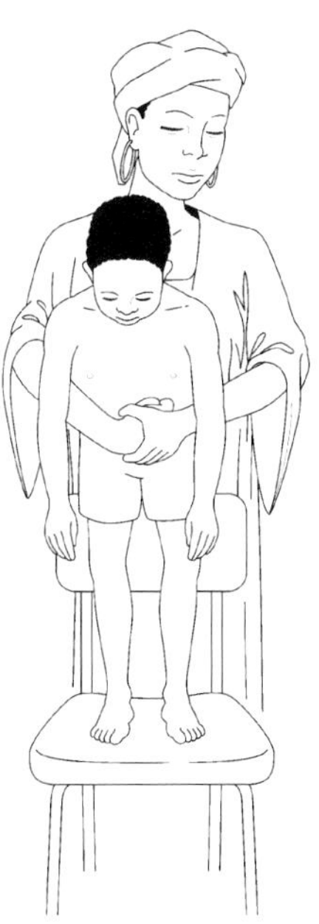

Heimlich manoeuvre in a choking older child

CHART 4. How to manage the airway in a child with obstructed breathing (or who has just stopped breathing) where no neck trauma is suspected

Child conscious

1. Inspect mouth and remove foreign body, if present
2. Clear secretions from throat
3. Let child assume position of maximal comfort

■ INFANT

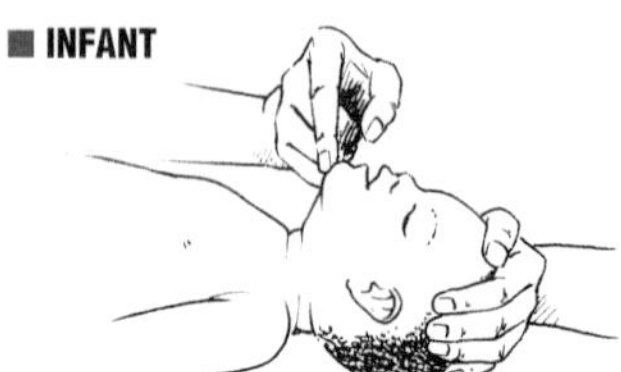

Neutral position to open the airway in an infant

Child unconscious

1. Tilt the head as shown
2. Inspect mouth and remove foreign body, if present
3. Clear secretions from throat
4. Check the airway by looking for chest movements, listening for breath sounds and feeling for breath

■ OLDER CHILD

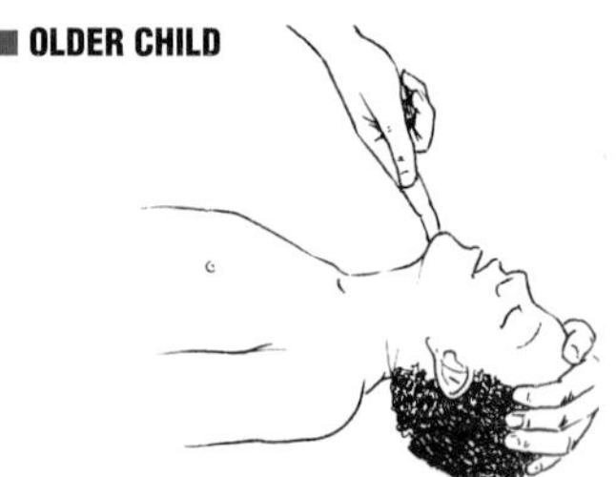

Sniffing position to open the airway in an older child

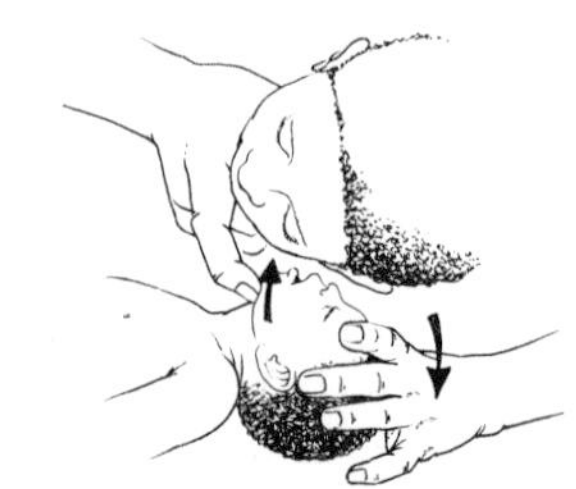

Look, listen and feel for breathing

CHART 4. How to manage the airway in a child with obstructed breathing (or who has just stopped breathing) where neck trauma or possible cervical spine injury is suspected

1. Stabilize the neck, as shown in Chart 6
2. Inspect mouth and remove foreign body, if present
3. Clear secretions from throat
4. Check the airway by looking for chest movements, listening for breath sounds, and feeling for breath

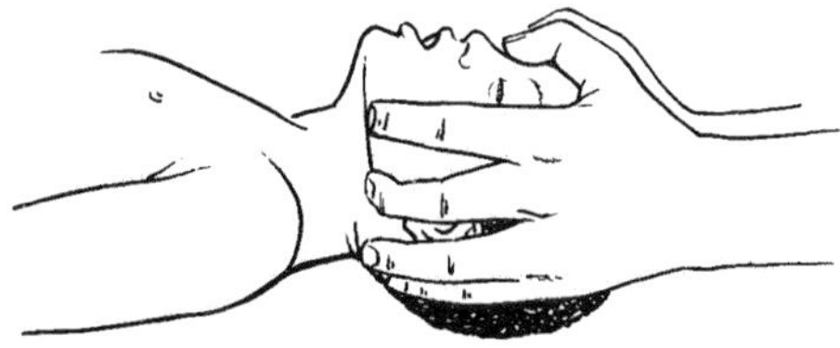

Use jaw thrust without head tilt. Place the 4th and 5th finger behind the angle of the jaw and move it upwards so that the bottom of the jaw is thrust forwards, at 90° to the body

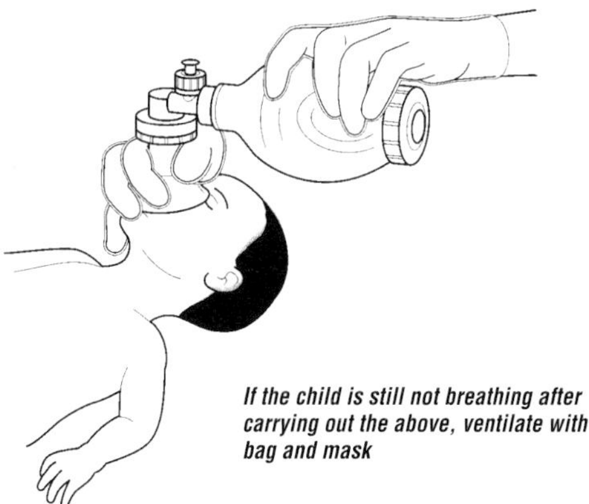

If the child is still not breathing after carrying out the above, ventilate with bag and mask

CHART 5. How to give oxygen

Give oxygen through nasal prongs or a nasal catheter

■ Nasal Prongs

➤ Place the prongs just inside the nostrils and secure with tape.

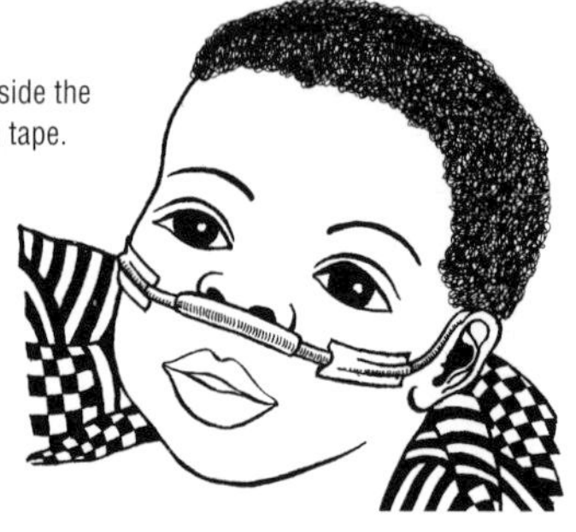

■ Nasal Catheter

➤ Use an 8 FG size tube

➤ Measure the distance from the side of the nostril to the inner eyebrow margin with the catheter

➤ Insert the catheter to this depth

➤ Secure with tape

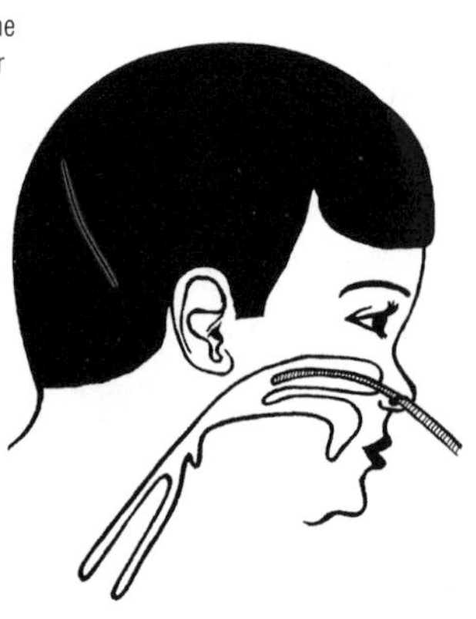

Start oxygen flow at 1–2 litres/minute (see pages 281–284)

CHART 6. How to position the unconscious child

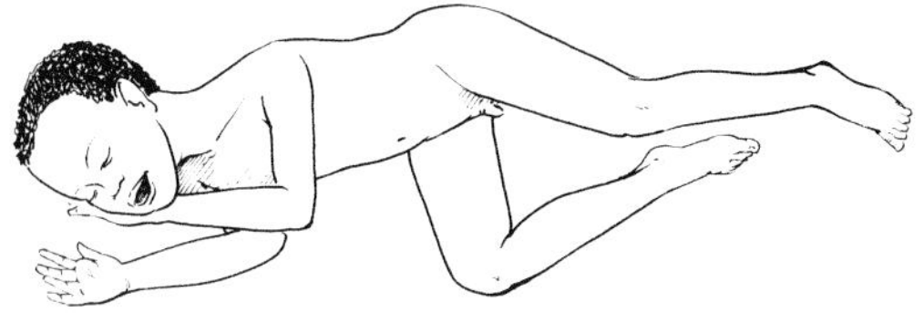

■ If neck trauma is not suspected:

- ➤ Turn the child on the side to reduce risk of aspiration.
- ➤ Keep the neck slightly extended and stabilize by placing cheek on one hand
- ➤ Bend one leg to stabilize the body position

■ If neck trauma is suspected:

- ➤ Stabilize the child's neck and keep the child lying on the back:
- ➤ Tape the child's forehead and chin to the sides of a firm board to secure this position
- ➤ Prevent the neck from moving by supporting the child's head (e.g. using litre bags of IV fluid on each side)
- ➤ If vomiting, turn on the side, keeping the head in line with the body.

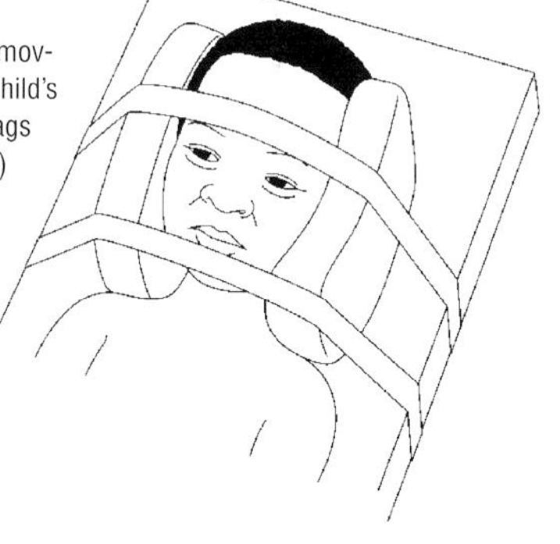

CHART 7. How to give IV fluids rapidly for shock in a child without severe malnutrition

➤ If the child is severely malnourished the fluid volume and rate are different, so check that the child is not severely malnourished

Shock in child without severe malnutrition—Chart 7
Shock in child with severe malnutrition—Chart 8 (and section 1.3, page 18)

➤ Insert an intravenous line (and draw blood for emergency laboratory investigations).

➤ Attach Ringer's lactate or normal saline—make sure the infusion is running well.

➤ Infuse 20 ml/kg as rapidly as possible.

Age/weight	Volume of Ringer's lactate or normal saline solution (20 ml/kg)
2 months (<4 kg)	75 ml
2–<4 months (4–<6 kg)	100 ml
4–<12 months (6–<10 kg)	150 ml
1–<3 years (10–<14 kg)	250 ml
3–<5 years (14–19 kg)	350 ml

Reassess child after appropriate volume has run in

Reassess after first infusion:	If no improvement, repeat 20 ml/kg as rapidly as possible.
Reassess after second infusion:	If no improvement, repeat 20 ml/kg as rapidly as possible.
Reassess after third infusion:	If no improvement, give blood 20 ml/kg over 30 minutes (if shock is not caused by profuse diarrhoea, in this case repeat Ringer's lactate or normal saline).
Reassess after fourth infusion:	If no improvement, see disease-specific treatment guidelines. You should have established a provisional diagnosis by now.

After improvement at any stage (pulse slows, faster capillary refill), go to Chart 11, page 16.

CHART 8. How to give IV fluids for shock in a child with severe malnutrition

Give this treatment only if the child has signs of shock ***and is lethargic or has lost consciousness***:

- Insert an IV line (and draw blood for emergency laboratory investigations)
- Weigh the child (or estimate the weight) to calculate the volume of fluid to be given
- Give IV fluid 15 ml/kg over 1 hour. Use one of the following solutions (in order of preference), according to availability:
  - Ringer's lactate with 5% glucose (dextrose); or
  - half-normal saline with 5% glucose (dextrose); or
  - half-strength Darrow's solution with 5% glucose (dextrose); or, if these are unavailable,
  - Ringer's lactate.

Weight	Volume IV fluid Give over 1 hour (15 ml/kg)	Weight	Volume IV fluid Give over 1 hour (15 ml/kg)
4 kg	60 ml	12 kg	180 ml
6 kg	90 ml	14 kg	210 ml
8 kg	120 ml	16 kg	240 ml
10 kg	150 ml	18 kg	270 ml

- Measure the pulse and breathing rate at the start and every 5–10 minutes.

  If there are signs of improvement (pulse and respiratory rates fall):
  - give repeat IV 15 ml/kg over 1 hour; then
  - switch to oral or nasogastric rehydration with ReSoMal (see page 179), 10 ml/kg/h up to 10 hours;
  - initiate refeeding with starter F-75 (see page 184).

  If the child fails to improve after the first 15ml/kg IV, assume the child has septic shock:
  - give maintenance IV fluid (4 ml/kg/h) while waiting for blood;
  - when blood is available, transfuse fresh whole blood at 10 ml/kg *slowly* over 3 hours (use packed cells if in cardiac failure); then
  - initiate refeeding with starter F-75 (see page 184);
  - start antibiotic treatment (see page 182).

  If the child deteriorates during the IV rehydration (breathing increases by 5 breaths/min or pulse by 15 beats/min), stop the infusion because IV fluid can worsen the child's condition.

CHART 9. How to give diazepam (or paraldehyde) rectally

■ **Give diazepam rectally:**

➤ Draw up the dose from an ampoule of diazepam into a tuberculin (1 ml) syringe. Base the dose on the weight of the child, where possible. Then remove the needle.

➤ Insert the syringe into the rectum 4 to 5 cm and inject the diazepam solution.

➤ Hold buttocks together for a few minutes.

	Diazepam given rectally 10 mg/2ml solution		Paraldehyde given rectally
Age/weight	**Dose 0.1ml/kg**		**Dose 0.3–0.4 ml/kg**
2 weeks to 2 months (<4 kg)*	0.3 ml	(1.5 mg)	1.0 ml
2–<4 months (4–<6 kg)	0.5 ml	(2.5 mg)	1.6 ml
4–<12 months (6–<10 kg)	1.0 ml	(5 mg)	2.4 ml
1–<3 years (10–<14 kg)	1.25 ml	(6.25 mg)	4 ml
3–<5 years (14–19 kg)	1.5 ml	(7.5 mg)	5 ml

If convulsion continues after 10 minutes, give a second dose of diazepam rectally (or give diazepam intravenously (0.05 ml/kg = 0.25 mg/kg) if IV infusion is running).

If convulsion continues after another 10 minutes, give a third dose of diazepam or give paraldehyde rectally (or phenobarbital IV or IM 15 mg/kg).

■ **If high fever:**

➤ Sponge the child with room-temperature water to reduce the fever.

➤ Do not give oral medication until the convulsion has been controlled (danger of aspiration).

* Use phenobarbital (200 mg/ml solution) in a dose of 20 mg/kg to control convulsions in infants <2 weeks of age:

Weight 2 kg—initial dose: 0.2 ml, repeat 0.1 ml after 30 minute } if convulsions continue

Weight 3 kg—initial dose: 0.3 ml, repeat 0.15 ml after 30 minute } if convulsions continue

CHART 10. How to give IV glucose

- ➤ Insert IV line and draw blood for emergency laboratory investigations
- ➤ Check blood glucose. If low (<2.5 mmol/litre (45 mg/dl) in a well nourished or <3 mmol/litre (54 mg/dl) in a severely malnourished child) or if dextrostix is not available:
- ➤ Give 5 ml/kg of 10% glucose solution rapidly by IV injection

Age/weight	Volume of 10% glucose solution to give as bolus (5 ml/kg)
Less than 2 months (<4 kg)	15 ml
2–<4 months (4–<6 kg)	25 ml
4–<12 months (6–<10 kg)	40 ml
1–<3 years (10–<14 kg)	60 ml
3–<5 years (14–<19 kg)	80 ml

- ➤ Recheck the blood glucose in 30 minutes. If it is still low, repeat 5 ml/kg of 10% glucose solution.
- ➤ Feed the child as soon as conscious.

  If not able to feed without danger of aspiration, give:

  - — milk or sugar solution via nasogastric tube (to make sugar solution, dissolve 4 level teaspoons of sugar (20 grams) in a 200-ml cup of clean water), or
  - — IV fluids containing 5–10% glucose (dextrose) (see App. 4, p. 357)

Note: 50% glucose solution is the same as 50% dextrose solution or D50.
If only 50% glucose solution is available: dilute 1 part 50% glucose solution to 4 parts sterile water, or dilute 1 part 50% glucose solution to 9 parts 5% glucose solution.

Note: For the use of dextrostix, refer to instruction on box. Generally, the strip must be stored in its box, at 2–3 °C, avoiding sunlight or high humidity. A drop of blood should be placed on the strip (it is necessary to cover all the reagent area). After 60 seconds, the blood should be washed off gently with drops of cold water and the colour compared with the key on the bottle or on the blood glucose reader. (The exact procedure will vary with different strips.)

CHART 11. How to treat severe dehydration in an emergency setting after initial management of shock

For children with severe dehydration but without shock, refer to diarrhoea treatment plan C, p.114.

If the child is in shock, first follow the instructions in Charts 7 and 8 (pages 12 and 13). Switch to the present chart when the child's pulse becomes slower or the capillary refill is faster.

➤ Give 70 ml/kg of Ringer's lactate solution (or, if not available, normal saline) over 5 hours in infants (aged <12 months) and over 2½ hours in children (aged 12 months to 5 years).

Weight	Total volume IV fluid (volume per hour)	
	Age <12 months Give over 5 hours	Age 12 months to 5 years Give over 2½ hours
<4 kg	200 ml (40 ml/h)	—
4–6 kg	350 ml (70 ml/h)	—
6–10 kg	550 ml (110 ml/h)	550 ml (220 ml/h)
10–14 kg	850 ml (170 ml/h)	850 ml (340 ml/h)
14–19 kg	—	1200 ml (480 ml/h)

Reassess the child every 1–2 hours. If the hydration status is not improving, give the IV drip more rapidly

Also give ORS solution (about 5 ml/kg/hour) as soon as the child can drink; this is usually after 3–4 hours (in infants) or 1–2 hours (in children).

Weight	Volume of ORS solution per hour
<4 kg	15 ml
4–6 kg	25 ml
6–10 kg	40 ml
10–14 kg	60 ml
14–19 kg	85 ml

Reassess after 6 hours (infants) and after 3 hours (children). Classify dehydration. Then choose the appropriate plan (A, B, or C, pages 120, 117, 114) to continue treatment.

If possible, observe the child for at least 6 hours after rehydration to be sure that the mother can maintain hydration by giving the child ORS solution by mouth.

1.2 Notes for the assessment of emergency and priority signs

■ Assess the airway and breathing (A, B)

Does the child's breathing appear obstructed? Look and listen to determine if there is poor air movement during breathing.

Is there severe respiratory distress? The breathing is very laboured, the child uses auxiliary muscles for breathing (shows head nodding), is breathing very fast, and the child appears to tire easily. Child is not able to feed because of respiratory distress.

Is there central cyanosis? There is a bluish/purplish discoloration of the tongue and the inside of the mouth.

■ Assess circulation (for shock) (C)

Check if the child's hand is cold? If so

Check if the capillary refill time is longer than 3 seconds. Apply pressure to whiten the nail of the thumb or the big toe for 3 seconds. Determine the time from the moment of release until total recovery of the pink colour.

If capillary refill takes longer than 3 seconds, check the pulse. Is it weak and fast? If the radial pulse is strong and not obviously fast, the child is ***not*** in shock. If you cannot feel a radial pulse of an infant (less than 1 year old), feel the brachial pulse or, if the infant is lying down, the femoral pulse. If you cannot feel the radial pulse of a child, feel the carotid. If the room is very cold, rely on the pulse to determine whether the child may be in shock.

■ Assess for coma or convulsions or other abnormal mental status (C)

Is the child in coma? Check the level of consciousness on the AVPU scale:

A alert,
V responds to voice,
P responds to pain,
U unconscious.

If the child is not awake and alert, try to rouse the child by talking or shaking the arm. If the child is not alert, but responds to voice, he is lethargic. If there is no response, ask the mother if the child has been abnormally sleepy or difficult to wake. Look if the child responds to pain, or if he is unresponsive to a painful stimulus. If this is the case, the child is in coma (unconscious) and needs emergency treatment.

Is the child convulsing? Are there spasmodic repeated movements in an unresponsive child?

■ Assess for severe dehydration if the child has diarrhoea (D)

Does the child have sunken eyes? Ask the mother if the child's eyes are more sunken than usual.

Does a skin pinch go back very slowly (longer than 2 seconds)? Pinch the skin of the abdomen halfway between the umbilicus and the side for 1 second, then release and observe.

■ Assess for priority signs

While assessing for emergency signs, you will have noted several possible priority signs:

Is there any respiratory distress (not severe)?
Is the child lethargic or continuously irritable or restless?

This was noted when you assessed for coma.

Note the other priority signs (see page 5).

1.3 Notes for giving emergency treatment to the child with severe malnutrition

During the triage process, all children with severe malnutrition will be identified as having *priority signs*, which means that they require prompt assessment and treatment.

A few children with severe malnutrition will be found during triage assessment to have ***emergency signs***.

- Those with emergency signs for "*airway and breathing*" and "*coma or convulsions*" should receive emergency treatment accordingly (see charts on pages 4–16).
- Those with signs of *severe dehydration* but not shock should **not** be rehydrated with IV fluids. This is because the diagnosis of severe dehydration is difficult in severe malnutrition and is often misdiagnosed. Giving IV fluids puts these children at risk of overhydration and death from heart failure. Therefore, these children should be rehydrated *orally* using the special rehydration solution for severe malnutrition (ReSoMal). See Chapter 7 (page 179).
- Those with signs of *shock* are assessed for further signs (*lethargic or unconscious*). This is because in severe malnutrition the usual emergency signs for shock may be present even when there is no shock.
  - — If the child is *lethargic or unconscious*, keep warm and give 10% glucose 5 ml/kg IV (see Chart 10, page 15), and then IV fluids (see Chart 8, page 13, and the Note given below).

— If the child is *alert*, keep warm and give 10% glucose (10 ml/kg) by mouth or nasogastric tube, and proceed to immediate full assessment and treatment. See Chapter 7 (page 173) for details.

Note: When giving IV fluids, treatment for shock differs from that for a well-nourished child. This is because shock from dehydration and sepsis are likely to coexist and these are difficult to differentiate on clinical grounds alone. Children with dehydration respond to IV fluids (breathing and pulse rates fall, faster capillary refill). Those with septic shock and no dehydration will not respond. The amount of fluid given should be guided by the child's response. Avoid overhydration. Monitor the pulse and breathing at the start and every 5–10 minutes to check if improving or not. Note that the type of IV fluid also differs in severe malnutrition, and the infusion rate is slower.

All severely malnourished children require prompt assessment and treatment to deal with serious problems such as hypoglycaemia, hypothermia, severe infection, severe anaemia and potentially blinding eye problems. It is equally important to take prompt action to prevent some of these problems, if they were not present at the time of admission to hospital.

1.4 **Diagnostic considerations of children presenting with emergency conditions**

The following text provides guidance for the approach to the diagnosis and the differential diagnosis of presenting conditions for which emergency treatment has been provided. After you have stabilized the child and provided emergency treatment, determine the underlying cause of the problem, to be able to provide specific curative treatment. The following lists and tables provide some guidance which help with the differential diagnosis, and are complemented by the tables in the symptom-specific chapters.

1.4.1 **Child presenting with an airway or severe breathing problem**

History

- Onset of symptoms: slowly developing or sudden onset
- Previous similar episodes
- Upper respiratory tract infection
- Cough
  — duration in days
- History of choking
- Present since birth, or acquired
- Immunization history
  — DTP, measles

(*continued on page 21*)

Table 1. Differential diagnosis of the child presenting with an airway or severe breathing problem

Diagnosis or underlying cause	In favour
Pneumonia	— Cough with fast breathing and fever — Development over days, getting worse — Crepitations on auscultation
Asthma	— History of recurrent wheezing — Prolonged expiration — Wheezing or reduced air entry — Response to bronchodilators
Foreign body aspiration	— History of sudden choking — Sudden onset of stridor or respiratory distress — Focal reduced air entry or wheeze
Retropharyngeal abscess	— Slow development over days, getting worse — Inability to swallow — High fever
Croup	— Barking cough — Hoarse voice — Associated with upper respiratory tract infection
Diphtheria	— Bull neck appearance of neck due to enlarged lymph nodes — Red throat — Grey pharyngeal membrane — No DTP vaccination

Table 2. Differential diagnosis of the child presenting with shock

Diagnosis or underlying cause	In favour
Bleeding shock	— History of trauma — Bleeding site
Dengue shock syndrome	— Known dengue outbreak or season — History of high fever — Purpura
Cardiac shock	— History of heart disease — Enlarged neck veins and liver
Septic shock	— History of febrile illness — Very ill child — Known outbreak of meningococcal infection
Shock associated with severe dehydration	— History of profuse diarrhoea — Known cholera outbreak

- Known HIV infection
- Family history of asthma

Examination

- Cough
  — quality of cough
- Cyanosis
- Respiratory distress
- Grunting
- Stridor, abnormal breath sounds
- Nasal flaring
- Swelling of the neck
- Crepitations
- Wheezing
  — generalized
  — focal
- Reduced air entry
  — generalized
  — focal

1.4.2 **Child presenting with shock**

History

- Acute or sudden onset
- Trauma
- Bleeding
- History of congenital or rheumatic heart disease
- History of diarrhoea
- Any febrile illness
- Known dengue outbreak
- Known meningitis outbreak
- Fever
- Able to feed

Examination

- Consciousness
- Any bleeding sites
- Neck veins
- Liver size
- Petechiae
- Purpura

1.4.3 Child presenting with lethargy, unconsciousness or convulsions

History

Determine if there is a history of:

- fever
- head injury
- drug overdose or toxin ingestion
- convulsions: How long do they last? Have there been previous febrile convulsions? Epilepsy?

In the case of an infant less than 1 week old, consider:

- birth asphyxia
- birth injury.

Examination

General

- jaundice
- severe palmar pallor
- peripheral oedema
- level of consciousness
- petechial rash.

Head/neck

- stiff neck
- signs of head trauma, or other injuries
- pupil size and reactions to light
- tense or bulging fontanelle
- abnormal posture.

Laboratory investigations

If meningitis is suspected and the child has no signs of raised intracranial pressure (unequal pupils, rigid posture, paralysis of limbs or trunk, irregular breathing), perform a lumbar puncture.

In a malarious area, prepare a blood smear.

If the child is unconscious, check the blood glucose. Check the blood pressure (if a suitable paediatric cuff is available) and carry out urine microscopy if possible.

It is important to determine the length of time a child has been unconscious and his/her AVPU score (see page 17). This coma scale score should be monitored

Table 3. Differential diagnosis of the child presenting with lethargy, unconsciousness or convulsions

Diagnosis or underlying cause	In favour
Meningitis [a,b]	— Very irritable — Stiff neck or bulging fontanelle — Petechial rash (meningococcal meningitis only)
Cerebral malaria (only in children exposed to *P. falciparum* transmission; often seasonal)	— Blood smear positive for malaria parasites — Jaundice — Anaemia — Convulsions — Hypoglycaemia
Febrile convulsions (not likely to be the cause of unconsciousness)	— Prior episodes of short convulsions when febrile — Associated with fever — Age 6 months to 5 years — Blood smear normal
Hypoglycaemia (always seek the cause, e.g. severe malaria, and treat the cause to prevent a recurrence)	— Blood glucose low; responds to glucose treatment [c]
Head injury	— Signs or history of head trauma
Poisoning	— History of poison ingestion or drug overdose
Shock (can cause lethargy or unconsciousness, but is unlikely to cause convulsions)	— Poor perfusion — Rapid, weak pulse
Acute glomerulonephritis with encephalopathy	— Raised blood pressure — Peripheral or facial oedema — Blood in urine — Decreased or no urine
Diabetic ketoacidosis	— High blood sugar — History of polydipsia and polyuria — Acidotic (deep, laboured) breathing

[a] The differential diagnosis of meningitis may include encephalitis, cerebral abscess or tuberculous meningitis. If these are common in your area, consult a standard textbook of paediatrics for further guidance.

[b] A lumbar puncture should not be done if there are signs of raised intracranial pressure (see pages 148, 316). A positive lumbar puncture is one where there is cloudy CSF on direct visual inspection. CSF examination shows an abnormal number of white cells (>100 polymorphonuclear cells per ml). A cell count should be carried out, if possible. However, if this is not possible, then a cloudy CSF on direct visual inspection could be considered positive. Confirmation is given by a low CSF glucose (<1.5 mmol/litre), high CSF protein (>0.4 g/litre), organisms identified by Gram stain or a positive culture, where these are available.

[c] Low blood glucose is <2.5 mmol/litre (<45 mg/dl), or <3.0 mmol/litre (<54 mg/dl) in a severely malnourished child.

regularly. In young infants (less than 1 week old), note the time between birth and the onset of unconsciousness.

Other causes of lethargy, unconsciousness or convulsions in some regions of the world include Japanese encephalitis, dengue haemorrhagic fever, typhoid, and relapsing fever.

Table 4. Differential diagnosis of the young infant (less than 2 months) presenting with lethargy, unconsciousness or convulsions

Diagnosis or underlying cause	In favour
Birth asphyxia Hypoxic ischaemic encephalopathy Birth trauma	— Onset in first 3 days of life — History of difficult delivery
Intracranial haemorrhage	— Onset in first 3 days of life in a low-birth-weight or preterm Infant
Haemolytic disease of the newborn, kernicterus	— Onset in first 3 days of life — Jaundice — Pallor — Serious bacterial infection
Neonatal tetanus	— Onset at age 3–14 days — Irritability — Difficulty in breastfeeding — Trismus — Muscle spasms — Convulsions
Meningitis	— Lethargy — Apnoeic episodes — Convulsions — High-pitched cry — Tense/bulging fontanelle
Sepsis	— Fever or hypothermia — Shock — Seriously ill with no apparent cause

1.5 **Common poisonings**

Suspect poisoning in any unexplained illness in a previously healthy child. Consult standard textbook of paediatrics for management of exposure to specific poisons and/or any local sources of expertise in the management of poisoning, for example a poison centre. The principles of the management of ingestion of a few of the more common poisons only is given here. Note that traditional medicines can be a source of poisoning.

Diagnosis

This is made from the history by the child or carer, from clinical examination, and the results of investigations, where appropriate.

- Find out full details of the poisoning agent, the amount ingested and the time of ingestion.

Attempt to identify the exact agent involved requesting to see the container, where relevant. Check that no other children were involved. Symptoms and signs depend on the agent ingested and therefore vary widely—see below.

- Check for signs of burns in or around the mouth or of stridor (laryngeal damage) suggesting ingestion of corrosives.

➤ Admit all children who have ingested iron, pesticides, paracetamol or aspirin, narcotics, antidepressant drugs; children who have ingested deliberately and those who may have been given the drug or poison intentionally by another child or adult.

➤ Children who have ingested corrosives or petroleum products should not be sent home without observation for 6 hours. Corrosives can cause oesophageal burns which may not be immediately apparent and petroleum products, if aspirated, can cause pulmonary oedema which may take some hours to develop.

1.5.1 **Principles for ingested poisons**

Gastric decontamination (removal of poison from stomach) is most effective within one hour of ingestion, and after this time there is usually little benefit, except with agents that delay gastric emptying or in patients who are deeply unconscious. The decision on whether to attempt this has to consider each case separately and must weigh the likely benefits against the risks with each method. Gastric decontamination will not guarantee that all of the substance has been removed, so the child may still be in danger.

Contraindications to gastric decontamination are:

— an unprotected airway in an unconscious child
— ingestion of corrosives or petroleum products unless there is the risk of serious toxicity.

➤ Check the child for emergency signs (see page 2) and check for hypoglycaemia (page 177).

➤ Identify the specific agent and remove or adsorb it as soon as possible. Treatment is most effective if given as quickly as possible after the poisoning event, ideally within 1 hour.

- If the child has swallowed kerosene, petrol or petrol-based products (note that most pesticides are in petrol-based solvents) or if the child's mouth and throat have been burned (for example with bleach, toilet cleaner or battery acid), then **do not** make the child vomit but give water orally.

➤ **Never** use salt as an emetic as this can be fatal.

➤ If the child has swallowed other poisons

➤ Give activated charcoal, if available, and **do not** induce vomiting; give by mouth or NG tube according to table below. If giving by NG tube, be particularly careful that the tube is in the stomach.

Table 5. Amount of activated charcoal per dose

Children up to one year of age:	1 g/kg
Children 1 to 12 years of age:	25 to 50 g
Adolescents and adults:	25 to 100 g

- Mix the charcoal in 8–10 times the amount of water, e.g. 5 g in 40 ml of water.
- If possible, give the whole amount at once; if the child has difficulty in tolerating it, the charcoal dose can be divided.

➤ If charcoal is not available, then induce vomiting *but only if the child is conscious* by rubbing the back of the child's throat with a spatula or spoon handle; if this does not work, give an emetic such as paediatric ipecacuanha (10 ml for 6 months to 2 year-olds or 15 ml for over 2 years); if this does not work, then try rubbing the back of the child's throat again. *Note:* ipecacuanha can cause repeated vomiting, drowsiness and lethargy which can confuse the diagnosis of poisoning.

Gastric lavage

Only do it in health care facilities if staff has experience in the procedure, and if the ingestion was only a few hours ago and is life threatening, and there has been no ingestion of corrosives or petroleum derivatives. Make sure a suction apparatus is available in case the child vomits. Place the child in the left lateral/ head down position. Measure the length of tube to be inserted. Pass a 24–28 French gauge tube through the mouth into the stomach, as a smaller size nasogastric tube is not sufficient to let particles such as tablets pass. Ensure the tube is in the stomach. Perform lavage with 10 ml/kg body weight of warm normal saline (0.9%). The volume of lavage fluid returned should approximate to the amount of fluid given. Lavage should be continued until the recovered lavage solution is clear of particulate matter.

Note that tracheal intubation may be required to reduce risk of aspiration.

- Give specific antidote if this is indicated
- Give general care.
- Keep the child under observation for 4–24 hours depending on the poison swallowed
- Keep unconscious children in recovery position.
- Consider transferring child to next level referral hospital, where appropriate and where this can be done safely, if the child is unconscious or has deteriorating conscious level, has burns to mouth and throat, is in severe respiratory distress, is cyanosed or is in heart failure.

1.5.2 **Principles for poisons in contact with skin or eyes**

Skin contamination

- Remove all clothing and personal effects and thoroughly flush all exposed areas with copious amounts of tepid water. Use soap and water for oily substances. Attending staff should take care to protect themselves from secondary contamination by wearing gloves and apron. Removed clothing and personal effects should be stored safely in a see-through plastic bag that can be sealed, for later cleansing or disposal.

Eye contamination

- Rinse the eye for 10–15 minutes with clean running water or saline, taking care that the run-off does not enter the other eye. The use of anaesthetic eye drops will assist irrigation. Evert the eyelids and ensure that all surfaces are rinsed. In the case of an acid or alkali irrigate until the pH of the eye returns to, and remains, normal (re-check pH 15–20 minutes after stopping irrigation). Where possible, the eye should be thoroughly examined under fluorescein staining for signs of corneal damage. If there is significant conjunctival or corneal damage, the child should be seen urgently by an ophthalmologist.

1.5.3 **Principles of inhaled poisons**

- Remove from the source of exposure.
- Administer supplemental oxygen if required.

Inhalation of irritant gases may cause swelling and upper airway obstruction, bronchospasm and delayed pneumonitis. Intubation, bronchodilators and ventilatory support may be required.

1.5.4 **Specific poisons**

Corrosive compounds

Examples—sodium hydroxide, potassium hydroxide, acids, bleaches or disinfectants

- **Do not** induce vomiting or use activated charcoal when corrosives have been ingested as this may cause further damage to the mouth, throat, airway, oesophagus and stomach.
- Give milk or water as soon as possible to dilute the corrosive agent.
- Then give the child nothing by mouth and arrange for surgical review to check for oesophageal damage/rupture, if severe.

Petroleum compounds

Examples—kerosene, turpentine substitutes, petrol

- **Do not** induce vomiting or give activated charcoal as inhalation can cause respiratory distress with hypoxaemia due to pulmonary oedema and lipoid pneumonia. Ingestion can cause encephalopathy.
- Specific treatment includes oxygen therapy if respiratory distress (see page 281).

Organo-phosphorus and carbamate compounds

Examples: organophosphorus – malathion, parathion, TEPP, mevinphos (Phosdrin); and carbamates – methiocarb, carbaryl

These can be absorbed through the skin, ingested or inhaled.

The child may complain of vomiting, diarrhoea, blurred vision or weakness. Signs are those of excess parasympathetic activation: salivation, sweating, lacrimation, slow pulse, small pupils, convulsions, muscle weakness/twitching, then paralysis and loss of bladder control, pulmonary oedema, respiratory depression.

Treatment involves:

- Remove poison by irrigating eye or washing skin (if in eye or on skin).
- Give activated charcoal if ingested and within 1 hour of the ingestion.
- **Do not** induce vomiting because most pesticides are in petrol-based solvents.
- In a serious ingestion where activated charcoal cannot be given, consider careful aspiration of stomach contents by NG tube (the airway should be protected).
- If the child has signs of excess parasympathetic activation (see above), then give atropine 15–50 micrograms/kg IM (i.e. 0.015–0.05 mg/kg) or by intravenous infusion over 15 minutes. The main aim is to reduce bronchial secretions whilst avoiding atropine toxicity. Auscultate the chest for signs of respiratory secretions and monitor respiratory rate, heart rate and coma score (if appropriate). Repeat atropine dose every 15 minutes until no chest signs of secretions, and pulse and respiratory rate returns to normal.
- Check for hypoxaemia with pulse oximetry, if possible, if giving atropine as it can cause heart irregularities (ventricular arrythmias) in hypoxic children. Give oxygen if oxygen saturation is less that 90%.
- If muscle weakness, give pralidoxime (cholinesterase reactivator) 25–50 mg/kg diluted with 15 ml water by IV infusion over 30 minutes repeated once or twice, or followed by an intravenous infusion of 10 to 20 mg/kg/hour, as necessary.

Paracetamol

- If within 1 hour of ingestion give activated charcoal, if available, or induce vomiting UNLESS an oral antidote may be required (see below).
- Decide if antidote is required to prevent liver damage: ingestions of 150 mg/kg or more, or toxic 4 hour paracetamol level where this is available. Antidote is more often required for older children who deliberately ingest paracetamol or when parents overdose children by mistake.
- If within 8 hours of ingestion give oral methionine or IV acetylcysteine. Methionine can be used if the child is conscious and not vomiting (<6 years: 1 gram every 4 hours for 4 doses; 6 years or older: 2.5 grams every 4 hours for 4 doses).
- If more than 8 hours after ingestion, or the child cannot take oral treatment, give IV acetylcysteine. Note that the fluid volumes used in the standard regimen are too large for young children.

For children <20 kg give the loading dose of 150 mg/kg in 3 ml/kg of 5% glucose over 15 minutes, followed by 50 mg/kg in 7 ml/kg of 5% glucose over 4 hours, then 100 mg/kg IV in 14 ml/kg of 5% glucose over 16 hours. The volume of glucose can be scaled up for larger children.

Aspirin and other salicylates

This can be very serious in young children because they rapidly become acidotic and are consequently more likely to suffer the severe CNS effects of toxicity. Salicylate overdose can be complex to manage.

■ These cause acidotic-like breathing, vomiting and tinnitus.

➤ Give activated charcoal if available. Note that salicylate tablets tend to form a concretion in the stomach leading to delayed absorption, so it is worthwhile giving several doses of charcoal. If charcoal is not available and a severely toxic dose has been given, then perform gastric lavage or induce vomiting, as above.

➤ Give IV sodium bicarbonate 1 mmol/kg over 4 hours to correct acidosis and to raise the pH of the urine to above 7.5 so that salicylate excretion is increased. Give supplemental potassium too. Monitor urine pH hourly.

➤ Give IV fluids at maintenance requirements unless child shows signs of dehydration in which case give adequate rehydration (see chapter 5).

➤ Monitor blood glucose every 6 hours and correct as necessary (see page 321).

➤ Give vitamin K 10mg IM or IV.

Iron

■ Check for clinical features of iron poisoning: nausea, vomiting, abdominal pain and diarrhoea. The vomit and stools are often grey or black. In severe poisoning there may be gastrointestinal haemorrhage, hypotension, drowsiness, convulsions and metabolic acidosis. Gastrointestinal features usually appear in the first 6 hours and a child who has remained asymptomatic for this time probably does not require antidote treatment.

➤ Activated charcoal does not bind to iron salts, therefore consider giving a gastric lavage if potentially toxic amounts of iron were taken.

➤ Decide whether to give antidote treatment. Since this can have side-effects it should only be used if there is clinical evidence of poisoning (see above).

➤ If you decide to give antidote treatment, give deferoxamine (50 mg/kg IM up to a maximum of 1 g) by deep IM injection repeated every 12 hours; if very ill, give IV infusion 15 mg/kg/hour to a maximum of 80 mg/kg in 24 hours.

Carbon monoxide poisoning

- Give 100% oxygen to accelerate removal of carbon monoxide (note patient can look pink but still be hypoxaemic) until signs of hypoxia disappear.
- Monitor with pulse oximeter but be aware that these can give falsely high readings. If in doubt, be guided by presence or absence of clinical signs of hypoxaemia.

Prevention

- Teach the parents to keep drugs and poisons in proper containers and out of reach of children
- Advise parents on first aid if this happens again in the future
  - Do not make child vomit if child has swallowed kerosene, petrol or petrol-based products or if child's mouth and throat have been burned, nor if the child is drowsy.
  - Try to make the child vomit if other drugs or poisons have been taken by stimulating the back of the throat.
  - Take the child to a health facility as soon as possible, together with information about the substance concerned e.g. the container, label, sample of tablets, berries etc.

1.6 Snake bite

- Snake bite should be considered in any severe pain or swelling of a limb or in any unexplained illness presenting with bleeding or abnormal neurological signs. Some cobras spit venom into the eyes of victims causing pain and inflammation.

Diagnosis of envenoming

- General signs include shock, vomiting and headache. Examine bite for signs such as local necrosis, bleeding or tender local lymph node enlargement.
- Specific signs depend on the venom and its effects. These include:
  - Shock
  - Local swelling that may gradually extend up the bitten limb
  - Bleeding: external from gums, wounds or sores; internal especially intracranial

— Signs of neurotoxicity: respiratory difficulty or paralysis, ptosis, bulbar palsy (difficulty swallowing and talking), limb weakness

— Signs of muscle breakdown: muscle pains and black urine

■ Check haemoglobin (where possible, blood clotting should be assessed).

Treatment

First aid

➤ Splint the limb to reduce movement and absorption of venom. If the bite was likely to have come from a snake with a neurotoxic venom, apply a firm bandage to affected limb from fingers or toes to proximal of site of bite.

➤ Clean the wound.

➤ If any of the above signs, transport to hospital which has antivenom as soon as possible. If snake has already been killed, take this with child to hospital.

➤ Avoid cutting the wound or applying tourniquet.

Hospital care

Treatment of shock/respiratory arrest

➤ Treat shock, if present (see pages 3, 15 and 16).

➤ Paralysis of respiratory muscles can last for days and requires intubation and mechanical ventilation or manual ventilation (with a mask or endotracheal tube and bag) by relays of staff and/or relatives until respiratory function returns. Attention to careful securing of endotracheal tube is important. An alternative is to perform an elective tracheostomy.

Antivenom

■ If there are systemic signs or severe local signs (swelling of more than half of the limb or severe necrosis), give antivenom, if available.

➤ Prepare IM epinephrine and IV chlorpheniramine and be ready if allergic reaction occurs (see below).

➤ Give monovalent antivenom if the species of snake is known. Give polyvalent antivenom if the species is not known. Follow the directions given on the antivenom preparation. The dose for children is the same as for adults.

— Dilute the antivenom in 2–3 volumes of 0.9% saline and give intravenously over 1 hour. Give more slowly initially and monitor closely for anaphylaxis or other serious adverse reactions.

- ➤ If itching/urticarial rash, restlessness, fever, cough or difficult breathing develop, then stop antivenom and give epinephrine 0.01 ml/kg of 1/1000 or 0.1 ml/kg of 1/10,000 solution subcutaneously and IM or IV/SC chlorpheniramine 250 micrograms/kg. When the child is stable, re-start antivenom infusion slowly.
- ➤ More antivenom should be given after 6 hours if there is recurrence of blood incoagulability, or after 1–2 hr if the patient is continuing to bleed briskly or has deteriorating neurotoxic or cardiovascular signs.

Blood transfusion should not be required if antivenom is given. Clotting function returns to normal only after clotting factors are produced by the liver. Response of abnormal neurological signs to antivenom is more variable and depends on type of venom.

- ➤ If there is no reponse to antivenom infusion this should be repeated.
- ➤ Anticholinesterases can reverse neurological signs in some species of snake (see standard textbooks of paediatrics for further details).

Other treatment

Surgical opinion

Seek surgical opinion if there is severe swelling in a limb, it is pulseless or painful or there is local necrosis.

Surgical care will include:

- — Excision of dead tissue from wound
- — Incision of fascial membranes to relieve pressure in limb compartments, if necessary
- — Skin grafting, if extensive necrosis
- — Tracheostomy (or endotracheal intubation) if paralysis of muscles involved in swallowing occurs

Supportive care

- ➤ Give fluids orally or by NG tube according to daily requirements (see page 273). Keep a close record of fluid intake and output.
- ➤ Provide adequate pain relief
- ➤ Elevate limb if swollen
- ➤ Give antitetanus prophylaxis
- ➤ Antibiotic treatment is not required unless there is tissue necrosis at wound site

➤ Avoid intramuscular injections

➤ Monitor very closely immediately after admission, then hourly for at least 24 hours as envenoming can develop rapidly.

1.7 Scorpion sting

Scorpion stings can be very painful for days. Systemic effects of venom are much more common in children than adults.

Diagnosis of envenoming

Signs of envenoming can develop within minutes and are due to autonomic nervous system activation. They include:

- shock
- high or low BP
- fast and/or irregular pulse
- nausea, vomiting, abdominal pain
- breathing difficulty (due to heart failure) or respiratory failure
- muscle twitches and spasms.

➤ Check for low BP or raised BP and treat if signs of heart failure (see page 107).

Treatment

First aid

➤ Transport to hospital as soon as possible.

Hospital care

Antivenom

➤ If signs of severe envenoming give scorpion antivenom, if available (as above for snake antivenom infusion).

Other treatment

➤ Treat heart failure, if present (see page 106).

➤ Consider use of prazosin if there is pulmonary oedema (see standard textbooks of paediatrics).

Supportive care

➤ Give oral paracetamol or oral or IM morphine according to severity. If very severe, infiltrate site with 1% lignocaine, without epinephrine.

1.8 **Other sources of envenoming**

➤ Follow the same principles of treatment, as above. Give antivenom, where available, if severe local or any systemic effects.

In general, venomous spider bites can be painful but rarely result in systemic envenoming. Antivenom is available for some species such as widow and banana spiders. Venomous fish can give very severe local pain but, again, systemic envenoming is rare. Box jellyfish stings are occasionally rapidly life-threatening. Apply vinegar on cotton wool to denature the protein in the skin. Adherent tentacles should be carefully removed. Rubbing the sting may cause further discharge of venom. Antivenom may be available. The dose of antivenom to jellyfish and spiders should be determined by the amount of the venom injected. Higher doses are required for multiple bites, severe symptoms or delayed presentation.

Notes

CHAPTER 2

Diagnostic approach to the sick child

2.1 Relationship to the IMCI approach

The pocket book is symptom-based in its approach, with the symptoms following the sequence of the IMCI guidelines: cough, diarrhoea, fever. The diagnoses also closely match the IMCI classifications, except that the expertise and investigative capabilities that are available in a hospital setting allow classifications like "very severe disease" or "very severe febrile disease" to be defined more precisely, making possible such diagnoses as very severe pneumonia, severe malaria, and meningitis. Classifications for conditions such as pneumonia and dehydration follow the same principles as the IMCI. Young infants (up to 2 months) are considered separately (see Chapter 3), as in the IMCI approach, but the guidelines cover conditions arising at birth such as birth asphyxia. The severely malnourished child is also considered separately (see Chapter 7), because these children require special attention and treatment if the high mortality is to be reduced.

2.2 Taking the history

Taking the history generally should start with the presenting complaint:

Why did you bring the child?

Then it progresses to the history of the present illness. The symptom-specific chapters give some guidance on specific questions which are important to ask concerning these specific symptoms, and which help in the differential diagnosis of the illness. This includes the personal history, family and social and environmental history. The latter might link to important counselling messages such as sleeping under a bednet for a child with malaria, breastfeeding or sanitary practices in a child with diarrhoea, or reducing exposure to indoor air pollution in a child with pneumonia.

Especially for younger infants, the history of pregnancy and birth is very important. In the infant and younger child, feeding history becomes essential. The older the child, the more important is information of the milestones of development and behaviour of the child. Whereas the history is obtained from a parent or caretaker in the younger child, an older child will contribute important information.

2.3 Approach to the sick child and clinical examination

All children must be examined fully so that no important sign will be missed. However, in contrast to the systematic approach in adults, the examination of the child needs to be organized in a way to upset the child as little as possible.

- Do not upset the child unnecessarily.
- Leave the child in the arms of the mother or carer.
- Observe as many signs as possible before touching the child. These include
  - Is the child alert, interested and looking about?
  - Does the child appear drowsy?
  - Is the child irritable?
  - Is the child vomiting?
  - Is the child able to suck or breastfeed?
  - Is the child cyanosed or pale?
  - Are there signs of respiratory distress?
    - Does the child use auxiliary muscles?
    - Is there lower chest wall indrawing?
    - Does the child appear to breath fast?
    - Count the respiratory rate.

These and other signs should all be looked for and recorded before the child is disturbed. You might ask the mother or caretaker to cautiously reveal part of the chest to look for lower chest wall indrawing or to count the respiratory rate. If a child is distressed or crying, it might need to be left for a brief time with its mother in order to settle, or the mother could be ask to breastfeed, before key signs such as respiratory rate can be measured.

Then proceed to signs which require touching the child but are little disturbing, such as listening to the chest. You get little useful information if you listen to the chest of a crying child. Therefore, signs that involve interfering with the child, such as recording the temperature or testing for skin turgor, should be done last.

2.4 Laboratory investigations

Laboratory investigations are targeted based on the history and examination, and help narrow the differential diagnosis. The following basic laboratory investigations should be available in all small hospitals which provide paediatric care in developing countries:

- haemoglobin or packed cell volume (PCV)
- blood smear for malaria parasites
- blood glucose
- microscopy of CSF and urine
- blood grouping and cross-matching
- HIV testing.

In the care of sick newborns (under 1 week old), blood bilirubin is also an essential investigation.

Indications for these tests are outlined in the appropriate sections of this pocket book. Other investigations, such as pulse oximetry, chest X-ray, blood cultures and stool microscopy, can help in complicated cases.

2.5 Differential diagnoses

After the assessment has been completed, consider the various conditions that could cause the child's illness and make a list of possible differential diagnoses. This helps to ensure that wrong assumptions are not made, a wrong diagnosis is not chosen, and rare problems are not missed. Remember that a sick child might have more than one diagnosis or clinical problem requiring treatment.

Section 1.4 and Tables 1–4 (pages 19–24) present the differential diagnoses for emergency conditions encountered during triage. Further tables of symptom-specific differential diagnoses for common problems are found at the beginning of each chapter and give details of the symptoms, examination findings and results of laboratory investigations, which can be used to determine the main diagnosis and any secondary diagnoses.

After the main diagnosis and any secondary diagnoses or problems have been determined, treatment should be planned and started. Once again, if there is more than one diagnosis or problem, the treatment recommendations for all of them may have to be taken together. It is necessary to review the list of differential diagnoses again at a later stage after observing the response to treatment, or in the light of new clinical findings. The diagnosis might be revised at this stage, or additional diagnoses included in the considerations.

Notes

CHAPTER 3

Problems of the neonate and young infant

This chapter provides guidance for the management of problems in neonates and young infants from birth to 2 months of age. This includes neonatal resuscitation, the recognition and management of neonatal sepsis and other bacterial infections, and the management of low and very low birth weight (VLBW) infants. Drug tables for commonly used drugs in neonates and young infants are included at the end of this chapter, also providing dosages for low birth weight and premature babies.

3.1 Routine care of the newborn at delivery

Most babies require only simple supportive care at and after delivery.

➤ Dry the baby with a clean towel.

➤ Observe baby (see chart 12) while drying.

➤ Give the baby to the mother as soon as possible, place on chest/abdomen.

➤ Cover the baby to prevent heat loss.

➤ Encourage initiation of breastfeeding within the first hour.

Skin-to-skin contact and early breastfeeding are the best ways to keep a baby warm and prevent hypoglycaemia.

3.2 Neonatal resuscitation

For some babies the need for resuscitation may be anticipated: those born to mothers with chronic illness, where the mother had a previous fetal or neonatal death, a mother with pre-eclampsia, in multiple pregnancies, in preterm delivery, in abnormal presentation of the fetus, with a prolapsed cord, or where there is prolonged labour or rupture of membranes, or meconium-stained liquor.

However, for many babies the need for resuscitation cannot be anticipated before delivery. Therefore,

- be prepared for resuscitation at every delivery,
- follow the assessment steps of chart 12.

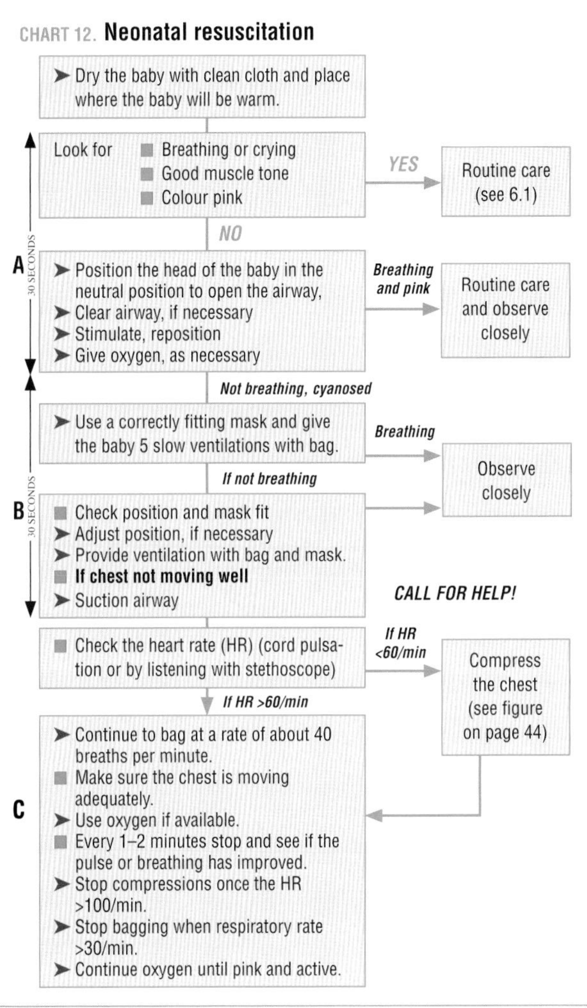
CHART 12. Neonatal resuscitation
➤ Dry the baby with clean cloth and place where the baby will be warm.
Look for ■ Breathing or crying ■ Good muscle tone ■ Colour pink
YES
Routine care (see 6.1)
NO
A
30 SECONDS
➤ Position the head of the baby in the neutral position to open the airway,
➤ Clear airway, if necessary
➤ Stimulate, reposition
➤ Give oxygen, as necessary
Breathing and pink
Routine care and observe closely
Not breathing, cyanosed
➤ Use a correctly fitting mask and give the baby 5 slow ventilations with bag.
Breathing
Observe closely
If not breathing
B
30 SECONDS
■ Check position and mask fit
➤ Adjust position, if necessary
➤ Provide ventilation with bag and mask.
■ If chest not moving well
➤ Suction airway
CALL FOR HELP!
■ Check the heart rate (HR) (cord pulsation or by listening with stethoscope)
If HR <60/min
Compress the chest (see figure on page 44)
If HR >60/min
C
➤ Continue to bag at a rate of about 40 breaths per minute.
■ Make sure the chest is moving adequately.
➤ Use oxygen if available.
■ Every 1–2 minutes stop and see if the pulse or breathing has improved.
➤ Stop compressions once the HR >100/min.
➤ Stop bagging when respiratory rate >30/min.
➤ Continue oxygen until pink and active.

CHART 12. Neonatal resuscitation

There is no need to slap the baby, drying is enough for stimulation.

A. Airway

- Suction airway—if there is meconium stained fluid AND baby is NOT crying and moving limbs:
  - — Suck the mouth, nose and oropharynx, do not suck right down the throat as this can cause apneoa/bradycardia.

B. Breathing

- Choosing mask size: Size 1 for normal weight baby, size 0 for small (less than 2.5 kg) baby
- Ventilation with bag and mask at 40–60 breaths/minute
- Make sure the chest moves up with each press on the bag and in a very small baby make sure the chest does not move too much.

C. Circulation

- 90 compressions coordinated with 30 breaths/min (3 compressions: 1 breath every 2 seconds).
- Place thumbs just below the line connecting the nipples on the sternum (see below).
- Compress 1/3 the A-P diameter of the chest.

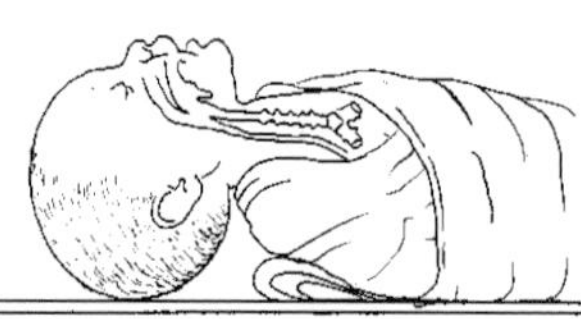

Correct head position to open up airways and for bag ventilation.

Do not hyperextend the neck

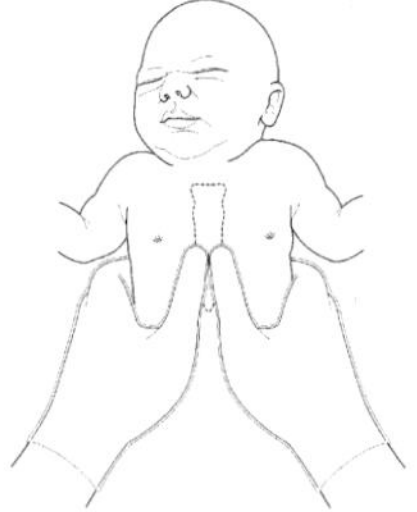

Correct position of hands for cardiac massage in a neonate. The thumbs are used for compression over the sternum

CHART 12. Neonatal resuscitation

Neonatal self-inflating resuscitation bag with round mask

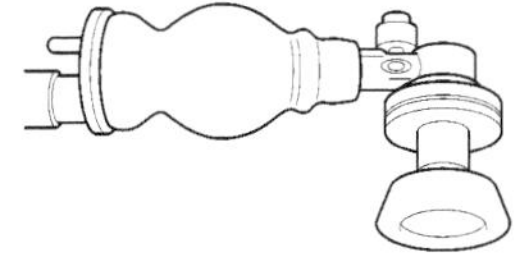

Fitting mask over face:

right size and position of mask	*mask held too low*	*mask too small*	*mask too large*
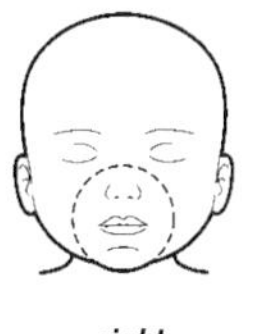	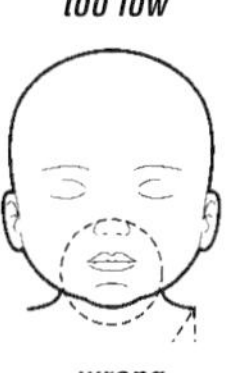	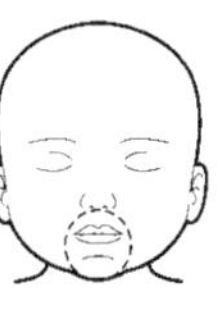	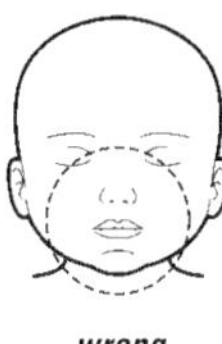
right	*wrong*	*wrong*	*wrong*

Ventilating a neonate with bag and mask

Pull the jaw forward towards the mask with the third finger of the hand holding the mask

Do not hyperextend the neck

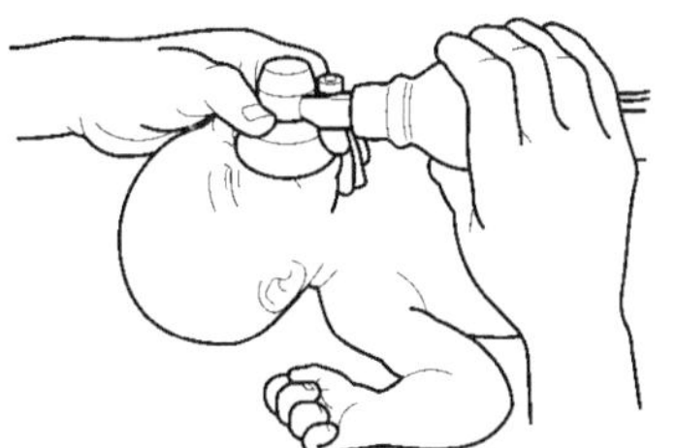

Inadequate seal

If you hear air escaping from the mask, form a better seal. The most common leak is between the nose and the cheeks.

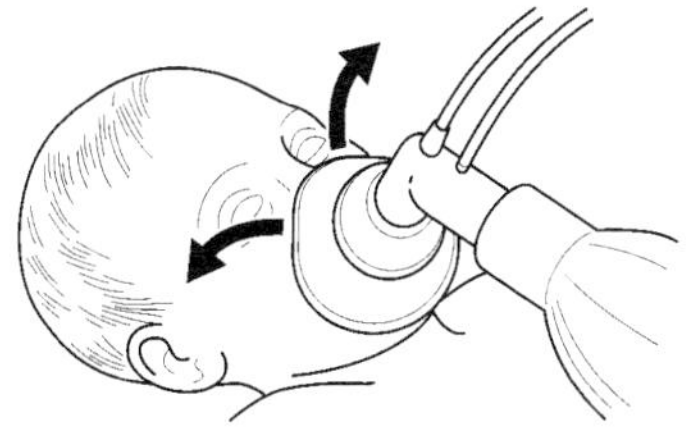

3.2.1 Cessation of resuscitation

If after 20 minutes of resuscitation the baby is:

- Not breathing and pulse is absent: cease efforts.
- Explain to the mother that the baby has died, and give it to her to hold if she wishes.

3.3 Routine care for all newborn babies after delivery (and for neonates born outside and brought to the hospital)

➤ Keep dry in a warm room away from drafts, well covered

➤ Keep the baby with the mother, rooming in

➤ Initiate breastfeeding within the first hour

➤ Let the baby breastfeed on demand if able to suck

➤ Give vitamin K (phytomenadione), according to national guidelines
1 ampoule (1 mg/0.5ml or 1 mg/ml) IM once
(Do NOT use 10 mg/ml ampoule)

➤ Keep umbilical cord clean and dry

➤ Apply antiseptic ointment or antibiotic eye drops/ointment (e.g. tetracycline eye ointment) to both eyes once, according to national guidelines

➤ Give oral polio, hepatitis B and BCG vaccines, depending on national guidelines

3.4 Prevention of neonatal infections

Many early neonatal infections can be prevented by:

- Good basic hygiene and cleanliness during delivery of the baby
- Special attention to cord care
- Eye care

Many late neonatal infections are acquired in hospitals. These can be prevented by:

- Exclusive breastfeeding
- Strict procedures for hand washing for all staff and for families before and after handling babies
- Not using water for humidification in incubators (where *Pseudomonas* will easily colonize) or by avoiding incubators (using kangaroo mother care instead).

- Strict sterility for all procedures
- Clean injection practices
- Removing intravenous drips when they are no longer necessary
- Avoiding unnecessary blood transfusion

3.5 Management of the child with perinatal asphyxia

May be the result of a lack of oxygen supply to organs before, during or immediately after birth. Initial treatment is effective resuscitation (see above).

Problems in the days after birth:

➤ *Convulsions*: treat with phenobarbital (see page 49), check glucose.

➤ *Apnoea*: common after severe birth asphyxia. Sometimes associated with convulsions. Manage with oxygen by nasal catheter and resuscitation with bag and mask.

➤ *Inability to suck*: feed with milk via a nasogastric tube. Beware of delayed emptying of the stomach which may lead to regurgitation of feeds.

➤ *Poor motor tone*. May be floppy or have limb stiffening (spasticity).

Prognosis: can be predicted by recovery of motor function and sucking ability. A baby who is normally active will usually do well. A baby who, a week after birth, is still floppy or spastic, unresponsive and cannot suck has a severe brain injury and will do poorly. The prognosis is less grim for babies who have recovered some motor function and are beginning to suck. The situation should be sensitively discussed with parents throughout the time the baby is in hospital.

3.6 Danger signs in newborns and young infants

Neonates and young infants often present with non-specific symptoms and signs which indicate severe illness. These signs might be present at or after delivery, or in a newborn presenting to hospital, or develop during hospital admission. Initial management of the neonate presenting with these signs is aimed at stabilizing the child and preventing deterioration. Signs include:

- Unable to breastfeed
- Convulsions
- Drowsy or unconscious
- Respiratory rate less than 20/min or apnoea (cessation of breathing for >15 secs)
- Respiratory rate greater than 60/min

- Grunting
- Severe chest indrawing
- Central cyanosis

EMERGENCY MANAGEMENT of danger signs:

- ➤ Give oxygen by nasal prongs or nasal catheter if the young infant is cyanosed or in severe respiratory distress.
- ➤ Give bag and mask ventilation (page 45), with oxygen (or room air if oxygen is not available) if respiratory rate too slow (<20).
- ➤ Give ampicillin (or penicillin) and gentamicin (see below).
- ➤ If drowsy, unconscious or convulsing, check blood glucose.

  If glucose <1.1 mmol/l (<20 mg/100 ml), give glucose IV.

  If glucose 1.1–2.2 mmol/l (20–40 mg/100 ml), feed immediately and increase feeding frequency.

  If you cannot check blood glucose quickly, assume hypoglycaemia and give glucose IV. If you cannot insert an IV drip, give expressed breast milk or glucose through a nasogastric tube.
- ➤ Give phenobarbital if convulsing (see page 49).
- ➤ Admit, or refer urgently if treatment is not available at your hospital
- ➤ Give vitamin K (if not given before).
- ➤ Monitor the baby frequently (see below).

3.7 Serious bacterial infection

Risk factors for serious bacterial infections are:

- Maternal fever (temperature >37.9 °C before delivery or during labour)
- Membranes ruptured more than 24 hours before delivery
- Foul smelling amniotic fluid

All of the DANGER SIGNS are signs of serious bacterial infection, but there are others:

- Deep jaundice
- Severe abdominal distension

Localizing signs of infection are:

- Painful joints, joint swelling, reduced movement, and irritability if these parts are handled

- Many or severe skin pustules
- Umbilical redness extending to the peri-umbilical skin or umbilicus draining pus.
- Bulging fontanelle (see below)

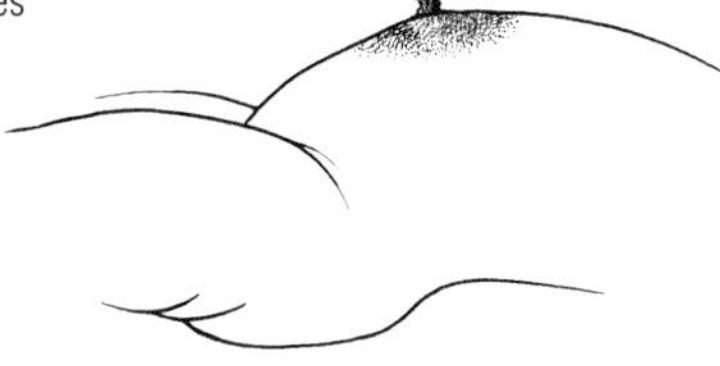

Peri-umbilical flare in umbilical sepsis. The inflammation extends beyond the umbilicus to the abdominal wall.

Treatment

Antibiotic therapy

- ➤ Admit to hospital
- ➤ Where blood cultures are available, obtain blood cultures before starting antibiotics
- ➤ For any of these signs, give ampicillin (or penicillin) and gentamicin (for dosages see pages 62–66)
- ➤ Give cloxacillin (if available) instead of penicillin if extensive skin pustules or abscesses as these might be signs of Staphylococcus infecton
- ➤ Most serious bacterial infections in neonates should be treated with antibiotics for at least 10 days
- ➤ If not improving in 2–3 days the antibiotic treatment may need to be changed, or the baby referred

Other treatment

- ➤ Give all sick infants aged <2 weeks 1 mg of vitamin K (IM)
- ➤ Treat *convulsions* with IM phenobarbital (1 dose of 15 mg/kg). If needed, continue with phenobarbital 5 mg/kg once daily
- ➤ For management of pus draining from eyes, see page 59
- ➤ If child is from malarious area and has fever, take blood film to check for malaria also. Neonatal malaria is very rare. If confirmed, treat with quinine (see page 140)
- ➤ For supportive care, see page 51

3.8 Meningitis

Clinical signs

Suspect if signs of serious bacterial infection are present, or any one of the following signs of meningitis.

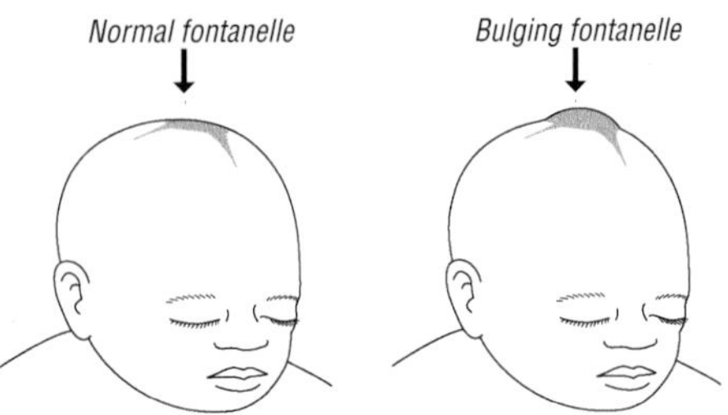

Bulging fontanelle – sign of meningitis in young infants with an open fontanelle

General signs

- Drowsy, lethargic or unconscious
- Reduced feeding
- Irritable
- High pitched cry
- Apnoeic episodes

More specific signs

- Convulsion
- Bulging fontanelle

Do a lumbar puncture (LP) if you suspect meningitis, unless the baby is having apnoea or there is no motor response to stimuli.

Treatment

Antibiotics

➤ Give ampicillin and gentamicin or a third generation cephalosporin, such as ceftriaxone (50 mg/kg every 12 hours (might cause biliary sludge leading to jaundice)) or cefotaxime (50 mg/kg every 6 hours) for 3 weeks.

➤ Alternative antibiotics are penicillin and gentamicin (see pages 65–66). Chloramphenicol is an alternative but should not be used in premature/low weight neonates (see page 64).

➤ If there are signs of hypoxaemia, give oxygen (see page 52).

Convulsions/fits

➤ Treat convulsions with phenobarbital (loading dose of 15 mg/kg). If convulsion persists, give further doses of 10 mg/kg phenobarbital up to a maximum of 40 mg/kg (see page 49). Watch for apnoea. If needed, continue with phenobarbital at a maintenance dose of 5 mg/kg/day. Check for hypoglycaemia.

3.9 Supportive care for the sick neonate

3.9.1 Thermal environment

- Keep the young infant dry and well wrapped.
- A bonnet or cap is helpful to reduce heat loss. Keep the room warm (at least 25 °C). Keeping the young infant in close skin-to-skin contact with the mother ("kangaroo mother care") for 24 hours a day is as effective as using an incubator or external heating device to avoid chilling.
- Pay special attention to avoid chilling the infant during examination or investigation.
- Regularly check that the infant's temperature is maintained in the range 36.5–37.5 °C (97.7–99.5 °F) rectal, or 36.0–37.0 °C (96.8–98.6 °F) axillary.

3.9.2 Fluid management

Encourage the mother to breastfeed frequently to prevent hypoglycaemia. If unable to feed, give expressed breast milk by nasogastric tube.

- Withhold oral feeding if there is bowel obstruction, necrotizing enterocolitis or the feeds are not tolerated, e.g. indicated by increasing abdominal distension or vomiting everything.
- Withhold oral feeding in the acute phase in babies who are lethargic or unconscious, or having frequent convulsions.

If IV fluids are given, reduce the IV fluid rates as the volume of milk feeds increases.

Babies who are suckling well but need an IV drip for antibiotics should be on minimal IV fluids to avoid fluid overload, or flush cannula with 0.5 ml NaCl 0.9% and cap.

Increase the amount of fluid given over the first 3–5 days (total amount, oral and IV).

Day 1	60 ml/kg/day
Day 2	90 ml/kg/day
Day 3	120 ml/kg/day
Then increase to	150 ml/kg/day

When babies are tolerating oral feeds well, this might be increased to 180 ml/kg/day after some days. But be careful with parenteral fluids, which can quickly overhydrate a child. When giving IV fluids, do not exceed this volume unless the baby is dehydrated or under phototherapy or a radiant heater. This amount is the TOTAL fluid intake a baby needs and oral intake must be taken into account when calculating IV rates.

- Give more fluid if under radiant heater (x 1.2–1.5)

Do NOT use IV glucose and water (without sodium) AFTER the first 3 days of life. Babies over 3 days of age need some sodium (for example, 0.18% saline/5% glucose).

Monitor the IV infusion very carefully.

- Use a monitoring sheet.
- Calculate drip rate
- Check drip rate and volume infused every hour
- Weigh baby daily
- Watch for facial swelling: if this occurs, reduce the IV fluid to minimal levels or take out the IV. Introduce milk feeding by nasogastric tube or breastfeeding as soon as it is safe to do so.

3.9.3 Oxygen therapy

➤ Give *oxygen treatment* to young infants with any of the following:

- central cyanosis
- grunting with every breath
- difficulty in feeding due to respiratory distress
- severe lower chest wall indrawing
- head nodding (i.e. a nodding movement of the head, synchronous with the respiration and indicating severe respiratory distress)

Where a pulse oximeter is available, this should be used to guide oxygen therapy. Oxygen should be given if the oxygen saturation is below 90%, and the oxygen flow should be regulated to have a saturation between 92% and 95%. Oxygen can be discontinued once the child can maintain a saturation above 90% in room air.

Nasal prongs are the preferred method for delivery of oxygen to this age group, with a flow rate of 0.5 litre per minute. Thick secretions from the throat may be cleared by intermittent suction, if they are troublesome and the young infant is too weak to clear them. Oxygen should be stopped when the infant's general condition improves and the above signs are no longer present.

3.9.4 High fever

Do *not* use antipyretic agents such as paracetamol for controlling fever in young infants. Control the environment. If necessary, undress the child.

3.10 Babies with low birth weight

3.10.1 Babies with birth weight between 2.25 and 2.5 kg

These babies are normally strong enough to start feeding themselves after delivery. They need to be kept warm and attention for infection control, but otherwise no special care.

3.10.2 Babies with birth weight between 1.75 and 2.25 kg

Sometimes these babies need extra care, but can normally stay with their mothers to provide feeding and warmth, especially if skin-to skin contact can be maintained.

Feeding. Start feeds within 1 hour of delivery. Many of these babies will be able to suck. Babies who can suck should be breastfed. Those who cannot breastfeed should be given expressed breast milk with a cup and spoon. When the baby is sucking well from the breast and gaining weight, reduce the cup and spoon feeds.

See the babies at least twice a day to assess feeding ability, fluid intake, or presence of any DANGER SIGNS (page 47) or signs of serious bacterial infection (page 48). If any of these signs are present, they should be closely monitored in the neonatal nursery in a similar way to very low birth weight babies (see below).

The risk of keeping the child in hospital (e.g. acquiring nosocomial infections), should be balanced with the potential benefit of obtaining better care.

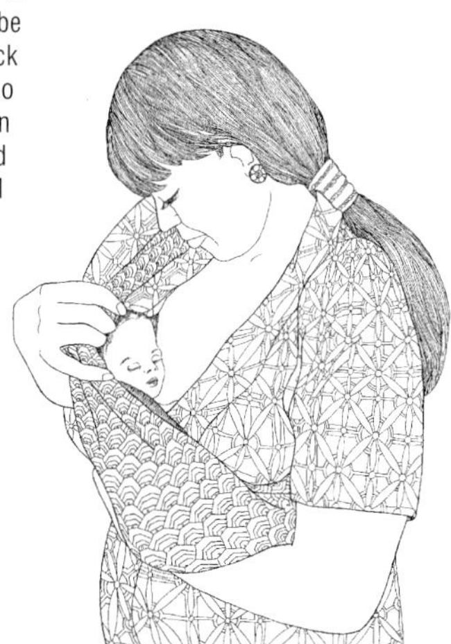

Keeping a child warm: the child has skin contact with the mother, is wrapped in her clothes, and the head is covered to prevent heat loss.

3.10.3 Babies with birth weight below 1.75 kg

These babies are at risk of hypothermia, apnoea, hypoxaemia, sepsis, feed intolerance and necrotizing enterocolitis. The risks increase the smaller the baby is. All low birth weight babies should be admitted to the Special Care or Neonatal Unit.

Treatment

➤ Give oxygen by nasal catheter or nasal prongs if any signs of hypoxaemia

Temperature

- Nurse skin-to-skin between the mother's breasts, or clothed in a warm room, or in a humidicrib if the staff have experience in using them. A hot water bottle wrapped in a towel can be useful for keeping the baby warm if no power for heating is available. Aim for a core body temperature of 36–37 °C with the feet warm and pink.

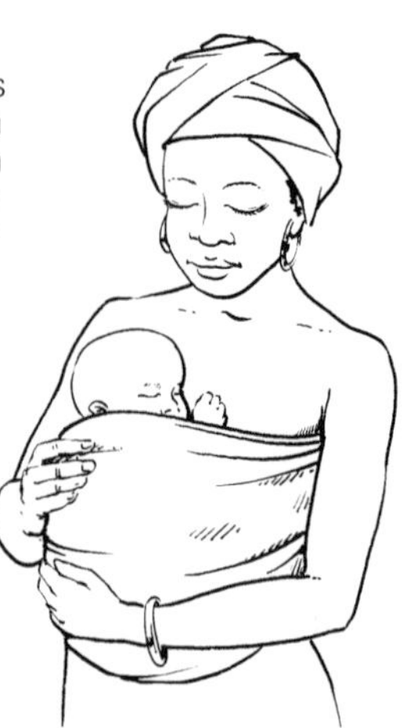

Position for kangaroo mother care of young infant. Note: after wrapping the child, the head needs to be covered with a cap or bonnet to prevent heat loss.

Fluids and feeds

- If possible give intravenous fluids at 60 ml/kg/day for the first day of life. Best to use a paediatric (100 ml) intravenous burette where 60 drops = 1 ml and therefore 1 drop per minute = 1 ml per hour. If the baby is well and active, give 2–4 ml of expressed breast milk every 2 hours through a nasogastric tube, depending on the weight of the baby (see page 51).
- If very small babies are under a radiant heater or phototherapy they need more fluid than the "usual maintenance" volumes (see page 51), but great care must be taken to accurately run the intravenous fluid as overhydration may be fatal.
- If possible, check blood sugar every 6 hours until enteral feeds established, especially if baby is having apnoea, lethargy or convulsions. VLBW babies may need a 10% glucose solution. Add 10 ml of 50% glucose to every 90 ml of 4.3% glucose + 1/5 normal saline or use a 10% glucose in water solution.

- Start feeding when the condition of the baby is stable (usually on the second day, might be possible in more mature babies on day 1). Start feeds if there is no abdominal distension or tenderness, bowel sounds are present, meconium passed and no apnoea.
- Use a prescription chart.
- Calculate exact amounts for feeding and the timing of feeds.
- Increase on a daily basis if well tolerated.
- When commencing milk feeds, start with 2–4 ml every 1–2 hours by nasogastric tube. Some active VLBW babies can be fed with a cup and spoon or an eyedropper, which must be sterilized before each feed. Use only expressed breast milk if possible. If 2–4 ml volume is tolerated with no vomiting, abdominal distension, or gastric aspirates of more than half the feed, the volume can be increased by 1–2 ml per feed each day. Reduce or withhold feeds if signs of poor tolerance occur. Aim to have feeding established in the first 5–7 days so that the IV drip can be removed, to avoid infection.
- The feeds may be increased over the first 2 weeks of life to 150–180 ml/kg/day (three-hourly feeds of 19–23 ml for a 1 kg baby and 28–34 ml for a 1.5 kg baby). As the baby grows, recalculate the feed volume based on the higher weight.

Antibiotics and sepsis

Risk factors for sepsis are: babies born outside hospital or born to unwell mothers, rupture of membranes >24 hours, smaller babies (closer to 1 kg).

Presence of any DANGER SIGNS (page 47) or other signs of serious bacterial infection (page 48).

➤ Initiate antibiotic treatment.

Apnoea

- Caffeine citrate and aminophylline prevent apnoea in premature babies. Caffeine is preferred if it is available. The loading dose of caffeine citrate is 20 mg/kg orally or IV (given slowly over 30 minutes). A maintenance dose should be prescribed (see page 63).

  If caffeine is not available give a loading dose of aminophylline of 10 mg/kg orally or by intravenous injection over 15–30 minutes (see page 63). A maintenance dose should be prescribed.
- If an apnoea monitor is available this should be used.

Discharge and follow-up of low birth weight babies

Low birth weight babies can be discharged when:

- they have no DANGER signs or signs of serious infection
- they are gaining weight on breastfeeding alone
- they can maintain their temperature in the normal range (36–37 °C) in an open cot
- the mother is confident and able to take care.

Low birth weight babies should be given all scheduled vaccines at the time of birth, and any second doses that are due by the time of discharge.

Counselling on discharge

Counsel parents before discharge on

- exclusive breastfeeding
- keeping the baby warm
- danger signs for seeking care

Low birth weight babies should be followed up weekly for weighing, assessment of feeding, and general health until they have reached 2.5 kg.

3.11 Necrotizing enterocolitis

Necrotizing enterocolitis (NEC, a bowel infection) may occur in low birth weight babies, especially after enteral feeds are started. It is more common in low birth weight babies fed artificial formulae, but may occur in breastfed babies.

Common signs of NEC are:

- Abdominal distension or tenderness
- Intolerance of feeding
- Bile-stained vomit or bile-stained fluid up the nasogastric tube
- Blood in the stools

General signs of systemic upset include

- Apnoeas
- Drowsy or unconscious
- Fever or hypothermia

Treatment

- ➤ Stop enteral feeds.
- ➤ Pass a nasogastric tube and leave it on free drainage.
- ➤ Start an IV infusion of glucose/saline (see page 51 for rate of infusion).
- ➤ Start antibiotics: give ampicillin (or penicillin) plus gentamicin plus metronidazole (if available) for 10 days.

If the baby has apnoea or other danger signs, give oxygen by nasal catheter. If apnoea continues give aminophylline or caffeine IV (see pages 62, 63).

If the baby is pale, check the haemoglobin and transfuse if Hb<10 g/dL.

Take a supine and lateral decubitus abdominal X-ray. If there is gas in the abdominal cavity outside the bowel there may be a bowel perforation. Ask a surgeon to see the baby urgently.

Examine the baby carefully each day. Reintroduce expressed breast milk feeds by nasogastric tube when the abdomen is soft and not tender, the baby is passing normal stools with no blood and is not having bilious vomiting. Start feeds slowly and increase slowly by 1–2 ml per feed each day.

3.12 Other common neonatal problems

3.12.1 Jaundice

More than 50% of normal newborns, and 80% of preterm infants, have some jaundice. Jaundice can be divided into abnormal or normal:

Abnormal (non physiological)

- Jaundice started on the first day of life
- Jaundice lasting longer than 14 days in term, 21 days in preterm infants
- Jaundice with fever
- Deep jaundice: palms and soles of the baby deep yellow

Normal (physiological)

- Skin and eyes yellow but none of the above

Abnormal jaundice may be due to

- Serious bacterial infection
- Haemolytic disease due to blood group incompatibility or G6PD deficiency
- Congenital syphilis (page 60) or other intrauterine infection

- Liver disease such as hepatitis or biliary atresia
- Hypothyroidism

Investigations for abnormal jaundice

The clinical impression of jaundice should be confirmed by a bilirubin measurement, where possible. The investigations depend on the likely diagnosis and what tests are available, but may include:

- Haemoglobin or PCV
- Full blood count to look for signs of serious bacterial infection (high or low neutrophil count with >20% band forms), and to look for signs of haemolysis
- Blood type of baby and mother, and Coombs test
- Syphilis serology such as VDRL tests
- G6PD screen, thyroid function tests, liver ultrasound

Treatment

➤ Phototherapy if

- Jaundice on day 1
- Deep jaundice involving palms and soles of the feet
- Prematurity and jaundice
- Jaundice due to haemolysis

Treatment of jaundice based on serum bilirubin level

	Phototherapy				Exchange transfusion[a]			
	Healthy term baby		Preterm or any risk factors[b]		Healthy term baby		Preterm or any risk factors	
	mg/dl	µmol/l	mg/dl	µmol/l	mg/dl	µmol/l	mg/dl	µmol/l
Day1	Any visible jaundice[c]				15	260	13	220
Day 2	15	260	13	220	25	425	15	260
Day 3	18	310	16	270	30	510	20	340
Day 4 and thereafter	20	340	17	290	30	510	20	340

[a] Exchange transfusion is not described in this pocket book. These serum bilirubin levels are included in case exchange transfusion is possible or in case the baby can be transferred quickly and safely to another facility where exchange transfusion can be performed.

[b] Risk factors include small size (less than 2.5 kg at birth or born before 37 weeks gestation), haemolysis, and sepsis.

[c] Visible jaundice anywhere on the body on day 1.

Continue phototherapy until serum bilirubin level is lower than threshold range or until baby is well and there is no jaundice of palms and soles.

If the bilirubin level is very elevated (see table) and you can safely do exchange transfusion, consider doing so.

Antibiotics

➤ If suspected infection or syphilis (page 60), treat for serious bacterial infection (page 61)

Antimalarials

➤ If fever is present and the baby is from a malarious area, check blood films for malaria parasites and give antimalarials, if positive

Encourage breastfeeding

3.12.2 Conjunctivitis

Sticky eyes and mild conjunctivitis

➤ Treat as outpatient

➤ Show the mother how to wash the eyes with water or breast milk and how to put eye ointment in the eyes. The mother must wash her hands before and after.

➤ Tell the mother to wash the eyes and put in eye ointment 4 times a day for 5 days

Give the mother a tube of

- Tetracycline eye ointment OR
- Chloramphenicol eye ointment

To treat the child. Review 48 hours after starting treatment, if not improving.

Severe conjunctivitis (a lot of pus and/or swelling of the eyelids) is often due to gonococcal infection. Treat as inpatient as there is a risk of blindness and it needs twice-daily review.

➤ Wash the eyes to clear as much pus as possible.

➤ Ceftriaxone (50 mg/kg up to total of 150 mg IM ONCE) *OR* Kanamycin (25 mg/kg up to total of 75 mg IM ONCE) according to national guidelines.

ALSO use as described above:

➤ Tetracycline eye ointment *OR*

➤ Chloramphenicol eye ointment

Also treat the mother and her partner for STDs: amoxicillin, spectinomycin or ciprofloxacin (for gonorrhoea) and tetracycline (for Chlamydia) depending on the resistance pattern in the country. Refer to the STD control guidelines.

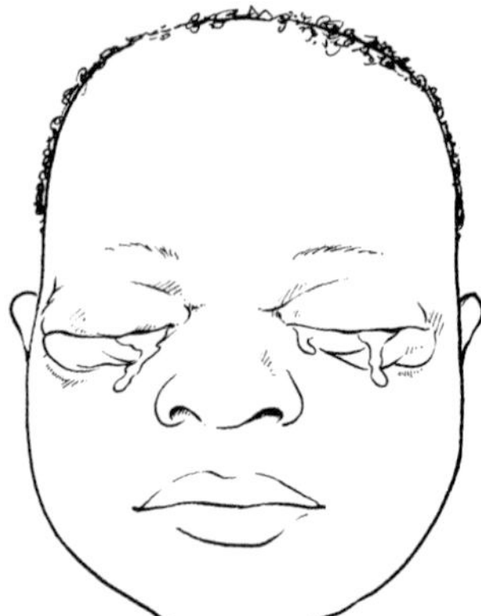

Ophthalmia neonatorum. Swollen, red eyelids with pus

3.12.3 Congenital malformations

See Chapter 9 (page 227) for:

- Cleft lip and palate
- Bowel obstruction
- Abdominal wall defects
- Meningomyelocele
- Congenital dislocation of the hip
- Talipes equinovarus (club foot)

3.13 Babies of mothers with infections

3.13.1 Congenital syphilis

Clinical signs

- Often low birth weight
- Palms and soles: red rash, grey patches, blisters or skin peeling
- 'Snuffles': rhinitis with nasal obstruction which is highly infectious
- Abdominal distension due to big liver and spleen
- Jaundice
- Anaemia
- Some VLBW babies with syphilis have signs of severe sepsis with lethargy, respiratory distress, skin petechiae or other bleeding

If you suspect syphilis, do VDRL test if possible

Treatment

- Asymptomatic neonates born to VDRL or RPR-positive women should receive 50 000 units/kg of benzathine benzyl penicillin in a single intramuscular dose.
- Symptomatic infants require treatment with:
  - procaine benzyl penicillin 50 000 units/kg as a single dose daily for 10 days

  or

  - benzyl penicillin 50 000 units/kg every 12 hours IM or IV for the first 7 days of life and then every 8 hours for a further 3 days.
- Treat the mother and partner for syphilis and check for other sexually transmitted infections.

3.13.2 Baby of a mother with tuberculosis

If the **mother has active lung tuberculosis and was treated for less than two months before birth or was diagnosed with tuberculosis after birth**:

- Reassure the mother that it is safe for her to breastfeed her baby;
- Do not give the tuberculosis vaccine (BCG) at birth;
  Give prophylactic isoniazid 5 mg/kg body weight by mouth once daily;
- At the age of six weeks, re-evaluate the baby, noting weight gain and taking an X-ray of the chest, if possible;
- If there are **any findings suggestive of active disease**, start full anti-tuberculosis treatment according to national guidelines;
- If the **baby is doing well and tests are negative**, continue prophylactic isoniazid to complete six months of treatment;
- Delay BCG vaccine until two weeks after treatment is completed. If **BCG was already given**, repeat BCG two weeks after the end of the isoniazid treatment.

3.13.3 Baby of a mother with HIV

See Chapter 8 (page 199) for guidance.

Drug doses of common drugs for neonates and low birth weight babies

			Weight of baby in kg						
Drug	**Dosage**	**Form**	**1–<1.5kg**	**1.5–<2kg**	**2–<2.5kg**	**2.5–<3kg**	**3–<3.5kg**	**3.5–<4kg**	**4–<4.5kg**
Aminophylline *for apnoea prevention*	*Calculate the EXACT oral maintenance dose*								
	Loading dose: Oral or IV over 30 minutes 10mg/kg, then	250 mg/10 ml vial Dilute loading dose to 5 ml with sterile water, give slowly over 15–30 min	0.4–0.6 ml	0.6–0.8 ml	0.8–1.0 ml	AMINOPHYLLINE IS NOT USUALLY USED FOR TERM BABIES WITH APNOEA			
	Maintenance dose: First week of life: Oral: 2.5mg/kg/dose 12 hourly		0.1–0.15 ml	0.15–0.2 ml	0.2–0.25 ml				
	Weeks 2–4 of life Oral: 4mg/kg/dose 12 hourly		0.15–0.25 ml	0.25–0.3 ml	0.3–0.4 ml				
Ampicillin	IM/IV: 50 mg/kg every 12 hours (1st week of life) Every 8 hours (weeks 2–4 of life)	Vial of 250 mg mixed with 1.3 ml sterile water to give 250 mg/1.5 ml	0.3–0.6 ml	0.6–0.9 ml	0.9–1.2 ml	1.2–1.5 ml	1.5–2.0 ml	2.0–2.5 ml	2.5–3.0 ml

Drug	Dosage	Form	Weight of baby in kg						
			1–<1.5kg	1.5–<2kg	2–<2.5kg	2.5–<3kg	3–<3.5kg	3.5–<4kg	4–<4.5kg
Caffeine citrate	*Calculate the EXACT oral maintenance dose*								
	Loading dose: Oral: 20 mg/kg (or IV over 30 minutes)		20–30 mg	30–40 mg	40–50 mg	50–60mg	60–70 mg	70–80 mg	80–90 mg
	Maintenance dose: 5 mg/kg daily oral (or IV over 30 minutes)		5–7.5 mg	7.5–10 mg	10–12.5 mg	12.5–15 mg	15–17.5 mg	17.5–20 mg	20–22.5 mg
Cefotaxime	IV: 50 mg/kg Premature babies: every 12 hours 1st week of life every 8 hours Weeks 2–4 of life every 6 hours	Vial of 500 mg mixed with 2 ml sterile water to give 250 mg/1 ml	0.3 ml	0.4 ml	0.5 ml	0.6 ml	0.7 ml	0.8 ml	0.9 ml

Drug	Dosage	Form	Weight of baby in kg						
			1–<1.5kg	1.5–<2kg	2–<2.5kg	2.5–<3kg	3–<3.5kg	3.5–<4kg	4–<4.5kg
Ceftriaxone									
For meningitis	IV: 50mg/kg every 12 hours	1g vial mix with 9.6 ml sterile water to give 1g/10 ml	0.5–0.75 ml	0.75 –1 ml	1–1.25 ml	1.25–1.5 ml	1.5–1.75 ml	1.75–2 ml	2–2.5 ml
	IM/IV: 100mg/kg once daily		1–1.5 ml	1.5–2 ml	2–2.5 ml	2.5–3 ml	3–3.5 ml	3.5–4 ml	4–4.5 ml
For pus draining from eye	50mg/kg once IM (max 125mg)								
Chloramphenicol	*Preferably calculate EXACT dose based on the infant's weight*								
	IV: 25 mg/kg/dose twice daily	Vial 1g mixed with 9.2 ml sterile saline to give 1g/10 ml	DO NOT USE IN PREMATURE BABIES			0.6–0.75 ml	0.75–0.9 ml	0.9–1.0 ml	1.0–1.1 ml
Cloxacillin	25–50mg/kg/dose 12 hourly (1st week of life)	250mg vial mixed with 1.3 ml sterile water to give 250 mg/1.5 ml	**25mg/kg:** 0.15–0.3 ml	0.3–0.5 ml	0.5–0.6 ml	0.6–0.75 ml	0.75–1.0 ml	1.0–1.25 ml	1.25–1.5 ml
	8 hourly (weeks 2–4 of life)		**50mg/kg:** 0.3–0.6 ml	0.6–0.9 ml	0.9–1.2 ml	1.2–1.5 ml	1.5–2.0 ml	2–2.5 ml	2.5–3.0 ml

Drug	Dosage	Form	Weight of baby in kg						
			1–<1.5kg	1.5–<2kg	2–<2.5kg	2.5–<3kg	3–<3.5kg	3.5–<4kg	4–<4.5kg
Gentamicin	*Preferably calculate EXACT dose based on the infant's weight*								
	1st week of life:	Vial 20 mg/2 ml							
	Low birth weight babies: IM/IV: 3mg/kg/dose once daily	Vial 80 mg/2 ml dilute to 8 ml with sterile water to give 10 mg/ml	0.3– 0.5 ml	0.5– 0.6 ml	0.6– 0.75 ml				
	Normal birth weight: IM/IV: 5mg/kg/dose once daily					1.25– 1.5 ml	1.5– 1.75 ml	1.75– 2 ml	2– 2.25 ml
	Weeks 2–4 of life: IM/IV: 7.5 mg/kg/dose once daily		0.75– 1.1 ml	1.1– 1.5 ml	1.5– 1.8 ml	1.8– 2.2 ml	2.2– 2.6 ml	2.6– 3.0 ml	3.0– 3.3 ml
Note: To use vial 80mg/2ml, dilute to 8ml with sterile water to give 10mg/ml, then use exactly the same dose as in the table above.									
Kanamycin	IM/IV: 20 mg/kg (one dose for pus draining from eyes)	2ml vial to make 125 mg/ml	0.2– 0.3 ml	0.3– 0.4 ml	0.4– 0.5 ml	0.5– 0.6 ml	0.6– 0.7 ml	0.7– 0.8 ml	0.8– 1.0 ml
Naloxone	0.1 mg/kg	Vial 0.4 mg/ml	$\frac{1}{4}$ ml	$\frac{1}{4}$ ml	$\frac{1}{2}$ ml	$\frac{1}{2}$ ml	$\frac{3}{4}$ ml	$\frac{3}{4}$ ml	1 ml

Drug	Dosage	Form	Weight of baby in kg						
			1–<1.5kg	1.5–<2kg	2–<2.5kg	2.5–<3kg	3–<3.5kg	3.5–<4kg	4–<4.5kg
PENICILLIN **Benzylpenicillin**	50,000 units/kg/dose 1st week of life 12 hourly Weeks 2–4 and older: 6 hourly	Vial of 600 mg (1 000 000 units) dilute with 1.6 ml sterile water to give 500 000 units/ml	0.2 ml	0.2 ml	0.3 ml	0.5 ml	0.5 ml	0.6 ml	0.7 ml
Benzathine benzylpenicillin	50 000 units/kg once a day	IM: vial of 1.2 million units mixed with 4 ml sterile water	0.2 ml	0.3 ml	0.4 ml	0.5 ml	0.6 ml	0.7 ml	0.8 ml
Procaine benzylpenicillin	IM: 50 000 units/kg once a day	3 g vial (3 000 000 units) mixed with 4 ml sterile water	0.1 ml	0.15 ml	0.2 ml	0.25 ml	0.3 ml	0.3 ml	0.35 ml
Phenobarbital	**Loading dose:** IM/IV or oral: 15 mg/kg.	Vial 200 mg/ml diluted with 4 ml sterile water	*Calculate the EXACT dose*						
		30 mg tabs	1/2	3/4	1	1 1/4	1 1/2	1 3/4	2
	Maintenance dose: Oral: 5 mg/kg/day	30 mg tabs	1/4	1/4	1/2	1/2	1/2	3/4	3/4

Notes

Notes

CHAPTER 4

Cough or difficult breathing

Cough and difficult breathing are common problems in young children. The causes range from a mild, self-limited illness to severe, life-threatening disease. This chapter provides guidelines for managing the most important conditions that cause cough, difficult breathing, or both in children aged 2 months to 5 years. The differential diagnosis of these conditions is described in Chapter 2. Management of these problems in infants <2 months of age is described in Chapter 3, and in severely malnourished children in Chapter 7.

Most episodes of cough are due to the common cold, with each child having several episodes a year. The commonest severe illness presenting with cough or difficult breathing is pneumonia, which should be considered first in any differential diagnosis (Table 6, page 71).

4.1 **Child presenting with cough**

History

Pay particular attention to the following:

- cough
  - — duration in days
  - — paroxysms with whoops or vomiting or central cyanosis

- exposure to someone with tuberculosis (or chronic cough) in the family
- history of choking or sudden onset of symptoms
- known HIV infection
- immunization history: BCG, DPT, measles, Hib
- personal or family history of asthma.

Examination

General

- central cyanosis
- grunting, nasal flaring, wheeze, stridor
- head nodding (a movement of the head synchronous with inspiration indicating severe respiratory distress)
- raised jugular venous pressure (JVP)
- severe palmar pallor.

Chest

- respiratory rate (make a count during 1 minute when the child is calm)

fast breathing:	<2 months old:	≥60 breaths
	aged 2–11 months:	≥50 breaths
	aged 1–5 years:	≥40 breaths

- lower chest wall indrawing
- apex beat displaced / trachea shifted from midline
- auscultation—coarse crackles or bronchial breath sounds.
- gallop rhythm of heart on auscultation
- percussion signs of pleural effusion (stony dullness) or pneumothorax (hyper-resonance)

Note: lower chest wall indrawing occurs when the lower chest wall goes in when the child breathes in; if only the soft tissue between the ribs or above the clavicle goes in when the child breathes, this is not lower chest wall indrawing

Abdomen

- abdominal masses (e.g. lymphadenopathy)
- enlarged liver and spleen.

Investigations

Pulse oximetry – to guide when to start and stop oxygen therapy

Chest X-ray – in children with very severe pneumonia, or severe pneumonia not responding to treatment or with complications, or associated with HIV

Table 6. Differential diagnosis of the child presenting with cough or difficult breathing

Diagnosis	In favour
Pneumonia	— Cough with fast breathing — Lower chest wall indrawing — Fever — Coarse crackles on auscultation — Nasal flaring — Grunting — Head nodding
Malaria	— Fast breathing in febrile child — Blood smear: high parasitaemia — Lives in or travelled to a malarious area — In severe malaria: deep (acidotic) breathing / lower chest wall indrawing — Chest clear on auscultation
Severe anaemia	— Severe palmar pallor — Haemoglobin <6 g/dl
Cardiac failure	— Raised jugular venous pressure — Apex beat displaced to the left — Gallop rhythm — Heart murmur — Basal fine crackles — Enlarged palpable liver
Congenital heart disease	— Cyanosis — Difficulty in feeding or breastfeeding — Enlarged liver — Heart murmur
Tuberculosis	— Chronic cough (more than 30 days) — Poor growth / wasting or weight loss — positive Mantoux test — Positive contact history with tuberculosis patient — Diagnostic chest X-ray may show primary complex or miliary tuberculosis — Sputum positive in older child
Pertussis	— Paroxysms of cough followed by whoop, vomiting, cyanosis or apnoea — Well between bouts of cough — No fever — No history of DPT immunization
Foreign body	— History of sudden choking — Sudden onset of stridor or respiratory distress — Focal areas of wheeze or reduced breath sounds
Effusion/ empyema	— Stony dullness to percussion — Air entry absent

Table 6. Continued

Diagnosis	In favour
Pneumothorax	— Sudden onset — Hyper-resonance on percussion on one side of the chest — Shift in mediastinum
Pneumocystis pneumonia	— 2–6-month-old child with central cyanosis — Hyper-expanded chest — Fast breathing — Finger clubbing — Chest X-ray changes, but chest clear on auscultation — Enlarged liver, spleen, lymph nodes — HIV test positive in mother or child

4.2 Pneumonia

Pneumonia is usually caused by viruses or bacteria. Most serious episodes are caused by bacteria. It is usually not possible, however, to determine the specific cause by clinical features or chest X-ray appearance. Pneumonia is classified as very severe, severe or non-severe, based on the clinical features, with specific treatment for each of them. Antibiotic therapy is needed in all cases. Severe and very severe pneumonia require additional treatment, such as oxygen, to be given in hospital.

Table 7. Classification of the severity of pneumonia

Sign or symptom	Classification	Treatment
■ Central cyanosis ■ Severe respiratory distress (e.g. head nodding) ■ Not able to drink	**Very severe pneumonia**	— Admit to hospital — Give recommended antibiotic — Give oxygen — Manage the airway — Treat high fever if present
■ Chest indrawing	**Severe pneumonia**	— Admit to hospital — Give recommended antibiotic — Manage the airway — Treat high fever if present
■ Fast breathing ≥60 breaths/minute in a child aged <2 months; ≥50 breaths/ minute in a child aged 2–11 months; ≥40 breaths/minute in a child aged 1–5 years	**Pneumonia**	— Home care — Give appropriate antibiotic for 5 days — Soothe the throat and relieve cough with a safe remedy — Advise the mother when to return immediately — Follow up in 2 days

Table 7. Continued

Sign or symptom	Classification	Treatment
■ Definite crackles on auscultation		
■ No signs of pneumonia, or severe or very severe pneumonia	**No pneumonia, cough or cold**	— Home care — Soothe the throat and relieve cough with safe remedy — Advise the mother when to return — Follow up in 5 days if not improving — If coughing for more than 30 days, follow chronic cough instructions (see page 96)

4.2.1 Very severe pneumonia

Diagnosis

Cough or difficult breathing plus *at least one* of the following:

- central cyanosis
- inability to breastfeed or drink, or vomiting everything
- convulsions, lethargy or unconsciousness
- severe respiratory distress.

In addition, *some or all* of the other signs of pneumonia or severe pneumonia *may* be present, such as:

- fast breathing: age <2 months: ≥60/minute
  age 2–11 months: ≥50/minute
  age 1–5 years: ≥40/minute
- nasal flaring
- grunting (in young infants)
- lower chest wall indrawing (lower chest wall goes in when the child breathes in; if only the soft tissue between the ribs or above the clavicle goes in when the child breathes, this is not lower chest wall indrawing)
- chest auscultation signs of pneumonia:
- decreased breath sounds
- bronchial breath sounds
- crackles
- abnormal vocal resonance (decreased over a pleural effusion, increased over lobar consolidation)
- pleural rub.

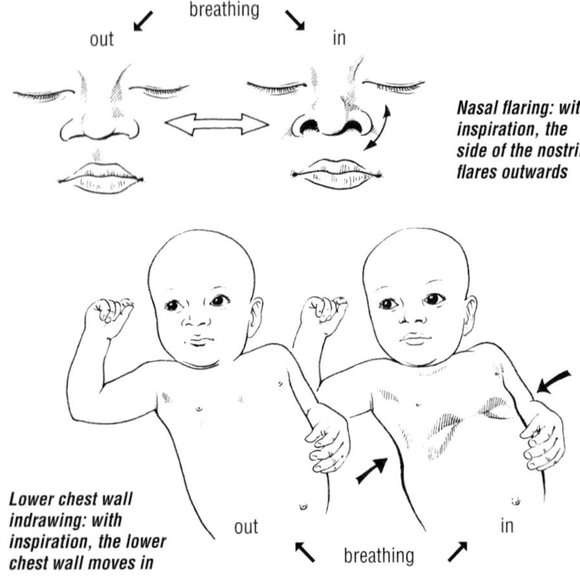

- If pulse oximetry is available, obtain an oxygen saturation measurement in all children suspected to have severe or very severe pneumonia
- If possible, obtain a chest X-ray to identify pleural effusion, empyema, pneumothorax, pneumatocoele, interstitial pneumonia and pericardial effusion.

Treatment

- Admit the child to hospital.

Antibiotic therapy

- Give ampicillin (50 mg/kg IM every 6 hours) and gentamicin (7.5 mg/kg IM once a day) for 5 days; then, if child responds well, complete treatment at home or in hospital with oral amoxicillin (15 mg/kg three times a day) plus IM gentamicin once daily for a further 5 days.

- Alternatively, give *chloramphenicol* (25 mg/kg IM or IV every 8 hours) until the child has improved. Then continue orally 4 times a day for a total course of 10 days. Or use ceftriaxone (80 mg/kg IM or IV once daily).
- If the child does not improve within 48 hours, switch to *gentamicin* (7.5 mg/kg IM once a day) and *cloxacillin* (50 mg/kg IM or IV every 6 hours), as described below for staphylococcal pneumonia. When the child improves, continue cloxacillin (or dicloxacillin) orally 4 times a day for a total course of 3 weeks.

Oxygen therapy

- Give oxygen to all children with very severe pneumonia
- Where pulse oximetry is available, use this to guide oxygen therapy (give to children with oxygen saturation less than 90%, where there is sufficient oxygen available)
- Use nasal prongs, a nasal catheter, or a nasopharyngeal catheter.

  Use of nasal prongs is the best method for delivering oxygen to young infants. Face masks or head masks are not recommended. Oxygen supplies need to be available continuously at all times. A comparison of the different methods of oxygen administration and diagrams showing their use is given in section 10.7, page 281.
- Continue with oxygen until the signs of hypoxia (such as severe lower chest wall indrawing or breathing rate of ≥70/minute) are no longer present.
- Where pulse oximetry is available, carry out a trial period without oxygen each day in stable children. Discontinue oxygen if the saturation remains stable above 90%. There is no value in giving oxygen after this time.

Nurses should check every 3 hours that the catheter or prongs are not blocked with mucus and are in the correct place and that all connections are secure.

The two main sources of oxygen are cylinders and oxygen concentrators. It is important that all equipment is checked for compatibility and properly maintained, and that staff are instructed in their correct use.

Supportive care

- If the child has fever (≥39 °C or ≥102.2 °F) which appears to be causing distress, give paracetamol.
- If wheeze is present, give a rapid-acting bronchodilator (see page 88).
- Remove by gentle suction any thick secretions in the throat, which the child cannot clear.

➤ Ensure that the child receives daily maintenance fluids appropriate for the child's age (see section 10.2, page 273), but avoid overhydration.

- — Encourage breastfeeding and oral fluids.
- — If the child cannot drink, insert a nasogastric tube and give maintenance fluids in frequent small amounts. *If the child is taking fluids adequately by mouth, do not use a nasogastric tube as it increases the risk of aspiration pneumonia.* If oxygen is given at the same time as nasogastric fluids, pass both tubes through the *same* nostril.

➤ Encourage the child to eat as soon as food can be taken.

Monitoring

The child should be checked by nurses at least every 3 hours and by a doctor at least twice a day. In the absence of complications, within two days there should be signs of improvement (breathing not so fast, less indrawing of the lower chest wall, less fever, and improved ability to eat and drink).

Complications

➤ If the child has not improved after two days, or if the child's condition has worsened, look for complications or other diagnoses. If possible, obtain a chest X-ray. The most common complications are given below.

Staphylococcal pneumonia. This is suggested if there is rapid clinical deterioration despite treatment, by a pneumatocoele or pneumothorax with effusion on chest X-ray, numerous Gram-positive cocci in a smear of sputum, or heavy growth of *S. aureus* in cultured sputum or empyema fluid. The presence of septic skin pustules supports the diagnosis.

➤ Treat with *cloxacillin* (50 mg/kg IM or IV every 6 hours) and *gentamicin* (7.5 mg/kg IM or IV once a day). When the child improves, continue cloxacillin orally 4 times a day for a total course of 3 weeks. Note that cloxacillin can be substituted by another anti-staphylococcal antibiotic such as oxacillin, flucloxacillin, or dicloxacillin.

Empyema. This is suggested by persistent fever, and physical and chest X-ray signs of pleural effusion.

➤ Diagnosis and management are described in section 4.2.4, page 81.

Tuberculosis. A child with persistent fever for more than 2 weeks and signs of pneumonia should be evaluated for tuberculosis. If another cause of the fever cannot be found, tuberculosis should be considered and treatment for tuberculosis, following national guidelines, may be initiated and response to anti-Tb treatment evaluated (see section 4.8, page 101).

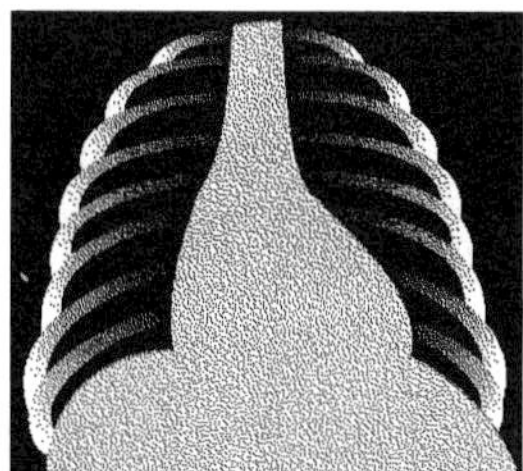

Normal chest X-ray

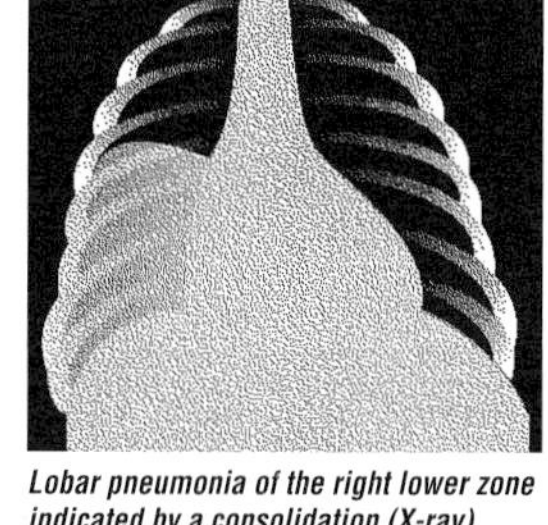

Lobar pneumonia of the right lower zone indicated by a consolidation (X-ray)

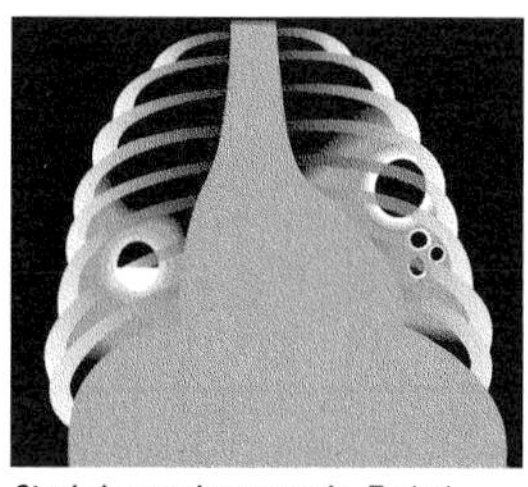

Staphylococcal pneumonia. *Typical features include pneumatocoeles on the right side of the illustration, and an abscess with an air-fluid level on the left side of the illustration (X-ray).*

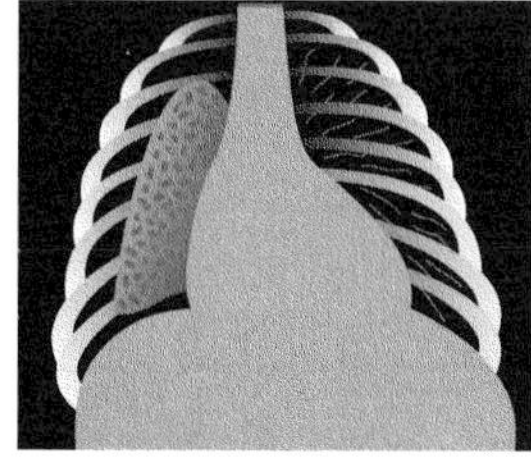

Pneumothorax. *The right lung (left side of the illustration) is collapsed towards the hilus, leaving a transparent margin around it without lung structure. In contrast, the right side (normal) demonstrates markings extending to the periphery (X-ray).*

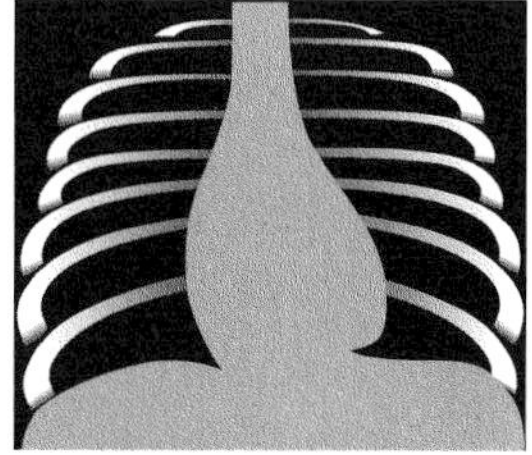

Hyperinflated chest. *Features are an increased transverse diameter, ribs running more horizontally, a small contour of the heart, and flattened diaphragms (X-ray).*

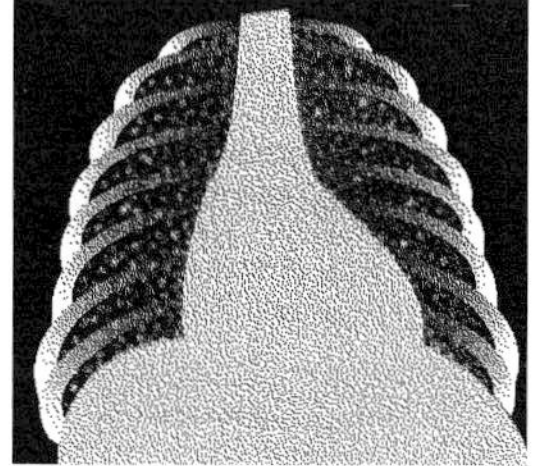

Appearance of miliary tuberculosis: *widespread small patchy infiltrates throughout both lungs: "snow storm appearance" (X-ray).*

Children who are HIV positive or in whom HIV is suspected. Some aspects of antibiotic treatment are different in children who are HIV positive or in whom HIV is suspected. Although the pneumonia in many of these children has the same aetiology as in children without HIV, PCP, often at the age of 4–6 months (see page 217) is an important additional cause which must be treated when present.

➤ Give ampicillin plus gentamicin for 10 days, as above

➤ If the child does not improve within 48 hours, a switch to ceftriaxone (80 mg/kg IV once daily over 30 minutes) if available. If it is not available, give gentamicin plus cloxacillin, as above.

➤ Also give high-dose cotrimoxazole (8 mg/kg of trimethoprim and 40 mg/kg of sulfamethoxazole IV every 8 hours or orally 3 times a day) for 3 weeks.

For the further management of the child, including PCP prophylaxis (see HIV Chapter, page 199).

4.2.2 **Severe pneumonia**

Diagnosis

Cough or difficult breathing plus *at least one* of the following signs:

- lower chest wall indrawing
- nasal flaring
- grunting (in young infants).
- Check that there are ***no*** signs of very severe pneumonia, such as:
  — central cyanosis
  — inability to breastfeed or drink
  — vomiting everything
  — convulsions, lethargy or unconsciousness
  — severe respiratory distress.

In addition, some or all of the other signs of pneumonia may also be present:

- fast breathing:
  - age <2 months: ≥60/minute
  - age 2–11 months: ≥50/minute
  - age 1–5 years: ≥40/minute
- chest auscultation signs of pneumonia:
  — decreased breath sounds
  — bronchial breath sounds
  — crackles
  — abnormal vocal resonance (decreased over a pleural effusion, increased over lobar consolidation)
  — pleural rub.

A routine chest X-ray rarely gives information which will change the management of severe pneumonia and is therefore not recommended.

Treatment

➤ Admit or refer the child to hospital.

Antibiotic therapy

➤ Give benzylpenicillin (50 000 units/kg IM or IV every 6 hours) for at least 3 days.

➤ When the child improves, switch to oral amoxicillin (25 mg/kg 2 times a day). The total course of treatment is 5 days.

➤ If the child does not improve within 48 hours, or deteriorates, look for complications and treat accordingly (see above, as described for very severe pneumonia, page 74, and below for suspected HIV). If there are no apparent complications, switch to chloramphenicol (25 mg/kg every 8 hours IM or IV) until the child has improved. Then continue orally for a total course of 10 days.

Oxygen therapy

➤ If readily available, give oxygen to any child with severe lower chest wall indrawing or a respiratory rate of ≥70/minute. See section 10.7 (page 281).

Supportive care

See above (page 75), as described for very severe pneumonia.

Monitoring

The child should be checked by nurses at least every 6 hours and by a doctor at least once a day. Record the respiratory rate and temperature, and note the child's level of consciousness and ability to drink or breastfeed. In the absence of complications, within two days there should be signs of improvement (slower breathing, less chest indrawing, less fever, and improved ability to eat and drink).

Complications

Children who are HIV positive or in whom HIV is suspected

➤ Give ampicillin plus gentamicin for 10 days, as for very severe pneumonia

➤ If the child does not improve within 48 hours, switch to ceftriaxone (80 mg/kg IV once daily over 30 minutes) if available. If it is not available give gentamicin plus cloxacillin, as for very severe pneumonia.

➤ *In child aged 2–11 months* also give high dose cotrimoxazole (8 mg/kg of trimethoprim and 40 mg/kg of sulfamethoxazole IV every 8 hours or orally 3 times a day) for 3 weeks. *In child aged 12–59 months*, give this only if there are clinical signs of PCP (such as chest X-ray findings of interstitial pneumonia).

For the further management of the child, including PCP prophylaxis (see HIV Chapter, page 199).

4.2.3 Pneumonia (non-severe)

Diagnosis

➤ On examination, the child has cough or difficult breathing and ***fast breathing***:
- — age 2–11 months: ≥50/minute
- — age 1–5 years: ≥40/minute.

➤ Check that the child has *none* of the signs of severe or very severe pneumonia given above in sections 4.1.2 and 4.1.1.

➤ In addition, other signs of pneumonia (on auscultation) may be present: crackles, reduced breath sounds, or an area of bronchial breathing.

Treatment

➤ Treat the child as an outpatient.

➤ Give cotrimoxazole (4 mg/kg trimethoprim / 20 mg/kg sulfamethoxazole twice a day) for 3 days ***or*** amoxicillin (25 mg/kg 2 times a day) for 3 days in non-HIV settings. In HIV settings, 5 days is recommended.

➤ Give the first dose at the clinic and teach the mother how to give the other doses at home.

Complications

Children who are HIV positive or in whom HIV is suspected

In children who are receiving PCP prophylaxis or live in a region in which this is commonly given to children, treat pneumonia with amoxicillin rather than co-trimoxazole where possible.

Follow-up

Encourage the mother to feed the child. Advise her to bring the child back after 2 days, or earlier if the child becomes more sick or is not able to drink or breastfeed. When the child returns:

- If the breathing has improved (slower), there is less fever, and the child is eating better, complete the 3 days of antibiotic treatment.

- If the breathing rate, fever and eating have not improved, change to the second-line antibiotic and advise the mother to return again in 2 days.
- If there are signs of severe or very severe pneumonia, *admit the child to hospital* and treat according to the guidelines above.

4.2.4 **Pleural effusion and empyema**

Diagnosis

A child with severe or very severe pneumonia may develop pleural effusion or empyema.

- On examination, the chest is dull to percussion and breath sounds are reduced or absent over the affected area.
- A pleural rub may be heard at an early stage before the effusion is fully developed.
- A chest X-ray shows fluid on one or both sides of the chest.
- When empyema is present, fever persists despite antibiotic therapy and the pleural fluid is cloudy or frankly purulent.

Treatment

Drainage

➤ Pleural effusions should be drained, unless they are very small. If effusions are present on both sides of the chest, drain both. It may be necessary to repeat drainage 2–3 times if fluid returns. See Appendix A1.5, page 318, for guidelines on chest drainage.

Subsequent management depends on the character of the fluid obtained.

Where possible, pleural fluid should be analysed for protein and glucose content, cell count and differential count, and examined after Gram and Ziehl-Neelsen staining, and bacterial and *Mycobacterium tuberculosis* culture.

Antibiotic therapy

➤ Give *chloramphenicol* (25 mg/kg IM or IV every 8 hours) until the child has improved. Then continue orally 4 times a day for a total of 4 weeks.

➤ If infection with *Staphylococcus aureus* is identified, give *cloxacillin* (dose: 50 mg/kg IM or IV every 6 hours) and gentamicin (dose: 7.5 mg/kg IM or IV once a day) instead. When the child improves, continue with cloxacillin orally, 4 times a day. Continue treatment for a total of 3 weeks.

Failure to improve

If fever and other signs of illness continue, despite adequate chest drainage and antimicrobial therapy, assess for possible tuberculosis.

➤ A trial of antituberculosis therapy may be required (see section 4.8, page 101).

4.3 Cough or cold

These are common, self-limited viral infections that require only supportive care. Antibiotics should not be given. Wheeze or stridor may occur in some children, especially infants. Most episodes end within 14 days. Cough lasting 30 days or more may be caused by tuberculosis, asthma, pertussis or symptomatic HIV infection (see Chapter 8, page 199).

Diagnosis

Common features:

- cough
- nasal discharge
- mouth breathing
- fever.
- The following are ***absent***:
  - — fast breathing
  - — lower chest wall indrawing
  - — stridor when the child is calm
  - — general danger signs.

Wheezing may occur in young children (see section 4.3, below).

Treatment

➤ Treat the child as an outpatient.

➤ Soothe the throat and relieve the cough with a safe remedy, such as a *warm, sweet drink*.

➤ Relieve high fever (≥39 °C or ≥102.2 °F) with *paracetamol*, if this is causing distress to the child.

➤ Clear secretions from the child's nose before feeds using a cloth soaked in water, which has been twisted to form a pointed wick.

➤ Do ***not*** give any of the following:

— an antibiotic (they are not effective and do not prevent pneumonia)

— remedies containing atropine, codeine or codeine derivatives, or alcohol (these may be harmful)
— medicated nose drops.

Follow-up

Advise the mother to:

- feed the child
- watch for *fast or difficult breathing* and return, if either develops
- *return* if the child becomes more sick, or is not able to drink or breastfeed.

4.4 Conditions presenting with wheeze

Wheeze is a high-pitched whistling sound near the end of each expiration. It is caused by spasmodic narrowing of the distal airways. To hear a wheeze, even in mild cases, place the ear next to the child's mouth and listen to the breathing while the child is calm, or use a stethoscope to listen for wheezes or rhonchi.

In the first 2 years of life, wheezing is mostly caused by acute viral respiratory infections such as bronchiolitis or coughs and colds. After 2 years of age, most wheezing is due to asthma (Table 8, page 84). Sometimes children with pneumonia present with wheeze. It is important always to consider pneumonia as a diagnosis, particularly in the first 2 years of life.

History

- previous episodes of wheeze
- response to bronchodilators
- asthma diagnosis or long-term treatment for asthma.

Examination

- wheezing on expiration
- prolonged expiration
- resonant percussion note
- hyperinflated chest
- rhonchi on auscultation.

Response to rapid-acting bronchodilator

➤ If the cause of the wheeze is not clear, or if the child has fast breathing or chest indrawing in addition to wheeze, give a rapid-acting bronchodilator and assess after 15 minutes. Response to a rapid-acting bronchodilator helps to determine the underlying diagnosis and treatment.

Table 8. Differential diagnosis of the child presenting with wheeze

Diagnosis	In favour
Asthma	— History of recurrent wheeze, some unrelated to coughs and colds — Hyperinflation of the chest — Prolonged expiration — Reduced air entry (if very severe, airway obstruction) — Good response to bronchodilators
Bronchiolitis	— First episode of wheeze in a child aged <2 years — Wheeze episode at time of seasonal bronchiolitis — Hyperinflation of the chest — Prolonged expiration — Reduced air entry (if very severe, airway obstruction) — Poor/no response to bronchodilators
Wheeze associated with cough or cold	— Wheeze always related to coughs and colds — No family or personal history of asthma/eczema/hay fever — Prolonged expiration — Reduced air entry (if very severe, airway obstruction) — Good response to bronchodilators — Tends to be less severe than wheeze associated with asthma
Foreign body	— History of sudden onset of choking or wheezing — Wheeze may be unilateral — Air trapping with hyper-resonance and mediastinal shift — Signs of lung collapse: reduced air entry and impaired percussion note — No response to bronchodilators
Pneumonia	— Cough with fast breathing — Lower chest wall indrawing — Fever — Coarse crackles — Nasal flaring — Grunting

Give the rapid-acting bronchodilator by one of the following methods:

- nebulized salbutamol
- salbutamol by a metered dose inhaler with spacer device
- if neither of the above methods is available, give a subcutaneous injection of epinephrine (adrenaline).

See page 88, for details of how to administer the above.

■ Assess the response after 15 minutes. Signs of improvement are:

— less respiratory distress (easier breathing)
— less lower chest wall indrawing
— improved air entry.

➤ Children who still have signs of hypoxia (i.e. central cyanosis, not able to drink due to respiratory distress, severe lower chest wall indrawing) or have fast breathing should be admitted to hospital for treatment.

4.4.1 **Bronchiolitis**

Bronchiolitis is a lower respiratory viral infection, which typically is most severe in young infants, occurs in annual epidemics, and is characterized by airways obstruction and wheezing. Respiratory syncytial virus is the most important cause. Secondary bacterial infection may occur and is common in some settings. The management of bronchiolitis associated with fast breathing or other signs of respiratory distress is therefore similar to that of pneumonia. Episodes of wheeze may occur for months after an attack of bronchiolitis, but eventually will stop.

Diagnosis

Typical features of bronchiolitis, on examination, include:

- wheezing which is *not* relieved by up to three doses of a rapid-acting bronchodilator
- hyperinflation of the chest, with increased resonance to percussion
- lower chest wall indrawing
- fine crackles or rhonchi on auscultation of the chest
- difficulty in feeding, breastfeeding or drinking owing to respiratory distress.

Treatment

Most children can be treated at home, but those with the following signs should be treated in hospital:

Signs of severe or very severe pneumonia (see sections 4.1.2 and 4.1.1):

- central cyanosis
- inability to breastfeed or drink, or vomiting everything
- convulsions, lethargy or unconsciousness
- lower chest wall indrawing
- nasal flaring
- grunting (in young infants).

OR signs of respiratory distress:

- obvious discomfort in breathing
- difficulty in drinking, feeding or talking.

Antibiotic treatment

- *If treated at home*, give cotrimoxazole (4 mg/kg trimethoprim/20 mg/kg sulfamethoxazole twice a day) or amoxicillin (25 mg/kg 2 times a day) orally for 3 days only if the child has fast breathing.
- If there is *respiratory distress*, such as lower chest wall indrawing, but the child is able to drink and there is no central cyanosis, give benzylpenicillin (50 000 units/kg IM or IV every 6 hours) for at least 3 days. When the child improves, switch to oral amoxicillin (25 mg/kg 2 times a day) for 3 days. (See p. 75.)
- If there are signs of *very severe pneumonia* (central cyanosis or inability to drink), give chloramphenicol (25 mg/kg IM or IV every 8 hours) until the child improves. Then continue by mouth 4 times a day for a total of 10 days.

Oxygen

- Give oxygen to all children with wheezing and severe respiratory distress (as for pneumonia: see sections 4.1.1 and 4.1.2).

The recommended methods for oxygen delivery are by nasal prongs or nasal catheter. It is also possible to use a nasopharyngeal catheter. Nasal prongs are the best oxygen delivery method for young infants: see page 282.

- Continue oxygen therapy until the signs of hypoxia are no longer present, after which there is no value in continuing with oxygen.

The nurse should check, every 3 hours, that the catheter or prongs are in the correct position and not blocked with mucus, and that all connections are secure.

Supportive care

- If the child has fever (≥39 °C or ≥102.2 °F) which appears to be causing distress, give paracetamol.
- Ensure that the hospitalized child receives daily maintenance fluids appropriate for the child's age (see section 10.2, page 273), but avoid overhydration. Encourage breastfeeding and oral fluids.
- Encourage the child to eat as soon as food can be taken.

Monitoring

A hospitalized child should be assessed by a nurse every 6 hours (or every 3 hours, if there are signs of very severe illness) and by a doctor at least once a day. Monitor oxygen therapy as described on page 283. Watch especially for signs of respiratory failure, i.e. increasing hypoxia and respiratory distress leading to exhaustion.

Complications

➤ If the child fails to respond to oxygen therapy, or the child's condition worsens suddenly, obtain a chest X-ray to look for evidence of pneumothorax.

Tension pneumothorax associated with severe respiratory distress and shift of the heart requires immediate relief by placing a needle in the affected area to allow the air that is under pressure to escape. (Following this, continuous air exit should be assured by inserting a chest tube with an underwater seal until the air leak closes spontaneously and the lung expands).

4.4.2 Asthma

Asthma is a chronic inflammatory condition with reversible airways obstruction. It is characterized by recurrent episodes of wheezing, often with cough, which respond to treatment with bronchodilators and anti-inflammatory drugs. Antibiotics should be given only when there are signs of pneumonia.

Diagnosis

History of recurrent episodes of wheezing, often with cough. Findings on examination may include:

- hyperinflation of the chest
- lower chest wall indrawing
- prolonged expiration with audible wheeze
- reduced air intake when obstruction is severe
- absence of fever
- good response to treatment with a bronchodilator.

If the diagnosis is uncertain, give a dose of a rapid-acting bronchodilator (see adrenaline/epinephrine (page 89) and salbutamol (page 88)). A child with asthma will usually improve rapidly, showing signs such as a decrease in the respiratory rate and in chest wall indrawing and less respiratory distress. A child with severe asthma may require several doses before a response is seen.

Treatment

➤ A child with the ***first episode of wheezing and no respiratory distress*** can usually be managed at home with supportive care only. A bronchodilator is not necessary.

➤ If the child is in ***respiratory distress or has recurrent wheezing***, give salbutamol by nebulizer or metered-dose inhaler. If salbutamol is not available, give subcutaneous epinephrine. Reassess the child after 30 minutes to determine subsequent treatment:

- *If respiratory distress has resolved*, and the child does not have fast breathing, advise the mother on home care with inhaled salbutamol or, when this is not available, oral salbutamol syrup or tablets (see page 89).
- *If respiratory distress persists*, admit to hospital and treat with oxygen, rapid-acting bronchodilators and other drugs, as described below.

➤ If the child has ***central cyanosis or is unable to drink***, admit to hospital and treat with oxygen, rapid-acting bronchodilators and other drugs, as described below.

➤ In children admitted to hospital, give oxygen, a rapid-acting bronchodilator, and a first dose of steroids promptly.

A positive response (less respiratory distress, better air entry on auscultation) should be seen in 15 minutes. If this does not occur, give the rapid-acting bronchodilator at up to 1-hourly intervals.

➤ If there is no response after 3 doses of rapid-acting bronchodilator, add IV aminophylline.

Oxygen

➤ Give oxygen to all children with asthma who are cyanosed or whose difficulty in breathing interferes with talking, eating or breastfeeding. See page 86.

Rapid-acting bronchodilators

➤ Give the child one of the three rapid-acting bronchodilators—nebulized salbutamol, salbutamol by metered-dose inhaler with a spacer device, or subcutaneous epinephrine (adrenaline), as described below.

(1) Nebulized salbutamol

The driving source for the nebulizer must deliver at least 6–9 litres/minute. Recommended methods are an air compressor or oxygen cylinder. If neither is available, use a durable and easy-to-operate foot-pump, although this is less effective.

➤ Place the bronchodilator solution and 2–4 ml of sterile saline in the nebulizer compartment and treat the child until the liquid is almost all used up. The dose of salbutamol is 2.5 mg (i.e. 0.5 ml of the 5 mg/ml nebulizer solution). This can be given 4-hourly, reducing to 6–8 hourly once the child's condition improves. If necessary in severe cases, it can be given hourly.

(2) Salbutamol by metered-dose inhaler with a spacer device

Spacer devices with a volume of 750 ml are commercially available.

➤ Introduce two puffs (200 micrograms) into the spacer chamber. Then place the child's mouth over the opening in the spacer and allow normal breathing for 3–5 breaths. This can be repeated 4-hourly, reducing to 6–8 hourly after the child's condition improves. If necessary in severe cases, it can be given up to several times an hour for a short period.

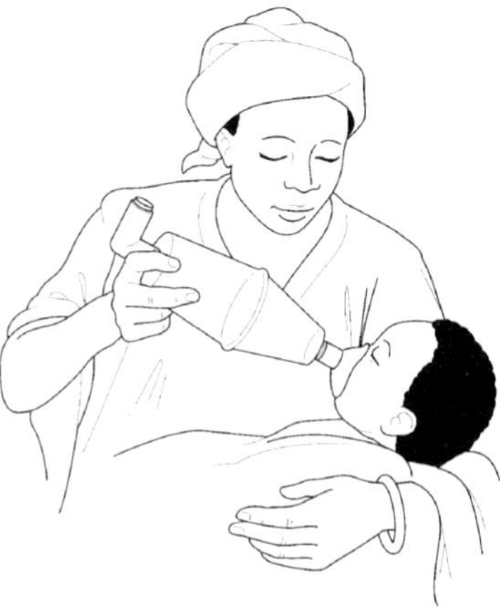

Use of spacer device and face mask to give bronchodilator treatment. A spacer can be made locally from a plastic soft drink bottle.

Some infants and young children cooperate better when a face mask is attached to the spacer instead of the mouthpiece.

If commercial devices are not available, a spacer device can be made from a plastic cup or a 1-litre plastic bottle. These require 3–4 puffs of salbutamol and the child should breathe from the device for up to 30 seconds.

(3) Subcutaneous epinephrine (adrenaline)

➤ If the above two methods of delivering salbutamol are not available, give a subcutaneous injection of epinephrine (adrenaline)—0.01 ml/kg of 1:1000 solution (up to a maximum of 0.3 ml), measured accurately with a 1 ml syringe (for injection technique, see page 305). If there is no improvement after 15 minutes, repeat the dose once.

Oral bronchodilators

➤ Once the child has improved sufficiently to be discharged home, if there is no inhaled salbutamol available or affordable, then oral salbutamol (in syrup or tablets) can be given. The dose is:

age 1–5 years: 2 mg 6–8 hourly.

Steroids

➤ If a child has a severe acute attack of wheezing *and* a history of recurrent wheezing, give oral prednisolone, 1 mg/kg, for 3 days. If the child remains very sick, continue the treatment until improvement is seen. Steroids are not usually required for the first episode of wheezing.

Aminophylline

➤ If a child does not improve after 3 doses of a rapid-acting bronchodilator given at short intervals plus oral prednisolone, give IV aminophylline—initial dose of 5–6 mg/kg (up to a maximum of 300 mg), followed by a maintenance dose of 5 mg/kg every 6 hours. Weigh the child carefully and give the IV dose over at least 20 minutes and preferably over 1 hour.

Intravenous aminophylline can be dangerous in an overdose or when given too rapidly. *Omit the initial dose if the child has already received any form of aminophylline in the previous 24 hours.*

➤ Stop giving it immediately if the child starts to vomit, has a pulse rate >180/min, develops a headache, or has a convulsion.

➤ If IV aminophylline is not available, aminophylline suppositories are an alternative.

Antibiotics

➤ Antibiotics should *not* be given routinely for asthma or to a child with asthma who has fast breathing *without* fever. Antimicrobial treatment is indicated, however, when there is persistent fever and other signs of pneumonia (see section 4.2, page 72).

Supportive care

➤ Ensure that the child receives daily maintenance fluids appropriate for his/her age (see page 273). Encourage breastfeeding and oral fluids. Encourage adequate complementary feeding for the young child, as soon as food can be taken.

Monitoring

A hospitalized child should be assessed by a nurse every 3 hours, or every 6 hours as the child shows improvement (i.e. decreased breathing rate, less lower chest wall indrawing, and less respiratory distress), and by a doctor at least once a day. Record the respiratory rate and watch especially for signs of respiratory failure—increasing hypoxia and respiratory distress leading to exhaustion. If the response to treatment is poor, give salbutamol more frequently, up to once every

60 minutes. If this is ineffective, give aminophylline. Monitor oxygen therapy as described on page 283.

Complications

➤ If the child fails to respond to the above therapy, or the child's condition worsens suddenly, obtain a chest X-ray to look for evidence of pneumothorax. Treat as described on page 87.

Follow-up care

Asthma is a chronic and recurrent condition.

➤ A long-term treatment plan should be made based on the frequency and severity of symptoms. This may include intermittent or regular treatment with bronchodilators, regular treatment with inhaled steroids or intermittent courses of oral steroids. See standard paediatric textbooks for more information.

4.4.3 Wheeze with cough or cold

Most first episodes of wheezing in children aged <2 years are associated with cough and cold. These children are not likely to have a family history of atopy (e.g. hay fever, eczema, allergic rhinitis) and their wheezing episodes become less frequent as they grow older. The wheezing, if troublesome, might respond to salbutamol treatment at home.

4.5 Conditions presenting with stridor

- Stridor is a harsh noise during inspiration, which is due to narrowing of the air passage in the oropharynx, subglottis or trachea. If the obstruction is severe, stridor may also occur during expiration.

The major causes of severe stridor are viral croup (caused by measles or other viruses), foreign body, retropharyngeal abscess, diphtheria and trauma to the larynx (Table 9 below).

History

- first episode or recurrent episode of stridor
- history of choking
- stridor present soon after birth.

Examination

- bull neck appearance
- blood-stained nasal discharge

- stridor present even when the child is quiet.
- grey pharyngeal membrane

Table 9. Differential diagnosis of the child presenting with stridor

Diagnosis	In favour
Viral croup	— Barking cough — Respiratory distress — Hoarse voice — If due to measles, signs of measles (see pages 154, 157)
Retropharyngeal abscess	— Soft tissue swelling — Difficulty in swallowing — Fever
Foreign body	— Sudden history of choking — Respiratory distress
Diphtheria	— Bull neck appearance due to enlarged cervical nodes and oedema — Red throat — Grey pharyngeal membrane — Blood-stained nasal discharge — No evidence of DTP vaccination
Congenital anomaly	— Stridor present since birth

4.5.1 **Viral croup**

Croup causes obstruction in the upper airway which, when severe, can be life-threatening. Most severe episodes occur in infants. This section deals with croup caused by various respiratory viruses. For croup associated with measles, see pages 154–157.

Diagnosis

Mild croup is characterized by:

- fever
- a hoarse voice
- a barking or hacking cough
- stridor that is heard only when the *child is agitated.*

Severe croup is characterized by:

- stridor when the *child is quiet*
- rapid breathing and indrawing of the lower chest wall.

Treatment

Mild croup can be managed at home with supportive care, including encouraging oral fluids, breastfeeding or feeding, as appropriate.

A child with ***severe croup*** should be admitted to hospital for treatment as follows:

➤ ***1. Steroid treatment***. Give one dose of oral dexamethasone (0.6 mg/kg) or equivalent dose of some other steroid—see pages 335 (dexamethasone) and 343 (prednisolone).

➤ ***2. Epinephrine (adrenaline)***. As a trial, give the child nebulized epinephrine (1:1000 solution). If this is effective, repeat as often as every hour, with careful monitoring. While this treatment can lead to improvement within 30 minutes in some children, it is often temporary and may last only about 2 hours.

➤ ***3. Antibiotics***. These are not effective and should *not* be given.

In a child with severe croup who is deterioriating, consider

1. Oxygen

➤ Avoid using oxygen unless there is incipient airway obstruction.

Signs such as severe indrawing of the lower chest wall and restlessness are more likely to indicate the need for tracheostomy (or intubation) than oxygen. Moreover, the use of nasal prongs or a nasal or nasopharyngeal catheter can upset the child and precipitate obstruction of the airway.

➤ However, oxygen should be given, if there is incipient airway obstruction and a tracheostomy is deemed necessary and is to be performed.

2. Intubation and tracheostomy

➤ If there are signs of incipient airway obstruction, such as severe indrawing of the lower chest wall and restlessness, intubate the child immediately.

➤ If this is not possible, transfer the child urgently to a hospital where intubation or emergency tracheostomy can be done.

➤ If this is not possible, monitor the child closely and ensure that facilities for an emergency tracheostomy are immediately available, as airway obstruction can occur suddenly.

Tracheostomy should only be done by experienced staff.

Supportive care

➤ Disturb as little as possible

➤ If the child has fever (≥39 °C or ≥102.2 °F) which appears to be causing distress, give paracetamol.

➤ Encourage breastfeeding and oral fluids. Avoid parenteral fluids, which are usually not required.

➤ Encourage the child to eat as soon as food can be taken.

Avoid using mist tents which are not effective. They separate the child from the parents and make observation of the child's condition very difficult.

Monitoring

The child's condition, especially respiratory status, should be assessed by nurses every 3 hours and by doctors twice a day. The child should occupy a bed close to the nursing station, so that any sign of incipient airway obstruction can be detected as soon as it develops.

4.5.2 Diphtheria

Diphtheria is a bacterial infection which can be prevented by immunization. Infection in the upper airway or nasopharynx produces a grey membrane which, when present in the larynx or trachea, can cause stridor and obstruction. Nasal involvement produces a bloody discharge. Diphtheria toxin causes muscular paralysis and myocarditis, which is associated with increased mortality.

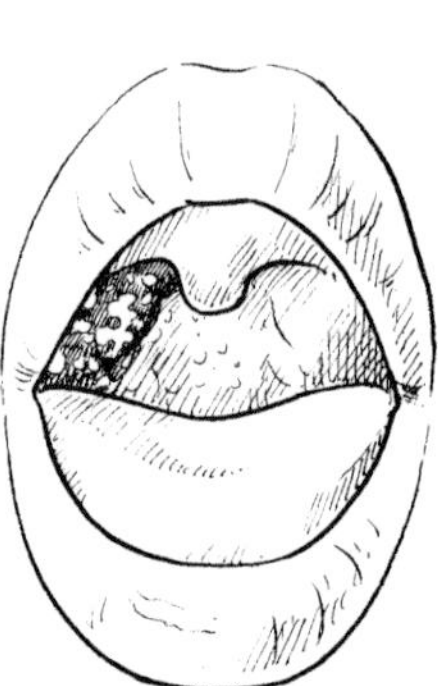

Pharyngeal membrane of diphtheria. Note: the membrane extends beyond the tonsils and covers the adjacent pharyngeal wall.

Diagnosis

- Carefully examine the child's nose and throat and look for a grey, adherent membrane, which cannot be wiped off with a swab. Great care is needed when examining the throat, as this may precipitate complete obstruction of the airway. A child with pharyngeal diphtheria may have an obviously swollen neck, termed a 'bull neck'.

Treatment

Antitoxin

➤ Give 40 000 units of diphtheria antitoxin (IM or IV) *immediately*, because delay can lead to increased mortality.

Antibiotics

➤ Any child with suspected diphtheria should be given procaine penicillin (50 000 units/kg IM) daily for 7 days.

As there is a small risk of a serious allergic reaction to the horse serum in the anti-toxin, an initial intradermal test to detect hypersensitivity should be carried out, as described in the instructions, and treatment for anaphylaxis be made available.

Oxygen

➤ Avoid using oxygen *unless* there is incipient airway obstruction.

Signs such as severe indrawing of the lower chest wall and restlessness are more likely to indicate the need for tracheostomy (or intubation) than oxygen. Moreover, the use of nasal prongs or a nasal or nasopharyngeal catheter can upset the child and precipitate obstruction of the airway.

➤ However, oxygen *should* be given, if there is incipient airway obstruction and a tracheostomy is deemed necessary and is to be performed.

Tracheostomy/intubation

➤ Tracheostomy should be performed only by experienced staff, if there are signs of incipient airway obstruction, such as severe lower chest wall indrawing and restlessness. If obstruction occurs, an emergency tracheostomy should be carried out. Orotracheal intubation is an alternative, but may dislodge the membrane and fail to relieve the obstruction.

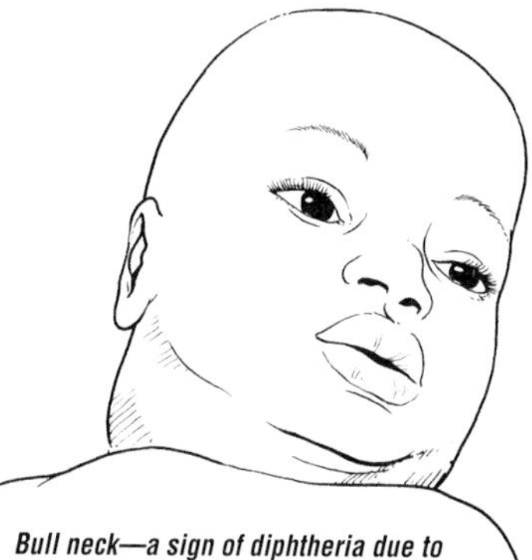

Bull neck—a sign of diphtheria due to enlarged lymph nodes in the neck

Supportive care

➤ If the child has fever (≥39 °C or ≥102.2 °F) which appears to be causing distress, give paracetamol.

➤ Encourage the child to eat and drink. If there is difficulty in swallowing, nasogastric feeding is required.

Avoid frequent examinations or disturbing the child unnecessarily.

Monitoring

The child's condition, especially respiratory status, should be assessed by nurses every 3 hours and by doctors twice a day. The child should occupy a bed close to the nursing station, so that any sign of incipient airway obstruction can be detected as soon as it develops.

Complications

Myocarditis and paralysis may occur 2–7 weeks after the onset of illness.

- Signs of *myocarditis* include a weak, irregular pulse and evidence of heart failure. Refer to standard paediatric textbooks for details of the diagnosis and management of myocarditis.

Public health measures

- ➤ Nurse the child in a separate room by staff who are fully immunized against diphtheria.
- ➤ Give all *immunized* household contacts a diphtheria toxoid booster.
- ➤ Give all *unimmunized* household contacts one IM dose of benzathine penicillin (600 000 units to those aged ≤5 years; 1 200 000 units to those aged >5 years). Immunize them with diphtheria toxoid and check daily for 5 days for any signs of diphtheria.

4.6 Conditions presenting with chronic cough

Chronic cough is one that lasts for 30 days or more.

History

Ask for

- duration of coughing
- nocturnal cough
- paroxysmal cough or associated severe bouts ending with vomiting or whooping
- weight loss (check growth chart, if available), night sweats
- persistent fever
- close contact with a known case of sputum-positive tuberculosis or with pertussis
- history of attacks of wheeze and a family history of allergy or asthma
- history of choking or inhalation of a foreign body
- child suspected or known to be HIV-infected
- treatment given and response.

Table 10. Differential diagnosis of the child presenting with chronic cough

Diagnosis	In favour
Tuberculosis	— Weight loss or failure to thrive — Anorexia, night sweats — Enlarged liver and spleen — Chronic or intermittent fever — History of exposure to infectious tuberculosis — Signs of fluid in chest (dull to percussion/reduced breath sounds)
Asthma	— History of recurrent wheeze, often unrelated to coughs and colds — Hyperinflation of the chest — Prolonged expiration — Reduced air entry (in very severe airway obstruction) — Good response to bronchodilators
Foreign body	— Sudden onset of choking or stridor — Unilateral chest signs (e.g. wheezing or hyperinflation) — Recurrent lobar consolidation — Poor response to medical treatment
Pertussis	— Paroxysms of cough followed by whoop, vomiting, cyanosis or apnoea — Subconjunctival haemorrhages — No history of DPT immunization — Afebrile
HIV	— Known or suspected maternal or sibling HIV infection — History of blood transfusion — Failure to thrive — Oral thrush — Chronic parotitis — Skin infection with herpes zoster (past or present) — Generalized lymphadenopathy — Chronic fever — Persistent diarrhoea — Finger clubbing
Bronchiectasis	— History of tuberculosis or aspirated foreign body — Poor weight gain — Purulent sputum, bad breath — Finger clubbing — Localized signs on X-ray
Lung abscess	— Reduced breath sounds over abscess — Poor weight gain / chronically ill child — Cystic or cavitating lesion on chest X-ray

Examination

- fever
- lymphadenopathy (generalized and localized, e.g. in the neck)
- wasting
- wheeze / prolonged expiration
- apnoeic episodes
- subconjunctival haemorrhages
- signs associated with foreign body aspiration:
  - unilateral wheeze
  - area of decreased breath sounds which is either dull or hyper-resonant on percussion
  - deviation of the trachea or apex beat.
- signs associated with HIV infection (see page 200).

Treatment guidelines for the causes of chronic cough are indicated below:

- tuberculosis (page 103)
- asthma (page 87)
- foreign body (page 105)
- pertussis (see below)
- HIV (pages 207–215).

4.7 Pertussis

Pertussis is most severe in young infants who have not yet been immunized. After an incubation period of 7–10 days, the child develops fever, usually with a cough and nasal discharge which clinically are indistinguishable from a common cough and cold. In the second week, there is paroxysmal coughing which can be recognized as pertussis. The episodes of coughing can continue for 3 months or longer. The child is infectious for a period of 2 weeks up to 3 months after the onset of illness.

Diagnosis

Suspect pertussis if a child has been having a severe cough for more than two weeks, especially if the disease is known to be occurring locally. The most useful diagnostic signs are:

- Paroxysmal coughing followed by a whoop when breathing in, often with vomiting
- Subconjunctival haemorrhages
- Child not immunized against pertussis.
- Young infants may not whoop; instead, the cough may be followed by

suspension of breathing (apnoea) or cyanosis, or apnoea may occur without coughing.

- Also, examine the child for signs of pneumonia and ask about convulsions.

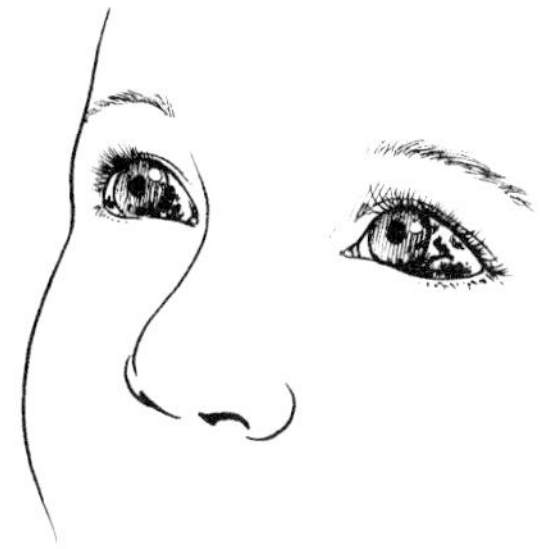

Subconjunctival haemorrhages prominent on the white sclera

Treatment

Treat mild cases in children aged ≥6 months at home with supportive care. Admit infants aged under 6 months to hospital; also admit any child with pneumonia, convulsions, dehydration, severe malnutrition, or prolonged apnoea or cyanosis after coughing.

Antibiotics

➤ Give oral erythromycin (12.5 mg/kg four times a day) for 10 days. This does not shorten the illness but reduces the period of infectiousness.

➤ If there is fever or if erythromycin is not available, give oral chloramphenicol (25 mg/kg three times a day) for 5 days to treat possible secondary pneumonia. Follow the other guidelines for severe pneumonia (see section 4.2.2, page 78). If chloramphenicol is not available, give cotrimoxazole, as described for pneumonia (non-severe) (see section 4.2.3, page 80).

Oxygen

➤ Give oxygen to children who have spells of apnoea or cyanosis, or severe paroxysms of coughing.

Use nasal prongs, *not* a nasopharyngeal catheter or nasal catheter which can provoke coughing. Place the prongs just inside the nostrils and secure with a piece of tape just above the upper lip. Care should be taken to keep the nostrils clear of mucus since this blocks the flow of oxygen. Set a flow rate of 1–2 litres/min (0.5 litre/min in young infants). Humidification is not required with nasal prongs.

➤ Continue oxygen therapy until the above signs are no longer present, after which there is no value in continuing with oxygen.

➤ The nurse should check, every 3 hours, that the prongs or catheter are in the correct place and not blocked with mucus, and that all connections are secure. See page 282 for further details.

Airway management

➤ During paroxysms of coughing, place the child head down and prone, or on the side, to prevent any inhaling of vomitus and to aid expectoration of secretions.

— If the child has *cyanotic* episodes, clear secretions from the nose and throat with brief, gentle suction.

— If *apnoea* occurs, clear the airway immediately with gentle suction, give manual respiratory stimulation or bag ventilation, and administer oxygen.

Supportive care

- Avoid, as far as possible, any procedure that could trigger coughing, such as application of suction, throat examination, and use of a nasogastric tube.
- Do *not* give cough suppressants, sedatives, mucolytic agents or antihistamines.

➤ If the child has fever (≥39 °C, ≥102.2 °F) which appears to be causing distress, give paracetamol.

➤ Encourage breastfeeding or oral fluids. If the child cannot drink, pass a nasogastric tube and give small, frequent amounts of fluid to meet the child's maintenance needs (see page 273). If there is respiratory distress, give maintenance fluids IV to avoid the risk of aspiration and reduce triggering of coughing. Ensure adequate nutrition by giving smaller, more frequent feeds. If there is continued weight loss despite theses measures, feed the child by nasogastric tube.

Monitoring

The child should be assessed by nurses every 3 hours and by the doctor once a day. To facilitate observation for early detection and treatment of apnoeic or cyanotic spells, or severe episodes of coughing, the child should occupy a bed in a place close to the nursing station where oxygen is available. Also, teach the child's mother to recognize apnoeic spells and to alert the nurse if this should occur.

Complications

Pneumonia. This most common complication of pertussis is caused by secondary bacterial infection or inhalation of vomited material.

■ Signs suggesting pneumonia include fast breathing between coughing episodes, fever, and the rapid onset of respiratory distress.

➤ Treat pneumonia in children with pertussis as follows:
  — Give chloramphenicol (dose: 25 mg/kg every 8 hours) for 5 days.
  — Give oxygen as described for the treatment of very severe pneumonia (see sections 4.1.1 and 10.7, pages 73 and 281).

Convulsions. These may result from anoxia associated with an apnoeic or cyanotic episode, or toxin-mediated encephalopathy.

➤ If a convulsion does not stop within two minutes, give an anticonvulsant (diazepam or paraldehyde), following guidelines in Chapter 1 (Chart 9, page 14).

Malnutrition. Children with pertussis may become malnourished as a result of reduced food intake and frequent vomiting.

➤ Prevent malnutrition by ensuring adequate feeding, as described above, under "supportive care".

Haemorrhage and hernias

■ Subconjunctival haemorrhage and epistaxis are common during pertussis.

➤ No specific treatment is needed.

■ Umbilical or inguinal hernias may be caused by violent coughing.

➤ Do not treat them unless there are signs of bowel obstruction, but refer the child for surgical evaluation after the acute phase.

Public health measures

➤ Give DPT immunization to any child in the family who is not fully immunized and to the child with pertussis.

➤ Give a DPT booster to previously immunized children.

➤ Give erythromycin estolate (12.5 mg/kg 4 times a day) for 10 days to any infant in the family who is aged under 6 months and has fever or other signs of a respiratory infection.

4.8 Tuberculosis

Most children infected with *Mycobacterium tuberculosis* do not develop tuberculosis disease. The only evidence of infection may be a positive skin test. The development of tuberculosis disease depends on the competence of the immune system to resist multiplication of the *M. tuberculosis* infection. This competence varies with age, being least in the very young. HIV and malnutrition lower the body's defences, and measles and whooping cough temporarily impair the strength of the immune system. In the presence of any of these conditions, tuberculosis disease can develop more easily.

Tuberculosis is most often severe when the disease is located in the lungs, meninges or kidney. Cervical lymph nodes, bones, joints, abdomen, ear, eye, and skin may also be affected. Many children present only with failure to grow normally, weight loss or prolonged fever. Cough for more than 30 days can also be a presenting sign; in children, however, sputum-positive pulmonary tuberculosis is rarely diagnosed.

Diagnosis

The risk of tuberculosis is increased when there is an active case (infectious, smear-positive pulmonary tuberculosis) in the same house, or when the child is malnourished, has HIV/AIDS, or has had measles in the past few months. Consider tuberculosis in any child with:

A ***history*** of:

- unexplained weight loss or failure to grow normally;
- unexplained fever, especially when it continues for more than 2 weeks;
- chronic cough (i.e. cough for more than 30 days, with or without a wheeze);
- exposure to an adult with probable or definite infectious pulmonary tuberculosis.

On ***examination***:

- fluid on one side of the chest (reduced air entry, stony dullness to percussion);
- enlarged non-tender lymph nodes or a lymph node abscess, especially in the neck;
- signs of meningitis, especially when these develop over several days and the spinal fluid contains mostly lymphocytes and elevated protein;
- abdominal swelling, with or without palpable lumps;
- progressive swelling or deformity in the bone or a joint, including the spine.

Investigations

- Try to obtain specimens for ***microscopic examination*** of acid-fast bacilli (Ziehl-Neelsen stain) and for ***culture*** of tubercle bacilli. Possible specimens include three consecutive early morning fasting gastric aspirates, CSF (if clinically indicated), and pleural fluid and ascites fluid. Owing to low detection rates by these methods, a positive result would confirm tuberculosis, but a negative result does not exclude the disease.
- Obtain a ***chest X-ray***. A diagnosis of tuberculosis is supported when a chest X-ray shows a miliary pattern of infiltrates or a persistent area of infiltrate or consolidation, often with pleural effusion, or a primary complex.

- Perform a ***PPD skin test***. The test is usually positive in children with pulmonary tuberculosis (reactions of >10 mm are suggestive of tuberculosis; <10 mm in a child, previously immunized with BCG, is equivocal). However, the PPD test may be negative in children with tuberculosis who have HIV/AIDS or when there is miliary disease, severe malnutrition or recent measles.

Treatment

➤ Give a full course of treatment to all confirmed or highly suspected cases.

➤ When in doubt, e.g. in a child highly suspected of tuberculosis or who fails to respond to treatment for other likely diagnoses, give treatment for tuberculosis.

Treatment failures for other diagnoses include antibiotic treatment for apparent bacterial pneumonia (when the child has pulmonary symptoms), or for possible meningitis (when the child has neurological symptoms), or for intestinal worms or giardiasis (when the child fails to thrive or has diarrhoea or abdominal symptoms).

➤ Follow the treatment recommended by the national tuberculosis programme. Inform this programme and arrange for adequate support and monitoring.

➤ If national recommendations are not available, follow the WHO guidelines which are given below.

1. **In the majority of cases of childhood tuberculosis (i.e. in the absence of smear-positive pulmonary tuberculosis or severe disease), give:**

   First 2 months (initial phase): *isoniazid + rifampicin + pyrazinamide daily or 3 times a week,*

   followed by EITHER

   Next 6 months (continuation phase): *isoniazid + ethambutol or isoniazid + thioacetazone daily;*

   OR

   Next 4 months (continuation phase): *isoniazid + rifampicin daily or 3 times a week.*

2. **In the case of smear-positive pulmonary tuberculosis or severe disease, give the following treatment:**

   First 2 months (initial phase): *isoniazid + rifampicin + pyrazinamide + ethambutol (or streptomycin) daily or 3 times a week,*

   followed by EITHER

   Next 6 months (continuation phase): *isoniazid + ethambutol daily;*

OR

Next 4 months (continuation phase): *isoniazid + rifampicin daily or 3 times a week.*

3. **In the case of tuberculous meningitis, miliary tuberculosis or spinal TB with neurological signs, give the following regimen:**

   First 2 months (initial phase): *isoniazid + rifampicin + pyrazinamide + ethambutol (or streptomycin) daily or 3 times a week,*

   followed by

   Next 7 months (continuation phase): *isoniazid + rifampicin daily.*

Details of the regimen and dosage for each of the above drugs is given in Appendix 2, page 352.

Precautions: Avoid streptomycin, where possible, in children because the injections are painful, irreversible auditory nerve damage may occur, and there is a risk of spreading HIV due to improper handling of the needle and syringe. Avoid thioacetazone in a child who is known to be HIV-infected or when the likelihood of HIV infection is high, because severe (sometimes fatal) skin reactions can occur.

Monitoring

Confirm that the medication is being taken as instructed, by *direct observation of each dose.* Monitor the child's weight gain (daily) and temperature (twice daily) in order to check for resolution of the fever. These are signs of the response to therapy. When treatment is given for suspected tuberculosis, improvement should be seen within one month. If this does not happen, review the patient, check compliance and reconsider the diagnosis.

Public health measures

- Notify the case to the responsible district health authorities. Ensure that treatment monitoring is carried out, as recommended by the national tuberculosis programme. Check all household members of the child (and, if necessary, school contacts) for undetected cases of tuberculosis and arrange treatment for any who are found.

4.9 Foreign body inhalation

Nuts, seeds or other small objects may be inhaled, most often by children under 4 years of age. The foreign body usually lodges in a bronchus (more often in the right) and can cause collapse or consolidation of the portion of lung distal to the site of blockage. Choking is a frequent initial symptom. This may be followed by a symptom-free interval of days or weeks before the child presents with persistent wheeze, chronic cough or pneumonia, which fails to respond to treatment. Small sharp objects can lodge in the larynx causing stridor or wheeze. Rarely, a large object lodging in the larynx could cause sudden death from asphyxia, unless an emergency tracheostomy is done.

Diagnosis

Inhalation of a foreign body should be considered in a child with the following signs:

- sudden onset of choking, coughing or wheezing; or
- segmental or lobar pneumonia which fails to respond to antibiotic therapy (note also differential diagnosis of tuberculosis—see page 97).

Examine the child for:

- unilateral wheeze;
- an area of decreased breath sounds which is either dull or hyper-resonant on percussion;
- deviation of the trachea or apex beat.

Obtain a chest X-ray at full expiration to detect an area of hyper-inflation or collapse, mediastinal shift (away from the affected side), or a foreign body if it is radio-opaque.

Treatment

Emergency first aid for the choking child. Attempt to dislodge and expel the foreign body. The management depends on the age of the child.

For infants:

- ➤ Lay the infant on one arm or on the thigh in a head-down position.
- ➤ Strike the infant's back five times with the heel of the hand.
- ➤ If the obstruction persists, turn the infant over and give five chest thrusts with two fingers, one finger's breadth below the nipple level in the midline.
- ➤ If the obstruction persists, check the infant's mouth for any obstruction which can be removed.
- ➤ If necessary, repeat this sequence with back slaps again.

For older children:

- ➤ While the child is sitting, kneeling or lying, strike the child's back five times with the heel of the hand.

➤ If the obstruction persists, go behind the child and pass your arms around the child's body; form a fist with one hand immediately below the sternum; place the other hand over the fist and thrust sharply upwards into the abdomen. Repeat this up to five times.

➤ If the obstruction persists, check the child's mouth for any obstruction which can be removed.

➤ If necessary, repeat the sequence with back slaps again.

Once this has been done, it is important to check the patency of the airway by:

- looking for chest movements
- listening for breath sounds, and
- feeling for breath.

If further management of the airway is required after the obstruction is removed, see Chart 4, pages 8–9. This describes actions which will keep the child's airway open and prevent the tongue from falling back to obstruct the pharynx while the child recovers.

➤ ***Later treatment of suspected foreign body aspiration.*** If a foreign body is suspected, refer the child to a hospital where diagnosis is possible and the object can be 'removed' by bronchoscopy. If there is evidence of pneumonia, begin treatment with ampicillin and gentamicin, as for very severe pneumonia (see page 74), before attempting to remove the foreign body.

4.10 **Heart failure**

Heart failure causes fast breathing and respiratory distress. Underlying causes include congenital heart disease (usually in the first months of life), acute rheumatic fever, myocarditis, suppurative pericarditis with constriction, infective endocarditis, acute glomerulonephritis, severe anaemia, very severe pneumonia and severe malnutrition. Heart failure can be precipitated or worsened by fluid overload, especially when giving salt-containing IV fluids.

Diagnosis

The most common signs of heart failure, on examination, are:

- Tachycardia (heart rate >160/minute in a child under 12 months old; >120/minute in a child aged 12 months to 5 years).
- Gallop rhythm with basal crackles on auscultation.
- Enlarged, tender liver.
- In *infants*—fast breathing (or sweating), especially when feeding (see section

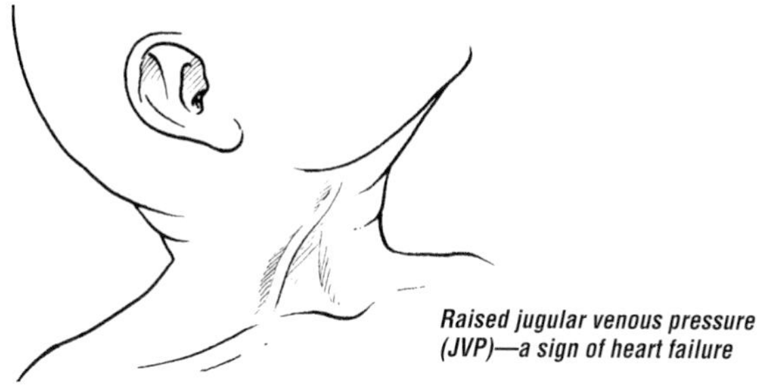

Raised jugular venous pressure (JVP)—a sign of heart failure

4.1.1, page 73, for definition of fast breathing); in *older children*—oedema of the feet, hands or face, or distended neck veins.

- Severe palmar pallor may be present if severe anaemia is the cause of the heart failure.
- If the diagnosis is in doubt, a chest X-ray can be taken and will show an enlarged heart.
- Measure blood pressure if possible. If raised consider acute glomerulonephritis (see standard paediatric textbook for treatment).

Treatment

For details on the treatment of the underlying heart disease, consult a standard paediatric textbook. The main measures for treatment of heart failure in non-severely malnourished children are as follows.

➤ **Diuretics**. Give furosemide (frusemide): a dose of 1 mg/kg should cause increased urine flow within 2 hours. For faster action, give the drug IV. If the initial dose is not effective, give 2 mg/kg and repeat in 12 hours, if necessary. Thereafter, a single daily dose of 1–2 mg/kg orally is usually sufficient.

➤ **Digoxin**. Consider giving digoxin (see Appendix 2, page 336).

➤ **Supplemental potassium**. Supplemental potassium is *not* required when furosemide is given alone for treatment lasting only a few days. When digoxin *and* furosemide are given, or if frusemide is given for more than 5 days, give oral potassium (3–5 mmol/kg/day).

➤ **Oxygen**. Give oxygen if the child has a respiratory rate of ≥70/min, shows signs of respiratory distress, or has central cyanosis. See page 281.

Supportive care

- Avoid the use of IV fluids, where possible.
- Support the child in a semi-seated position with head and shoulders elevated and lower limbs dependent.
- Relieve any fever with paracetamol to reduce the cardiac workload.

Monitoring

The child should be checked by nurses every 6 hours (3-hourly whilst on oxygen therapy) and by doctors once a day. Monitor both respiratory and pulse rates, liver size, and body weight to assess the response to treatment. Continue treatment until the respiratory and pulse rates are normal and the liver is no longer enlarged.

Notes

CHAPTER 5

Diarrhoea

This chapter gives treatment guidelines on the management of acute diarrhoea (with severe, some or no dehydration), persistent diarrhoea, and dysentery in children aged 1 week to 5 years. Assessment of severely malnourished children is described in sections 7.2 and 7.3 (pages 174, 176). The 3 essential elements in the management of all children with diarrhoea are **rehydration therapy**, **zinc supplementation**, and **continued feeding**.

During diarrhoea there is an increased loss of water and electrolytes (sodium, potassium and bicarbonate) in the liquid stool. Dehydration occurs when these losses are not adequately replaced and a deficit of water and electrolytes develops. The degree of dehydration is graded according to symptoms and signs that reflect the amount of fluid lost (see sections 2.3 (page 38) and 5.1 (below)). The rehydration regimen is selected according to the degree of dehydration.

Zinc is an important micronutrient for a child's overall health and development. Zinc is lost in greater quantity during diarrhoea. Replacing the lost zinc is important to help the child recover and to keep the child healthy in the coming months. It has been shown that zinc supplements given during an episode of diarrhoea reduce the duration and severity of the episode, and lower the incidence of diarrhoea in the following 2–3 months. For these reasons, all patients with diarrhoea should be given zinc supplements as soon as possible after the diarrhoea has started.

During diarrhoea, a decrease in food intake and nutrient absorption and increased nutrient requirements often combine to cause weight loss and failure to grow. In turn, malnutrition can make the diarrhoea more severe, more prolonged and more frequent, compared with diarrhoea in non-malnourished children. This vicious circle can be broken by giving nutrient-rich foods during the diarrhoea and when the child is well.

Antibiotics should not be used routinely. They are reliably helpful *only* for children with bloody diarrhoea (probable shigellosis), suspected cholera with severe dehydration, and other serious non-intestinal infections such as pneumonia. Antiprotozoal drugs are rarely indicated. "Antidiarrhoeal" drugs and anti-emetics should *not* be given to young children with acute or persistent diarrhoea or dysentery: they do not prevent dehydration or improve nutritional status and some have dangerous, sometimes fatal, side-effects.

5.1 Child presenting with diarrhoea

History

A careful feeding history is essential in the management of a child with diarrhoea. Also, inquire into the following:

- diarrhoea
  - — frequency of stools
  - — number of days
  - — blood in stools
- local reports of cholera outbreak
- recent antibiotic or other drug treatment
- attacks of crying with pallor in an infant.

Examination

Look for:

- signs of some dehydration or severe dehydration:
  - — restlessness or irritability
  - — lethargy/reduced level of consciousness
  - — sunken eyes
  - — skin pinch returns slowly or very slowly
  - — thirsty/drinks eagerly, or drinking poorly or not able to drink
- blood in stool
- signs of severe malnutrition
- abdominal mass
- abdominal distension.

There is no need for routine stool cultures in children with diarrhoea.

Table 11. Differential diagnosis of the child presenting with diarrhoea

Diagnosis	In favour
Acute (watery) diarrhoea	— More than 3 stools per day — No blood in stools
Cholera	— Diarrhoea with severe dehydration during cholera outbreak — Positive stool culture for *V. cholerae* 01 or 0139
Dysentery	— Blood in stool (seen or reported)
Persistent diarrhoea	— Diarrhoea lasting 14 days or longer
Diarrhoea with severe malnutrition	— Any diarrhoea with signs of severe malnutrition (see page 173)
Diarrhoea associated with recent antibiotic use	— Recent course of broad-spectrum oral antibiotics
Intussusception	— Blood in stool — Abdominal mass (check with rectal examination) — Attacks of crying with pallor in infant

5.2 Acute diarrhoea

Assessing dehydration

In all children with diarrhoea, decide if dehydration is present and give appropriate treatment (see Table 12 below).

For all children with diarrhoea, hydration status should be classified as **severe dehydration**, **some dehydration** or **no dehydration** (see below) and appropriate treatment given.

Table 12. Classification of the severity of dehydration in children with diarrhoea

Classification	Signs or symptoms	Treatment
Severe dehydration	***Two*** or more of the following signs: ■ lethargy/unconsciousness ■ sunken eyes ■ unable to drink or drinks poorly ■ skin pinch goes back very slowly (≥2 seconds)	➤ Give fluid for severe dehydration (see Diarrhoea Treatment Plan C in hospital, page 114)
Some dehydration	***Two*** or more of the following signs: ■ restlessness, irritability ■ sunken eyes ■ drinks eagerly, thirsty ■ skin pinch goes back slowly	➤ Give fluid and food for some dehydration (see Diarrhoea Treatment Plan B, page 117) ➤ After rehydration, advise mother on home treatment and when to return immediately (see pages 116, 118) ➤ Follow up in 5 days if not improving.

Table 12. Continued

Classification	Signs or symptoms	Treatment
No dehydration	Not enough signs to classify as some or severe dehydration	➤ Give fluid and food to treat diarrhoea at home (see Diarrhoea Treatment Plan A, page 120) ➤ Advise mother on when to return immediately (see page 119) ➤ Follow up in 5 days if not improving.

5.2.1 Severe dehydration

Children with severe dehydration require rapid IV rehydration with close monitoring, which is followed by oral rehydration once the child starts to improve sufficiently. In areas where there is a cholera outbreak, give an antibiotic effective against cholera (see page 113).

Diagnosis

If any *two* of the following signs are present in a child with diarrhoea, *severe dehydration* should be diagnosed:

- lethargy or unconsciousness
- sunken eyes
- skin pinch goes back very slowly (2 seconds or more)
- not able to drink or drinks poorly.

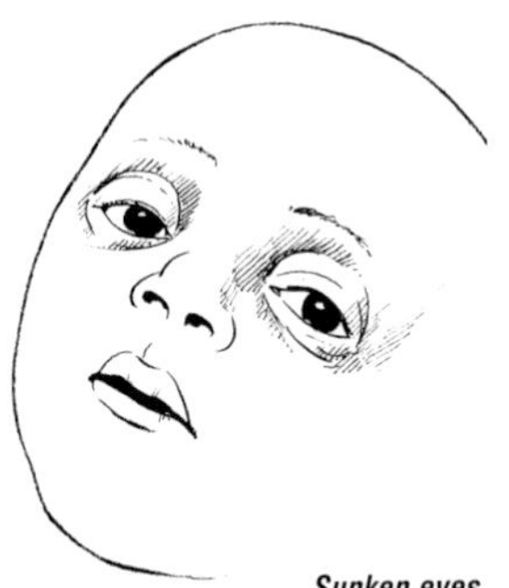

Sunken eyes

Treatment

Children with severe dehydration should be given rapid IV rehydration followed by oral rehydration therapy.

➤ *Start IV fluids immediately.* While the drip is being set up, give ORS solution if the child can drink.

Note: The best IV fluid solution is Ringer's lactate Solution (also called Hartmann's Solution for Injection). If Ringer's lactate is not available, normal saline solution (0.9% NaCl) can be used. 5% glucose (dextrose) solution on its own is **not** effective and should not be used.

➤ *Give 100 ml/kg of the chosen solution* divided as shown in Table 13.

Table 13. Administration of IV fluid to a severely dehydrated child

	First, give 30 ml/kg in:	**Then, give 70 ml/kg in:**
<12 months old	1 hour[a]	5 hours
≥12 months old	30 minutes[a]	2½ hours

[a] Repeat again if the radial pulse is still very weak or not detectable.

For more information, see Treatment Plan C in hospital, page 114. This includes guidelines for giving ORS solution by nasogastric tube or by mouth when IV therapy is not possible.

Cholera

- Suspect cholera in children over 2 years old who have acute watery diarrhoea and signs of severe dehydration, if cholera is occurring in the local area.
- ➤ Assess and treat dehydration as for other acute diarrhoea.
- ➤ Give an oral antibiotic to which strains of *Vibrio cholerae* in the area are known to be sensitive. Possible choices are: tetracycline, doxycycline, cotrimoxazole,

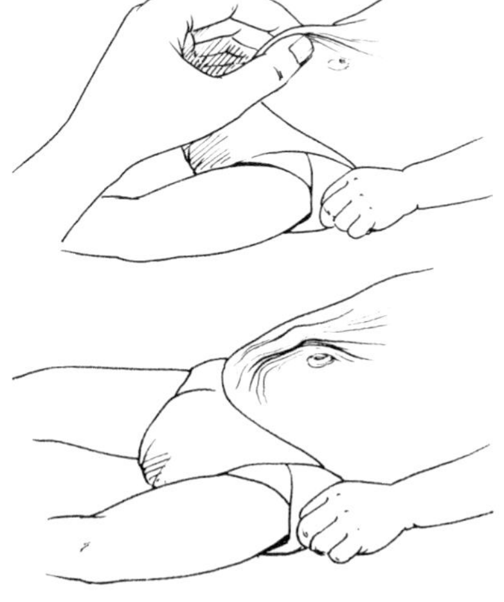

Pinching the child's abdomen to test for decreased skin turgor

Slow return of skin pinch in severe dehydration

CHART 13. **Diarrhoea Treatment Plan C: Treat severe dehydration quickly**

➥ **Follow the arrows. If answer is YES go across. If NO go down.**

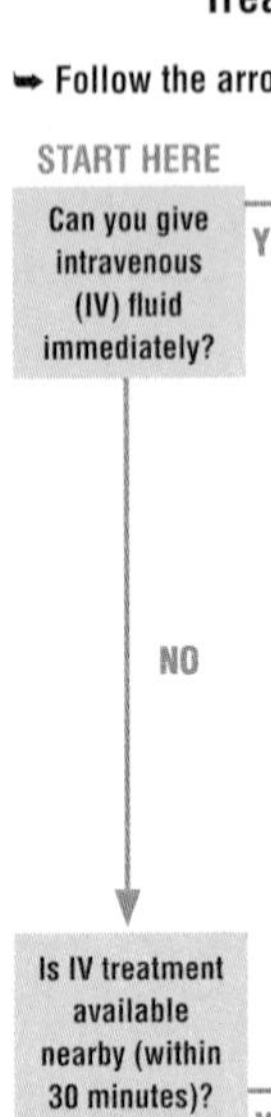

START HERE

Can you give intravenous (IV) fluid immediately? — YES →

➤ Start IV fluid immediately. If the child can drink, give ORS by mouth while the drip is set up. Give 100 ml/kg Ringer's lactate solution (or, if not available, normal saline), divided as follows:

AGE	First give 30 ml/kg in:	Then give 70 ml/kg in:
Infants (under 12 months)	1 hour*	5 hours
Children (12 months up to 5 years)	30 minutes*	2 1/2 hours

* Repeat once if radial pulse is still very weak or not detectable.

■ Reassess the child every 15–30 minutes. If hydration status is not improving, give the IV drip more rapidly.

➤ Also give ORS (about 5 ml/kg/hour) as soon as the child can drink: usually after 3–4 hours (infants) or 1–2 hours (children).

■ Reassess an infant after 6 hours and a child after 3 hours. Classify dehydration. Then choose the appropriate plan (A, B, or C) to continue treatment.

NO ↓

Is IV treatment available nearby (within 30 minutes)? — YES →

➤ Refer URGENTLY to hospital for IV treatment.

➤ If the child can drink, provide the mother with ORS solution and show her how to give frequent sips during the trip.

NO ↓

Are you trained to use a nasogastric (NG) tube for rehydration? — YES →

NO ↓

Can the child drink? — YES →

➤ Start rehydration by tube (or mouth) with ORS solution: give 20 ml/kg/hour for 6 hours (total of 120 ml/kg).

■ Reassess the child every 1–2 hours:

— If there is repeated vomiting or increasing abdominal distension, give the fluid more slowly.

— If hydration status is not improving after 3 hours, send the child for IV therapy.

■ After 6 hours, reassess the child. Classify dehydration. Then choose the appropriate plan (A, B, or C) to continue treatment.

NO ↓

Refer URGENTLY to hospital for IV or NG treatment

Note: If possible, observe the child for at least 6 hours after rehydration to be sure the mother can maintain hydration giving the child ORS solution by mouth.

erythromycin, and chloramphenicol (for dosages, see Appendix 2, page 325).

➤ Prescribe zinc supplementation as soon as vomiting stops (see page 118).

Monitoring

Reassess the child every 15–30 minutes until a strong radial pulse is present. If hydration is not improving, give the IV solution more rapidly. Thereafter, reassess the child by checking skin pinch, level of consciousness, and ability to drink, at least every hour, in order to confirm that hydration is improving. Sunken eyes recover more slowly than other signs and are less useful for monitoring.

When the full amount of IV fluid has been given, reassess the child's hydration status fully, using Chart 7 (page 12).

- *If signs of severe dehydration are still present*, repeat the IV fluid infusion as outlined earlier. Persistent severe dehydration after IV rehydration is unusual; it usually occurs only in children who pass large watery stools frequently during the rehydration period.
- *If the child is improving but still shows signs of some dehydration*, discontinue IV treatment and give ORS solution for 4 hours (see section 5.1.2 below and Treatment Plan B, page 117). If the child is normally breastfed, encourage the mother to continue breastfeeding frequently.
- *If there are no signs of dehydration*, follow the guidelines in section 5.1.3 below and Treatment Plan A, page 120. Where appropriate, encourage the mother to continue breastfeeding frequently. Observe the child for at least 6 hours before discharge, to confirm that the mother is able to maintain the child's hydration by giving ORS solution.

All children should start to receive some ORS solution (about 5ml/kg/hour) by cup when they can drink without difficulty (usually within 3–4 hours for infants, or 1–2 hours for older children). This provides additional base and potassium, which may not be adequately supplied by the IV fluid.

When severe dehydration is corrected, prescribe zinc (see page 118).

5.2.2 Some dehydration

In general, children with some dehydration should be given ORS solution, for the first 4 hours at a clinic while the child is monitored and the mother is taught how to prepare and give ORS solution.

Diagnosis

If the child has *two or more* of the following signs, the child has ***some dehydration***:

- restlessness/irritability
- thirsty and drinks eagerly
- sunken eyes
- skin pinch goes back slowly.

Note that if a child has only one of the above signs and one of the signs of severe dehydration (e.g. restless/irritable and drinking poorly), then that child also has some dehydration.

Treatment

➤ In the first 4 hours, give the child the following approximate amounts of ORS solution, according to the child's weight (or age if the weight is not known), as shown in chart 14.

However, if the child wants more to drink, give more.

➤ Show the mother how to give the child ORS solution, a teaspoonful every 1–2 minutes if the child is under 2 years; frequent sips from a cup for an older child.

➤ Check regularly to see if there are problems.

- *If the child vomits*, wait 10 minutes; then, resume giving ORS solution more slowly (e.g. a spoonful every 2–3 minutes).
- *If the child's eyelids become puffy*, stop ORS solution and give plain water or breast milk.

➤ Advise breastfeeding mothers to continue to breastfeed whenever the child wants.

➤ If the mother cannot stay for 4 hours, show her how to prepare ORS solution and give her enough ORS packets to complete the rehydration at home plus enough for 2 more days.

➤ *Reassess the child after 4 hours*, checking for signs of dehydration listed earlier.

(*Note:* Reassess the child before 4 hours if the child is not taking the ORS solution or seems to be getting worse.)

— *If there is no dehydration*, teach the mother the four rules of home treatment:

CHART 14. Diarrhoea Treatment Plan B: Treat some dehydration with ORS

GIVE RECOMMENDED AMOUNT OF ORS IN CLINIC OVER 4-HOUR PERIOD

➤ **Determine amount of ORS to give during first 4 hours.**

AGE*	Up to 4 months	4 months up to 12 months	12 months up to 2 years	2 years up to 5 years
WEIGHT	<6 kg	6–<10 kg	10–<12 kg	12–19 kg
In ml	200–400	400–700	700–900	900–1400

* *Use the child's age only when you do not know the weight. The approximate amount of ORS required (in ml) can also be calculated by multiplying the child's weight (in kg) by 75.*

— If the child wants more ORS than shown, give more.

➤ **Show the mother how to give ORS solution.**

— Give frequent small sips from a cup.

— If the child vomits, wait 10 minutes. Then continue, but more slowly.

— Continue breastfeeding whenever the child wants.

■ **After 4 hours:**

— Reassess the child and classify the child for dehydration.

— Select the appropriate plan to continue treatment.

— Begin feeding the child in clinic.

➤ **If the mother must leave before completing treatment:**

— Show her how to prepare ORS solution at home.

— Show her how much ORS to give to finish 4-hour treatment at home.

— Give her enough ORS packets to complete rehydration. Also give her 2 packets as recommended in Plan A.

— Explain the 4 Rules of Home Treatment:

1. Give extra fluid
2. Give zinc supplements
3. Continue feeding
3. When to return

} **See Diarrhoea Treatment Plan A** (page 120) and **Mother's Card** (page 294)

(i) give extra fluid

(ii) give zinc supplements for 10–14 days

(iii) continue feeding (see Chapter 10, page 261)

(iv) return if the child develops any of the following signs:

— drinking poorly or unable to drink or breastfeed
— becomes more sick
— develops a fever
— has blood in the stool.

— *If the child still has some dehydration*, repeat treatment for another 4 hours with ORS solution, as above, and start to offer food, milk or juice and breastfeed frequently.
— *If signs of severe dehydration have developed*, see section 5.2.1 (page 112) for treatment.

Treatment plans B and A on pages 120 and 117 give further details.

Give zinc supplements

➤ Tell the mother how much zinc to give

Up to 6 months	1/2 tablet (10 mg) per day
6 months and more	1 tablet (20 mg) per day

for 10–14 days

Feeding

Continuation of nutritious feeding is an important element in the management of diarrhoea.

➤ In the initial 4-hour rehydration period, do not give any food except breast milk. Breastfed children should continue to breastfeed frequently *throughout* the episode of diarrhoea.

➤ After 4 hours, if the child still has some dehydration and ORS continues to be given, give food every 3–4 hours.

➤ All children over 4–6 months old should be given some food before being sent home.

If the child is not normally breastfed, explore the feasibility of **relactation** (i.e. restarting breastfeeding after it was stopped—see page 264) or give the usual breast milk substitute. If the child is 6 months or older or already taking solid food, give freshly prepared foods—cooked, mashed or ground. The following are recommended:

- cereal or another starchy food mixed with pulses, vegetables and meat/fish, if possible, with 1–2 teaspoons of vegetable oil added to each serving
- local complementary foods recommended by IMCI in that area (see section 10.1, page 261)
- fresh fruit juice or mashed banana to provide potassium.

➤ Encourage the child to eat by offering food at least 6 times a day. Give the same foods after the diarrhoea stops and give an extra meal a day for 2 weeks.

5.2.3 No dehydration

Children with diarrhoea but no dehydration should receive extra fluids at home to prevent dehydration. They should continue to receive an appropriate diet for their age, including continued breastfeeding.

Diagnosis

Diarrhoea with no dehydration should be diagnosed if the child does ***not*** have two or more of the following signs which characterize some or severe dehydration:

- restlessness/irritability
- lethargy or unconsciousness
- not able to drink or drinks poorly
- thirsty and drinks eagerly
- sunken eyes
- skin pinch goes back slowly or very slowly.

Treatment

➤ Treat the child as an outpatient.

➤ Counsel the mother on the 4 rules of home treatment:

— give extra fluid
— give zinc supplements
— continue feeding
— give advice on when to return.

See Treatment plan A on page 120.

➤ *Give extra fluid, as follows:*

— If the child is being breastfed, advise the mother to breastfeed frequently and for longer at each feed. If the child is exclusively breastfed, give ORS

CHART 15. Diarrhoea Treatment Plan A: Treat diarrhoea at home

COUNSEL THE MOTHER ON THE 4 RULES OF HOME TREATMENT: GIVE EXTRA FLUID, CONTINUE FEEDING, WHEN TO RETURN

➤ **1. GIVE EXTRA FLUID (AS MUCH AS THE CHILD WILL TAKE)**

➤ **TELL THE MOTHER:**

— Breastfeed frequently and for longer at each feed.

— If the child is exclusively breastfed, give ORS or clean water in addition to breastmilk.

— If the child is not exclusively breastfed, give one or more of the following: ORS solution, food-based fluids (such as soup, rice water, and yoghurt drinks), or clean water.

It is especially important to give ORS at home when:

— the child has been treated with Plan B or Plan C during this visit.

— the child cannot return to a clinic if the diarrhoea gets worse.

➤ **TEACH THE MOTHER HOW TO MIX AND GIVE ORS. GIVE THE MOTHER 2 PACKETS OF ORS TO USE AT HOME.**

➤ **SHOW THE MOTHER HOW MUCH FLUID TO GIVE IN ADDITION TO THE USUAL FLUID INTAKE:**

Up to 2 years	50 to 100 ml after each loose stool
2 years or more	100 to 200 ml after each loose stool

Tell the mother to:

— Give frequent small sips from a cup.

— If the child vomits, wait 10 minutes. Then continue, but more slowly.

— *Continue giving extra fluid until the diarrhoea stops.*

➤ **2. GIVE ZINC SUPPLEMENTS**

➤ **TELL THE MOTHER HOW MUCH ZINC TO GIVE:**

Up to 6 months 1/2 tablet (10 mg) per day for 10–14 days

6 months and more 1 tablet (20 mg) per day for 10–14 days

➤ **SHOW THE MOTHER HOW TO GIVE THE ZINC SUPPLEMENTS:**

— Infants, dissolve the tablet in a small amount of clean water, expressed milk or ORS in a small cup or spoon.

— Older children, tablet can be chewed or dissolved in a small amount of clean water in a cup or spoon.

➤ **REMIND THE MOTHER TO GIVE THE ZINC SUPPLEMENTS FOR THE FULL 10–14 DAYS.**

➤ **3. CONTINUE FEEDING**
➤ **4. WHEN TO RETURN**
} **SEE MOTHER'S CARD** (page 294)

solution or clean water in addition to breast milk. After the diarrhoea stops, exclusive breastfeeding should be resumed, if appropriate to the child's age.

— In non-exclusively breastfed children, give one or more of the following:

- ORS solution
- food-based fluids (such as soup, rice water and yoghurt drinks)
- clean water.

To prevent dehydration from developing, advise the mother to give extra fluids—as much as the child will take:

- for children <2 years, about 50–100 ml after each loose stool
- for children 2 years or over, about 100–200 ml after each loose stool.

Tell the mother to give small sips from a cup. If the child vomits, wait 10 minutes and then give more slowly. She should continue giving extra fluid until the diarrhoea stops.

Teach the mother how to mix and give ORS solution and give her two packets of ORS to take home.

➤ Give zinc supplements

— Tell the mother how much zinc to give:

Up to 6 months	1/2 tablet (10 mg) per day
6 months and more	1 tablet (20 mg) per day

for 10–14 days

— Show the mother how to give the zinc supplements:

- Infants, dissolve the tablet in a small amount of clean water, expressed milk or ORS.
- Older children, tablet can be chewed or dissolved

— Remind the mother to give the zinc supplements for the full 10–14 days.

➤ Continue feeding—see nutrition counselling in Chapters 10 (page 261) and 12 (page 293).

➤ Advise the mother on when to return—see below.

Follow-up

➤ Advise the mother to return *immediately* to the clinic if the child becomes more sick, or is unable to drink or breastfeed, or drinks poorly, or develops a fever, or shows blood in the stool. If the child shows none of these signs but is still not improving, advise the mother to return for follow-up at 5 days.

Also explain that this same treatment should be given in the future as soon as diarrhoea develops. See Treatment plan A, page 120.

5.3 Persistent diarrhoea

Persistent diarrhoea is diarrhoea, with or without blood, which begins acutely and lasts for 14 days or longer. When there is some or severe dehydration, persistent diarrhoea is classified as "severe".

The following guidelines are for children with persistent diarrhoea who are *not* severely malnourished. Severely malnourished children with persistent diarrhoea require hospitalization and specific treatment, as described in Chapter 7 (section 7.5.4, page 192).

In areas where HIV is highly prevalent, suspect HIV if there are other clinical signs or risk factors (see Chapter 8, page 199). Do stool microscopy for isospora.

5.3.1 Severe persistent diarrhoea

Diagnosis

- Infants or children with diarrhoea lasting ≥14 days, with signs of dehydration (see page 112), have *severe* persistent diarrhoea and require hospital treatment.

Treatment

- ➤ *Assess the child for signs of dehydration and give fluids* according to Treatment Plans B or C, as appropriate (see pages 117, 114).

ORS solution is effective for most children with persistent diarrhoea. In a few, however, glucose absorption is impaired and ORS solution is not effective. When given ORS, their stool volume increases markedly, thirst increases, signs of dehydration develop or worsen, and the stool contains a large amount of unabsorbed glucose. These children require IV rehydration until ORS solution can be taken without causing the diarrhoea to worsen.

Routine treatment of persistent diarrhoea with antibiotics is not effective and should not be given. Some children, however, have non-intestinal or intestinal infections that require specific antibiotic therapy.

- *Examine every child with persistent diarrhoea for non-intestinal infections* such as pneumonia, sepsis, urinary tract infection, oral thrush, and otitis media and treat appropriately.

- ➤ *Give micronutrients and vitamins* according to box on page 125.
- ➤ *Treat persistent diarrhoea with blood in the stool with an oral antibiotic* effective for *Shigella* as described in section 5.4, page 127.

➤ *Give treatment for amoebiasis* (oral metronidazole: 7.5 mg/kg, 3 times a day, for 5 days) only if:

— microscopic examination of fresh faeces carried out in a reliable laboratory reveals trophozoites of *Entamoeba histolytica* within red blood cells; OR

— two different antibiotics, which are usually effective for *Shigella* locally, have been given without clinical improvement.

➤ *Give treatment for giardiasis* (metronidazole: 5 mg/kg, 3 times a day, for 5 days) if cysts or trophozoites of *Giardia lamblia* are seen in the faeces.

Feeding

Careful attention to feeding is *essential* for all children with persistent diarrhoea.

Breastfeeding should be continued for as often and as long as the child wants. Other food should be withheld for 4–6 hours—*only* for children with dehydration who are being rehydrated following Treatment Plans B or C.

Hospital diets

Children treated in hospital require special diets until their diarrhoea lessens and they are gaining weight. The goal is to give a daily intake of *at least* 110 calories/kg.

Infants aged under 6 months

- Encourage exclusive breastfeeding. Help mothers who are not breastfeeding exclusively to do so.
- If the child is not breastfeeding, give a breast milk substitute that is low in lactose, such as yoghurt, or is lactose-free. Use a spoon or cup, do *not* use a feeding bottle. Once the child improves, help the mother to re-establish lactation.
- If the mother is not breastfeeding because she is HIV-positive, she should receive appropriate counselling about the correct use of breast milk substitutes.

Children aged 6 months or older

Feeding should be restarted as soon as the child can eat. Food should be given 6 times a day to achieve a total intake of at least 110 calories/kg/day. Many children will eat poorly, however, until any serious infection has been treated for 24–48 hours. Such children may require nasogastric feeding initially.

Two recommended diets

Given below (Tables 14 and 15) are two diets recommended for children and infants aged >6 months with severe persistent diarrhoea. If there are signs of dietary failure (see below) or if the child is not improving after 7 days of treatment, the first diet should be stopped and the second diet given for 7 days.

Successful treatment with either diet is characterized by:

- adequate food intake
- weight gain
- fewer diarrhoeal stools
- absence of fever.

The most important criterion is weight gain. There should be at least *three* successive days of increasing weight before one can conclude that weight gain is occurring.

Give additional fresh fruit and well cooked vegetables to children who are responding well. After 7 days of treatment with the effective diet, they should resume an appropriate diet for their age, including milk, which provides at least 110 calories/kg/day. Children may then return home, but follow them up regularly to ensure continued weight gain and compliance with feeding advice.

Dietary failure is shown by:

- an increase in stool frequency (usually to >10 watery stools a day), often with a return of signs of dehydration (this usually occurs shortly after a new diet is begun), OR
- a failure to establish daily weight gain within 7 days.

Table 14. Diet for persistent diarrhoea, first diet: A starch-based, reduced milk concentration (low lactose) diet

The diet should contain at least 70 calories/100 g, provide milk or yoghurt as a source of animal protein, but no more than 3.7 g lactose/kg body weight/day, and should provide at least 10% of calories as protein. The following example provides 83 calories/100 g, 3.7 g lactose/kg body weight/day and 11% of calories as protein:

• full-fat dried milk (or whole liquid milk: 85 ml)	11 g
• rice	15 g
• vegetable oil	3.5 g
• cane sugar	3 g
• water to make	200 ml

Table 15. Diet for persistent diarrhoea, second diet: A no-milk (lactose-free) diet with reduced cereal (starch)

The second diet should contain at least 70 calories/100 g, and provide at least 10% of calories as protein (egg or chicken). The following example provides 75 calories/100 g:

• whole egg	64 g
• rice	3 g
• vegetable oil	4 g
• glucose	3 g
• water to make	200 ml

Finely ground, cooked chicken (12 g) can be used in place of egg to give a diet providing 70 calories/100 g.

Supplementary multivitamins and minerals

Give all children with persistent diarrhoea daily supplementary multivitamins and minerals for two weeks. These should provide as broad a range of vitamins and minerals as possible, including at least two recommended daily allowances (RDAs) of folate, vitamin A, zinc, magnesium and copper.

As a guide, one RDA for a child aged 1 year is:

- folate 50 micrograms
- zinc 10 mg
- vitamin A 400 micrograms
- iron 10 mg
- copper 1mg
- magnesium 80 mg.

Monitoring

Nurses should check the following daily:

- body weight
- temperature
- food taken
- number of diarrhoea stools.

5.3.2 Persistent diarrhoea (non-severe)

These children do not require hospital treatment but need special feeding and extra fluids at home.

Diagnosis

Children with diarrhoea lasting 14 days or longer who have no signs of dehydration and no severe malnutrition.

Treatment

- Treat the child as an outpatient.
- Give micronutrients and vitamins according to box on page 125.

Prevent dehydration

- Give fluids according to Treatment Plan A, page 120. ORS solution is effective for most children with persistent diarrhoea. In a few, however, glucose absorption is impaired and when given ORS solution their stool volume increases markedly, thirst increases, signs of dehydration develop or worsen, and the stool contains a large amount of unabsorbed glucose. These children require admission to hospital for IV rehydration until ORS solution can be taken without aggravating the diarrhoea.

Identify and treat specific infections

- *Do not routinely treat with antibiotics as they are not effective.* However, give antibiotic treatment to children with specific non-intestinal or intestinal infections. Until these infections are treated correctly, persistent diarrhoea will not improve.
- **Non-intestinal infections**. Examine every child with persistent diarrhoea for non-intestinal infections, such as pneumonia, sepsis, urinary tract infection, oral thrush and otitis media. Treat with antibiotics following the guidelines in this manual.
- **Intestinal infections**. Treat persistent diarrhoea with blood in the stool with an oral antibiotic which is effective for *Shigella*, as described in section 5.4 below.

Feeding

Careful attention to feeding is *essential* for all children with persistent diarrhoea. These children may have difficulty in digesting animal milk other than breast milk.

- ➤ Advise the mother to reduce the amount of animal milk in the child's diet temporarily.
- ➤ Continue breastfeeding and give appropriate complementary foods:
  - — If still breastfeeding, give more frequent, longer breastfeeds, by day and night.
  - — If taking other animal milk, explore the feasibility of replacing animal milk with fermented milk products (e.g. yoghurt), which contain less lactose and are better tolerated.
  - — If replacement of animal milk is not possible, limit animal milk to 50 ml/kg/day. Mix the milk with the child's cereal, but do not dilute it.
  - — Give other foods appropriate for the child's age to ensure an adequate caloric intake. Infants aged >4 months whose only food has been animal milk should begin to take solid foods.
  - — Give frequent small meals, at least 6 times a day.

Supplementary micronutrients, including zinc

See Box, page 125.

Follow-up

- ➤ Ask the mother to bring the child back for reassessment after five days, or earlier if the diarrhoea worsens or other problems develop.
- ➤ Fully reassess children who have not gained weight or whose diarrhoea has not improved in order to identify any problems, such as dehydration or infection, which need immediate attention or admission to hospital.

Those who have gained weight and who have less than three loose stools per day may resume a normal diet for their age.

5.4 Dysentery

Dysentery is diarrhoea presenting with loose frequent stools containing blood. Most episodes are due to *Shigella* and nearly all require antibiotic treatment.

Diagnosis

The diagnostic signs of dysentery are frequent loose stools with visible red blood.

Other findings on examination may include:

- abdominal pain

- fever
- convulsions
- lethargy
- dehydration (see section 5.1, page 111)
- rectal prolapse.

Treatment

Children with severe malnutrition and dysentery, and young infants (<2 months old) with dysentery should be admitted to hospital. In addition children who are toxic, lethargic, have abdominal distension and tenderness or convulsions are at high risk of sepsis and should be hospitalized. Others can be treated at home.

➤ Give an oral antibiotic (for 5 days), to which most strains of *Shigella* locally are sensitive.

Examples of antibiotics to which *Shigella* strains can be sensitive are ciprofloxacin, pivmecillinam, and other fluoroquinolones. Note that metronidazole, streptomycin, tetracyclines, chloramphenicol, sulfonamides, nitrofurans (e.g. nitrofurantoin, furazolidone), aminoglycosides (e.g. gentamicin, kanamycin), first and second-generation cephalosporins (e.g. cephalexin, cefamandole), and amoxycillin are not effective in the treatment of *Shigella*. Co-trimoxazole and ampicilin are not effective any more due to widespread resistance.

➤ Prescribe a zinc supplement as done for children with watery diarrhoea without dehydration.

Follow-up

Follow-up children after two days, look for *signs of improvement* such as no fever, fewer stools with less blood, improved appetite.

- If there is no improvement after two days,
  - ➤ check for other conditions (see Chapter 2),
  - ➤ stop the first antibiotic, and
  - ➤ give the child a second-line antibiotic which is known to be effective against *Shigella* in the area. See Appendix 2 for dosages).
- If the two antibiotics, which are usually effective for *Shigella* in the area, have each been given for 2 days and produced no signs of clinical improvement,

5. DIARRHOEA

- ➤ check for other conditions (refer to a standard paediatric textbook).
- ➤ Admit the child if there is another condition requiring hospital treatment.
- ➤ Otherwise treat as an outpatient for possible amoebiasis.
- ➤ Give the child metronidazole (10 mg/kg, 3 times a day) for 5 days.

➤ *Young infants (<2 months).* Examine the young infant for surgical causes of blood in the stools (for example, intussusception—see Chapter 9, page 253) and refer to a surgeon, if appropriate. Otherwise give the young infant IM/IV ceftriaxone (100 mg/kg) once daily for 5 days.

Severely malnourished children. See Chapter 7 for the general management of these children.

➤ Treat for *Shigella* first and then for amoebiasis.

➤ If microscopic examination of fresh faeces in a reliable laboratory is possible, check for trophozoites of *E. histolytica* within red blood cells and treat for amoebiasis, if present.

Supportive care

Supportive care includes the prevention or correction of dehydration and continued feeding. For guidelines on supportive care of severely malnourished children with bloody diarrhoea, see also Chapter 7 (page 173).

Never give drugs for symptomatic relief of abdominal pain and rectal pain, or to reduce the frequency of stools, as they can increase the severity of the illness.

Treatment of dehydration

➤ Assess the child for signs of dehydration and give fluids according to Treatment Plan A, B or C (see pages 120, 117, 114), as appropriate.

Nutritional management

Ensuring a good diet is very important as dysentery has a marked adverse effect on nutritional status. However, feeding is often difficult because of lack of appetite. Return of appetite is an important sign of improvement.

➤ Breastfeeding should be continued throughout the course of the illness, more frequently than normal, if possible, because the infant may not take the usual amount per feed.

➤ Children aged 6 months or more should receive their normal foods. Encourage the child to eat and allow the child to select preferred foods.

Complications

- *Potassium depletion.* This can be prevented by giving ORS solution (when indicated) or potassium-rich foods such as bananas, coconut water or dark green leafy vegetables.

➤ *High fever.* If the child has high fever (≥39 °C or ≥102.2 °F) which appears to be causing distress, give paracetamol.

➤ *Rectal prolapse.* Gently push back the rectal prolapse using a surgical glove or a wet cloth. Alternatively, prepare a warm solution of saturated magnesium sulphate and apply compresses with this solution to reduce the prolapse by decreasing the oedema.

➤ *Convulsions.* A single convulsion is the most common finding. However, if this is prolonged or is repeated, give anticonvulsant treatment with IM paraldehyde (see page 342). Avoid giving rectal paraldehyde or diazepam. If convulsions are repeated, check for hypoglycaemia.

➤ *Haemolytic-uraemic syndrome.* Where laboratory tests are not possible, suspect haemolytic-uraemic syndrome (HUS) in patients with easy bruising, pallor, altered consciousness, and low or no urine output.

Further details of treatment can be found in standard paediatric textbooks.

Notes

Notes

CHAPTER 6

Fever

This chapter gives treatment guidelines for the management of the most important conditions presenting with fever in children aged between 2 months and 5 years. Management of febrile conditions in young infants (<2 months old) is described in Chapter 3, page 41.

6.1 Child presenting with fever

Special attention should be paid to the following in children presenting with fever.

History

- duration of fever
- residence in or recent travel to an area with *Plasmodium falciparum* transmission
- skin rash
- stiff neck or neck pain
- headache
- pain on passing urine
- ear pain.

Examination

- stiff neck
- skin rash
  — haemorrhagic: purpura, petechiae
  — maculopapular: measles
- skin sepsis: cellulitis or skin pustules
- discharge from ear/red immobile ear-drum on otoscopy
- severe palmar pallor
- refusal to move joint or limb
- local tenderness
- fast breathing.

Laboratory investigations

- blood smear
- LP if signs suggest meningitis
- urine microscopy

Table 16. Differential diagnosis of fever without localizing signs

Diagnosis of fever	In favour
Malaria (only in children exposed to malaria transmission)	— Blood film positive — Anaemia — Enlarged spleen
Septicaemia	— Seriously and obviously ill with no apparent cause — Purpura, petechiae — Shock or hypothermia in young infant or severely malnourished child
Typhoid	— Seriously and obviously ill with no apparent cause — Abdominal tenderness — Shock — Confusion
Urinary tract infection	— Costo-vertebral angle or suprapubic tenderness — Crying on passing urine — Passing urine more frequently than usual — Incontinence in previously continent child — White blood cells and/or bacteria in urine on microscopy, or positive dipstick
Fever associated with HIV infection	— Signs of HIV infection (see Chapter 8, page 199)

Differential diagnosis

There are three major categories of children presenting with fever:

- fever due to infection with non-localized signs (no rash) (see Table 16 above)
- fever due to infection with localized signs (no rash) (see Table 17 below)
- fever with rash (see Table 18, page 136).

Table 17. Differential diagnosis of fever with localized signs

Diagnosis of fever	In favour
Meningitis	— LP positive — Stiff neck — Bulging fontanelle — Meningococcal rash (petechial or purpuric)
Otitis media	— Red immobile ear-drum on otoscopy — Pus draining from ear — Ear pain
Mastoiditis	— Tender swelling above or behind ear
Osteomyelitis	— Local tenderness — Refusal to move the affected limb — Refusal to bear weight on leg
Septic arthritis	— Joint hot, tender, swollen
Skin and soft tissue infection	— Cellulitis — Boils — Skin pustules — Pyomyositis (purulent infection of muscles)
Pneumonia (see section 4.2, pages 72–81, for other clinical findings)	— Cough with fast breathing — Lower chest wall indrawing — Fever — Coarse crackles — Nasal flaring — Grunting
Viral upper respiratory tract infection	— Symptoms of cough / cold — No systemic upset
Throat abscess	— Sore throat in older child — Difficulty in swallowing/drooling of saliva — Tender cervical nodes
Sinusitis	— Facial tenderness on percussion over affected sinus — Foul nasal discharge
Dengue	— Coming from epidemic areas in at-risk season — Joint and muscle pains

Some causes of fever are only found in certain regions (e.g. dengue haemorrhagic fever, relapsing fever). Other fevers are mainly seasonal (e.g. malaria, meningococcal meningitis) or can occur in epidemics (measles, meningococcal meningitis, typhus).

Table 18. Differential diagnosis of fever with rash

Diagnosis of fever	In favour
Measles	— Typical rash — Cough, runny nose, red eyes — Mouth ulcers — Corneal clouding — Recent exposure to a measles case — No documented measles immunization
Viral infections	— Mild systemic upset — Transient non-specific rash
Meningococcal infection	— Petechial or purpuric rash — Bruising — Shock — Stiff neck (if meningitis)
Relapsing fever	— Petechial rash / skin haemorrhages — Jaundice — Tender enlarged liver and spleen — History of relapsing fever — Positive blood smear for Borrelia
Typhus [a]	— Epidemic of typhus in region — Characteristic macular rash
Dengue haemorrhagic fever [b]	— Bleeding from nose or gums, or in vomitus — Bleeding in stools or black stools — Skin petechiae — Enlarged liver and spleen — Shock — Abdominal tenderness

[a] In some regions, other rickettsial infections may be relatively common.
[b] In some regions, other viral haemorrhagic fevers have a similar presentation to dengue.

6.1.1 Fever lasting longer than 7 days

As there are many causes of prolonged fever, it is important to know the most common causes in a given area. Investigations for the most likely cause can then be started and treatment decided. Sometimes there has to be a "trial of treatment", e.g. for highly suspected tuberculosis or salmonella infections; if the child improves, this supports the suspected diagnosis.

History

Take a history as for fever (see above, page 133). In addition, ask if the child has a chronic illness such as rheumatoid arthritis or malignancy which may cause persistent fever.

Examination

Fully undress the child and examine the whole body for any localizing signs of infection:

- stiff neck (meningitis)
- red tender joint (septic arthritis or rheumatic fever)
- fast breathing or chest indrawing (pneumonia or severe pneumonia)
- petechial rash (meningococcal disease or dengue)
- maculopapular rash (viral infection or drug reaction)
- throat and mucous membranes (throat infection)
- red/painful ear with immobile ear-drum (otitis media)
- jaundice or anaemia (malaria or septicaemia)
- spine and hips (septic arthritis)
- abdomen (suprapubic tenderness in urinary tract infection, masses, tender kidneys).

Some causes of persistent fever may have no localizing signs—septicaemia, salmonella infections, miliary tuberculosis, HIV infection or urinary infection.

Laboratory investigations

Where available, perform the following:

- blood films for malaria parasites
- full blood count, including platelet count, and examination of a thin film for cell morphology
- urinalysis
- Mantoux test (note: it is often negative in a child with tuberculosis who has severe malnutrition or miliary tuberculosis)
- chest X-ray
- blood culture
- HIV testing (if the fever has lasted for more than 30 days and there are other reasons to suspect HIV infection)
- lumbar puncture (if there are signs of meningitis).

Table 19. Additional differential diagnosis of fever lasting longer than 7 days

Diagnosis	In favour
Abscess	— Fever with no obvious focus of infection (deep abscess) — Tender or fluctuant mass — Local tenderness or pain — Specific signs depend on site—subphrenic, psoas, retroperitoneal, lung, renal, etc.
Salmonella infection (non-typhoidal)	— Child with sickle-cell disease — Osteomyelitis or arthritis in infant — Anaemia associated with malaria
Infective endocarditis	— Weight loss — Enlarged spleen — Anaemia — Heart murmur — Petechiae — Splinter haemorrhages in nail beds — Microscopic haematuria — Finger clubbing
Rheumatic fever	— Heart murmur which may change over time — Arthritis/arthralgia — Cardiac failure — Fast pulse rate — Pericardial friction rub — Chorea — Recent known streptococcal infection
Miliary tuberculosis	— Weight loss — Anorexia, night sweats — Enlarged liver and/or spleen — Cough — Tuberculin test negative — Family history of TB — Fine miliary pattern on chest X-ray (see p. 77)
Brucellosis (local knowledge of prevalence is important)	— Chronic relapsing or persistent fever — Malaise — Musculoskeletal pain — Lower backache or hip pain — Enlarged spleen — Anaemia — History of drinking unboiled milk
Borreliosis (relapsing fever) (local knowledge of prevalence important)	— Painful muscles and joints — Red eyes — Enlarged liver and spleen — Jaundice — Petechial rash — Decreased level of consciousness — Spirochaetes on blood film

Differential diagnosis

Review all the conditions included in Tables 16–18 (pages 134–136). *In addition*, consider the causes for a fever lasting longer than 7 days in Table 19 on page 138.

6.2 Malaria

6.2.1 Severe malaria

Severe malaria, which is due to *Plasmodium falciparum*, is serious enough to be an immediate threat to life. The illness starts with fever and often vomiting. Children can deteriorate rapidly over 1–2 days, going into coma (cerebral malaria) or shock, or manifesting convulsions, severe anaemia and acidosis.

Diagnosis

History. This will indicate a change of behaviour, confusion, drowsiness, and generalized weakness.

Examination. The main features are:

- fever
- lethargic or unconscious
- generalized convulsions
- acidosis (presenting with deep, laboured breathing)
- generalized weakness (prostration), so that the child can no longer walk or sit up without assistance
- jaundice
- respiratory distress, pulmonary oedema
- shock
- bleeding tendency
- severe pallor.

Laboratory investigations. Children with the following findings have severe malaria:

- severe anaemia (haematocrit <15%; haemoglobin <5 g/dl)
- hypoglycaemia (blood glucose <2.5 mmol/litre or <45 mg/dl).

In children with altered consciousness and/or convulsions, check:

- blood glucose.

In addition, in all children suspected of severe malaria, check:

- thick blood smears (and thin blood smear if species identification required)
- haematocrit.

In suspected cerebral malaria (i.e. children with unrousable coma for no obvious cause), perform a lumbar puncture to exclude bacterial meningitis—if there are no contra-indications to lumbar puncture (see page 316). If bacterial meningitis cannot be excluded, give treatment for this also (see page 150).

If severe malaria is suspected on clinical findings and the blood smear is negative, repeat the blood smear.

Treatment

Emergency measures—to be taken within the first hour:

➤ Check for hypoglycaemia and correct, if present (see below, page 143).

➤ Treat convulsions with rectal diazepam or paraldehyde (see Chart 9, page 14) or with IM paraldehyde (see Appendix 2, page 342).

➤ Restore the circulating blood volume (see fluid balance disturbances, page 141 below).

➤ If the child is unconscious, minimize the risk of aspiration pneumonia by inserting a nasogastric tube and removing the gastric contents by suction.

➤ Treat severe anaemia (see below, page 142).

➤ Start treatment with an effective antimalarial (see below).

Antimalarial treatment

➤ If blood smear confirmation of malaria is likely to take more than one hour, start antimalarial treatment before the diagnosis is confirmed.

- *Quinine* is the drug of choice in all African countries and most other countries, except in parts of south-east Asia and the Amazon basin. Give it preferably IV in normal saline or 5% glucose; if this is not possible, give it IM. Replace with oral administration as soon as possible.

➤ ***IV quinine.*** Give a loading dose of quinine (20 mg/kg of quinine dihydrochloride salt) in 10 ml/kg of IV fluid over a period of 4 hours. Some 8 hours after the start of the loading dose, give 10 mg/kg quinine salt in IV fluid over 2 hours, and repeat every 8 hours until the child is able to take oral treatment. Then, give oral quinine doses to complete 7 days of treatment **or** give one dose of sulfadoxine-pyrimethamine (SP) where there is no SP resistance. If there is resistance to SP, give a full therapeutic dose of artemisinin-based combination therapy. *It is essential that the loading dose of quinine is given only if there is close nursing supervision of the infusion and control of the infusion rate. If this is not possible, it is safer to give IM quinine.*

➤ ***IM quinine.*** If IV infusion is not possible, quinine dihydrochloride can be given in the same dosages by IM injection. Give 10 mg of quinine salt per kg IM and repeat after 4 hours. Then, give every 8 hours until the malaria is no longer severe. The parenteral solution should be diluted before use because it is better absorbed and less painful.

➤ ***IM artemether***. Give 3.2 mg/kg IM on the first day, followed by 1.6 mg/kg IM daily for a minimum of 3 days until the child can take oral treatment. Use a 1 ml tuberculin syringe to give the small injection volume.

➤ ***IV artesunate***. Give 2.4 mg/kg IV or IM on admission, followed by 1.2 mg/kg IV or IM after 12 hours, then daily for a minimum of 3 days until the child can take oral treatment of another effective antimalarial.

Complete treatment in severe malaria following parenteral artesunate or artemether administration by giving a full course of artemisinin-based combination therapy or oral quinine to complete 7 days of treatment. If available and affordable, quinine should be combined with clindamycin.

Supportive care

➤ Examine all children with convulsions for hyperpyrexia and hypoglycaemia. Treat hypoglycaemia (see below, page 143). If a temperature of ≥39 °C (≥102.2 °F) is causing the child distress or discomfort, give paracetamol.

➤ If meningitis is a possible diagnosis and cannot be excluded by a lumbar puncture (see above), give parenteral antibiotics immediately (see page 150).

- Avoid useless or harmful ancillary drugs like corticosteroids and other anti-inflammatory drugs, urea, invert glucose, low-molecular dextran, heparin, adrenaline (epinephrine), prostacyclin and cyclosporin.

In an unconscious child:

➤ Maintain a clear airway.

➤ Nurse the child on the side to avoid aspiration of fluids.

➤ Turn the patient every 2 hours.

- Do not allow the child to lie in a wet bed.
- Pay attention to pressure points.

Take the following precautions in the delivery of fluids:

- Check for dehydration (see page 111) and treat appropriately.
- During rehydration, examine frequently for signs of fluid overload. The most reliable sign is an enlarged liver. Additional signs are gallop rhythm, fine crackles at lung bases and/or fullness of neck veins when upright. Eyelid oedema is a useful sign in infants.

- If, after careful rehydration, the urine output over 24 hours is less than 4 ml/kg body weight, give IV furosemide, initially at 2 mg/kg body weight. If there is no response, double the dose at hourly intervals to a maximum of 8 mg/kg body weight (given over 15 minutes).
- In children with no dehydration, ensure that they receive their daily fluid requirements but take care not to exceed the recommended limits (see section 10.2, page 273). Be particularly careful in monitoring IV fluids.

Complications

Coma (cerebral malaria)

- Assess the level of consciousness according to the AVPU or another locally used coma scale for children (see page 17).
- Give meticulous nursing care and pay careful attention to the airway, eyes, mucosae, skin and fluid requirements.
- Exclude other treatable causes of coma (e.g. hypoglycaemia, bacterial meningitis). Perform a lumbar puncture if there are no signs of raised intracranial pressure (see above). If you cannot do a lumbar puncture and cannot exclude meningitis, give antibiotics as for bacterial meningitis.

➤ Convulsions are common before and after the onset of coma. When convulsions are present, give anticonvulsant treatment with rectal diazepam or paraldehyde (see Chart 9, page 14) or IM paraldehyde (see Appendix 2, page 342). Correct any possible contributing cause such as hypoglycaemia or very high fever. If there are repeated convulsions, give phenobarbital (see page 343).

Some children may have a cold, clammy skin. Some of them may be in shock (cold extremities, weak pulse, capillary refill longer than 3 seconds). These features are not usually due to malaria alone. Suspect an additional bacteraemia and give both an antimalarial and antibiotic treatment, as for septicaemia (see section 6.5, page 158).

Severe anaemia

This is indicated by severe palmar pallor, often with a fast pulse rate, difficult breathing, confusion or restlessness. Signs of heart failure such as gallop rhythm, enlarged liver and, rarely, pulmonary oedema (fast breathing, fine basal crackles on auscultation) may be present.

➤ Give a *blood transfusion* as soon as possible (see page 277) to:

— all children with a haematocrit of ≤12% or Hb of ≤4 g/dl

— less severely anaemic children (haematocrit >12–15%; Hb 4–5 g/dl) with any of the following:
— clinically detectable dehydration
— shock
— impaired consciousness
— deep and laboured breathing
— heart failure
— very high parasitaemia (>10% of red cells parasitized).

➤ Give *packed cells* (10 ml/kg body weight), if available, over 3–4 hours in preference to whole blood. If not available, give fresh whole blood (20 ml/kg body weight) over 3–4 hours.

- A diuretic is not usually indicated because many of these children have a low blood volume (hypovolaemia).
- Check the respiratory rate and pulse rate every 15 minutes. If one of them rises, transfuse more slowly. If there is any evidence of fluid overload due to the blood transfusion, give IV furosemide (1–2 mg/kg body weight) up to a maximum total of 20 mg.
- After the transfusion, if the Hb remains low, repeat the transfusion.
- In severely malnourished children, fluid overload is a common and serious complication. Give whole blood (10 ml/kg body weight rather than 20 ml/kg) once only and do not repeat the transfusion.

Hypoglycaemia

Hypoglycaemia (blood glucose: <2.5 mmol/litre or <45 mg/dl) is particularly common in children under 3 years old, in children with convulsions or hyper-parasitaemia, and in comatose patients. It is easily overlooked because clinical signs may mimic cerebral malaria.

➤ Give 5 ml/kg of 10% glucose (dextrose) solution IV rapidly (see Chart 10, page 15). Recheck the blood glucose in 30 minutes, and repeat the dextrose (5 ml/kg) if the level is low (<2.5 mmol/litre or <45 mg/dl).

Prevent further hypoglycaemia in an unconscious child by giving 10% glucose (dextrose) infusion (add 10 ml of 50% glucose to 90 ml of a 5% glucose solution, or 10 ml of 50% glucose to 40 ml of sterile water). Do not exceed maintenance fluid requirements for the child's weight (see section 10.2, page 273). If the child develops signs of fluid overload, stop the infusion; repeat the 10% glucose (5 ml/kg) at regular intervals.

Once the child is conscious, stop IV treatment. Feed the child as soon as it is possible. Breastfeed every 3 hours, if possible, or give milk feeds of 15 ml/kg if the child can swallow. If not able to feed without risk of aspiration, give sugar solution by nasogastric tube (see Chapter 1, page 4). Continue to monitor the blood glucose level, and treat accordingly (as above) if found to be <2.5 mmol/litre or <45 mg/dl.

Respiratory distress (acidosis)

This presents with deep, laboured breathing while the chest is clear—sometimes accompanied by lower chest wall indrawing. It is caused by systemic metabolic acidosis (frequently lactic acidosis) and may develop in a fully conscious child, but more often in children with cerebral malaria or severe anaemia.

- Correct reversible causes of acidosis, especially dehydration and severe anaemia.
  - *If Hb is ≥5 g/dl*, give 20 ml/kg of normal saline or an isotonic glucose-electrolyte solution IV over 30 minutes.
  - *If Hb is <5 g/dl*, give whole blood (10 ml/kg) over 30 minutes, and a further 10 ml/kg over 1–2 hours *without* diuretics. Check the respiratory rate and pulse rate every 15 minutes. If either of these shows any rise, transfuse more slowly to avoid precipitating pulmonary oedema (see guidelines on blood transfusion in section 10.6, page 277).

Aspiration pneumonia

Treat aspiration pneumonia immediately because it can be fatal.

➤ Place the child on his/her side. Give IM or IV chloramphenicol (25 mg/kg every 8 hours) until the child can take this orally, for a total of 7 days. Give oxygen if the SaO_2 is <90%, or, if you cannot do pulse oximetry, there is cyanosis, severe lower chest wall indrawing or a respiratory rate of ≥70/minute.

Monitoring

The child should be checked by nurses at least every 3 hours and by a doctor at least twice a day. The rate of IV infusion should be checked hourly. Children with cold extremities, hypoglycaemia on admission, respiratory distress, and/or deep coma are at highest risk of death. It is particularly important that these children be kept under very close observation.

- Monitor and report immediately any change in the level of consciousness, convulsions, or changes in the child's behaviour.

- Monitor the temperature, pulse rate, respiratory rate (and, if possible, blood pressure) every 6 hours, for at least the first 48 hours.
- Monitor the blood glucose level every 3 hours until the child is fully conscious.
- Check the rate of IV infusion regularly. If available, use a giving chamber with a volume of 100–150 ml. Be very careful about overinfusion of fluids from a 500 ml or 1 litre bottle or bag, especially if the child is not supervised all the time. Partially empty the IV bottle or bag. If the risk of overinfusion cannot be ruled out, rehydration using a nasogastric tube may be safer.
- Keep a careful record of fluid intake (including IV) and output.

6.2.2 Malaria (non-severe)

Diagnosis

The child has:

- fever (temperature ≥37.5 °C or ≥99.5 °F) or history of fever, and
- a positive blood smear or positive rapid diagnostic test for malaria.

None of the following is present, on examination:

— altered consciousness

— severe anaemia (haematocrit <15% or haemoglobin <5 g/dl)

— hypoglycaemia (blood glucose <2.5 mmol/litre or <45 mg/dl)

— respiratory distress

— jaundice.

Note: If a child in a malarious area has fever, but it is not possible to confirm with a blood film, treat the child as for malaria.

Treatment

Treat at home with a first-line antimalarial, as recommended in the national guidelines. WHO now recommends artemisinin-based combination therapy as first line treatment (see possible regimens below). Chloroquine and sulfadoxine-pyrimethamine are no longer the first- and second-line antimalarials due to high level of drug resistance to these medicines in many countries for falciparum malaria. However, chloroquine is the treatment for non-falciparum malaria (*P. vivax*, *P. ovale*, *P. malariae*).

Treat for 3 days with one of the following regimens recommended by WHO:

➤ ***Artemether/lumefantrine.*** *Combined tablets containing 20 mg of artemether and 120 mg of lumefantrine:*

Combined tablet: child 5–<15 kg: 1 tablet two times a day for 3 days; child 15–24 kg: 2 tablets two times a day for 3 days

➤ ***Artesunate plus amodiaquine.*** *Separate tablets of 50 mg artesunate and 153 mg base of amodiaquine:*

Artesunate: child 3–<10 kg: $^{1}/_{2}$ tablet once daily for 3 days; child 10 kg or over: 1 tablet once daily for 3 days.

Amodiaquine: child 3–<10 kg: $^{1}/_{2}$ tablet once daily for 3 days; child 10 kg or over: 1 tablet once daily for 3 days

➤ ***Artesunate plus sulfadoxine/pyrimethamine.*** *Separate tablets of 50 mg artesunate and 500 mg sulfadoxine/25 mg pyrimethamine:*

Artesunate: child 3–<10 kg: $^{1}/_{2}$ tablet once daily for 3 days; child 10 kg or over: 1 tablet once daily for 3 days.

Sulfadoxine/pyrimethamine: child 3–<10 kg: $^{1}/_{2}$ tablet once on day 1; child 10 kg or over: 1 tablet once on day 1

➤ ***Artesunate plus mefloquine.*** *Separate tablets of 50 mg artesunate and 250 mg base of mefloquine:*

Artesunate: child 3–<10 kg: $^{1}/_{2}$ tablet once daily for 3 days; child 10 kg or over: 1 tablet once daily for 3 days.

Mefloquine: child 3–<10 kg: $^{1}/_{2}$ tablet once on day 2; child 10 kg or over: 1 tablet once on day 2

➤ ***Amodiaquine plus sulfadoxine/pyrimethamine.*** *Separate tablets of 153 mg base of amodiaquine and 500 mg sulfadoxine/25 mg pyrimethamine*

Amodiaquine: child 3–<10 kg: $^{1}/_{2}$ tablet once daily for 3 days; child 10 kg or over: 1 tablet once daily for 3 days

Sulfadoxine/pyrimethamine: child 3–<10 kg: $^{1}/_{2}$ tablet once on day 1; child 10 kg or over: 1 tablet once on day 1.

Complications

Anaemia (not severe)

In any child with palmar pallor, determine the haemoglobin or haematocrit level. Check that severe anaemia is not present. Haemoglobin between 5 g/dl and 9.3 g/dl (equivalent to a haematocrit of between approximately 15% and 27%) indicates non-severe anaemia. Begin treatment (omit iron in any child with severe malnutrition).

➤ Give home treatment with a daily dose of iron/folate tablet or iron syrup for 14 days: see page 339). *Note: If the child is taking sulfadoxine-pyrimethamine for malaria, do not give iron tablets that contain folate until a follow-up visit in 2 weeks. The folate may interfere with the action of the antimalarial.*

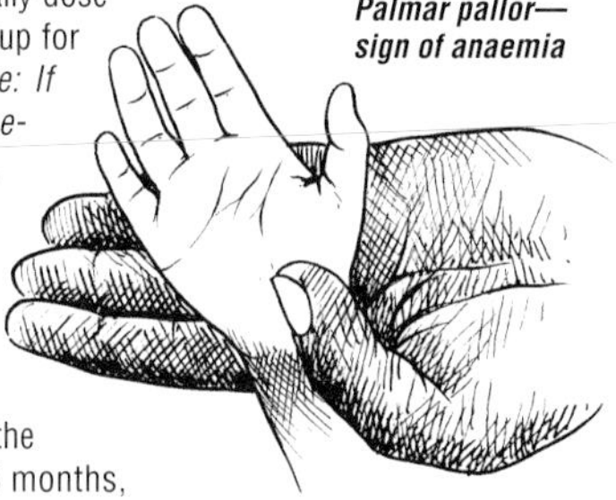

Palmar pallor—sign of anaemia

- Ask the parent to return with the child in 14 days. Treat for 3 months, where possible (it takes 2–4 weeks to correct the anaemia and 1–3 months to build up iron stores).

➤ If the child is over 1 year and has not had mebendazole in the previous 6 months, give one dose of mebendazole (500 mg) for possible hookworm or whipworm infestation (see page 340).

➤ Advise the mother about good feeding practices.

- Omit iron in any child with severe malnutrition in the acute phase.

Follow-up

Tell the mother to return if the fever persists for two days after starting treatment, or sooner if the child's condition gets worse. She should also return if the fever comes back.

If this happens: check if the child actually took the treatment and repeat a blood smear. If the treatment was not taken, repeat it. If it was taken but the blood smear is still positive, treat with a second-line antimalarial. Reassess the child to exclude the possibility of other causes of fever (see pages 133–139, and sections 6.3 to 6.10 below).

If the fever persists after two days of treatment with the second-line antimalarial, ask the mother to return with the child to reassess for other causes of fever.

6.3 Meningitis

Early diagnosis is essential for effective treatment. This section covers children and infants over 2 months old. See section 3.8 (page 49) for diagnosis and treatment of meningitis in young infants.

Diagnosis

Look for a *history* of:

- vomiting
- inability to drink or breastfeed
- a headache or pain in back of neck
- convulsions
- irritability
- a recent head injury.

On *examination*, look for:

- a stiff neck
- repeated convulsions
- lethargy
- irritability
- bulging fontanelle
- a petechial rash or purpura
- evidence of head trauma suggesting possibility of a recent skull fracture.

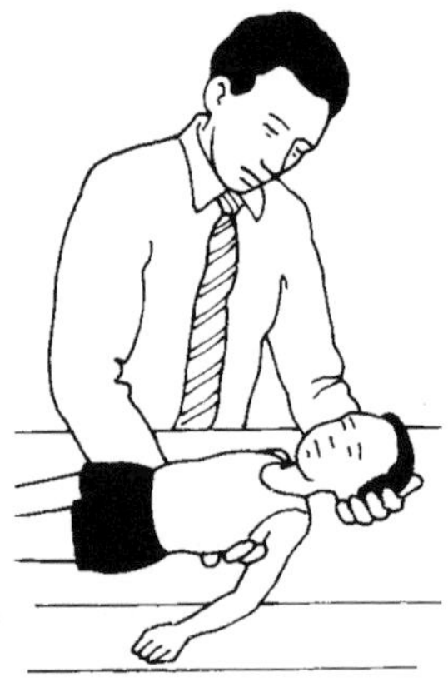

Looking and feeling for stiff neck in a child

Also, look for any of the following signs of raised intracranial pressure:

- unequal pupils
- rigid posture or posturing
- focal paralysis in any of the limbs or trunk
- irregular breathing.

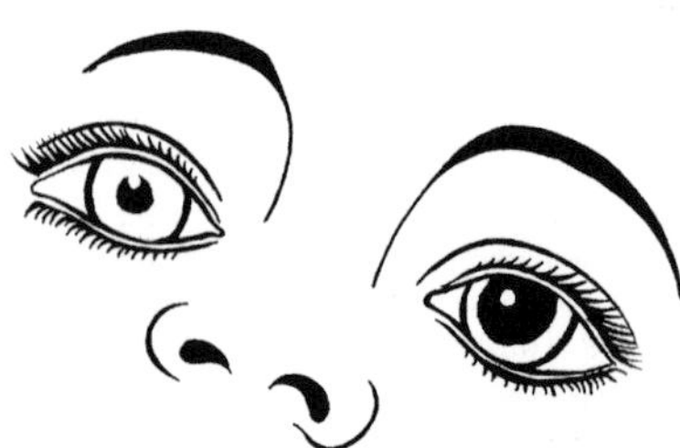

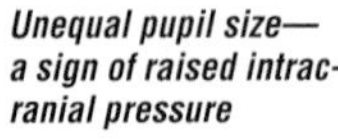

Unequal pupil size—a sign of raised intracranial pressure

Opisthotonus and rigid posture: a sign of meningeal irritation and raised intracranial pressure

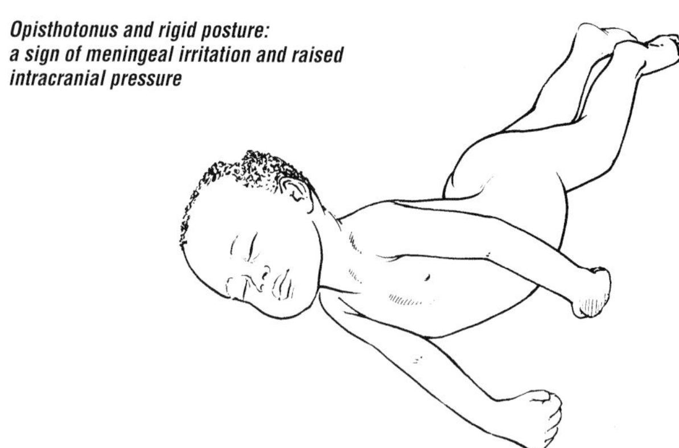

Laboratory investigations

If possible, confirm the diagnosis with a lumbar puncture and examination of the CSF. If the CSF is cloudy, assume meningitis and start treatment while waiting for laboratory confirmation. Microscopy should indicate the presence of meningitis in the majority of cases with the white cell (polymorph) count above 100/mm^3. Confirmatory information can be gained from the CSF glucose (low: <1.5 mmol/litre), CSF protein (high: >0.4 g/litre), and Gram staining and culture of the CSF, where possible. If there are signs of increased intracranial pressure, the potential value of the information gained from a lumbar puncture should be carefully weighed against the risk of the procedure. If in doubt, it might be better to start treatment for suspected meningitis, and delay performing a lumbar puncture (see p. 316).

Specific causes of meningitis

- During a *confirmed epidemic of meningococcal meningitis* it is not necessary to perform a lumbar puncture on children who have petechial or purpuric signs, which are characteristic of meningococcal infection. During such epidemics, give oily chloramphenicol (100 mg/kg IM as a single dose up to a maximum of 3 grams) for the treatment of meningococcal meningitis. The oily suspension is thick and may be difficult to push through the needle. If this problem is encountered, the dose can be divided into two parts and an injection given into each buttock of the child. This simplified treatment schedule is particularly useful in situations where there are limited resources to deal with the epidemic.

- Consider tuberculous meningitis if:
  - fever persists for 14 days
  - fever persists for more than 7 days and there is a family member with tuberculosis
  - a chest X-ray suggests tuberculosis
  - the patient remains unconscious
  - CSF continues to have moderately high white blood cell counts (typically, <500 white cells per ml, mostly lymphocytes), elevated protein levels (0.8–4 g/l) and low glucose levels (<1.5 mmol/litre).

In children known or suspected to be HIV-positive, tuberculous or cryptococcal meningitis should also be considered. For diagnosis of cryptococcus, do a CSF stain with India ink.

Treatment

If the CSF is obviously cloudy, treat immediately with antibiotics before the results of laboratory CSF examination are available. If the child has signs of meningitis and a lumbar puncture is not possible, treat immediately.

Antibiotic treatment

➤ Give antibiotic treatment as soon as possible. Choose one of the following two regimens:

1. Chloramphenicol: 25 mg/kg IM (or IV) every 6 hours
   plus ampicillin: 50 mg/kg IM (or IV) every 6 hours

   OR

2. Chloramphenicol: 25 mg/kg IM (or IV) every 6 hours
   plus benzylpenicillin: 60 mg/kg (100 000 units/kg) every 6 hours IM (or IV).

   Where there is known significant drug resistance of common pathogens (e.g. *Haemophilus influenzae* or Pneumococcus) to these antibiotics, follow the national guidelines. In many circumstances, the most appropriate treatment will be a third-generation cephalosporin such as:

   - ceftriaxone: 50 mg/kg IM/IV, over 30–60 minutes every 12 hours; or 100 mg/kg IM/IV, over 30–60 minutes once daily; or
   - cefotaxime: 50 mg/kg IM or IV, every 6 hours.

➤ Review therapy when CSF results are available. If the diagnosis is confirmed, give treatment parenterally for at least 5 days. Once the child has improved, give chloramphenicol orally unless there is concern about oral absorption (e.g. in severely malnourished children or in those with diarrhoea), in which cases the full treatment should be given parenterally. The total duration of treatment is 10 days.

- If there is a poor response to treatment:
  - Consider the presence of common complications, such as subdural effusions (persistent fever plus focal neurological signs or reduced level of consciousness) or a cerebral abscess. If these are suspected, refer the child to a central hospital with specialized facilities for further management (see a standard paediatrics textbook for details of treatment).
  - Look for other sites of infection which may be the cause of fever, such as cellulitis at injection sites, arthritis, or osteomyelitis.
  - Repeat the lumbar puncture after 3–5 days if the fever is still present and the child's overall condition is not improving, and look for evidence of improvement (e.g. fall in leukocyte count and rise in glucose level).
- Consult a standard paediatrics textbook for further details if tuberculous meningitis is suspected. Occasionally, when the diagnosis is not clear, a trial of treatment for tuberculous meningitis is added to the treatment for bacterial meningitis. Consult national tuberculosis programme guidelines. The optimal treatment regimen, where there is no drug resistance, comprises:
  - isoniazid (10 mg/kg) for 6–9 months; and
  - rifampicin (15–20 mg/kg) for 6–9 months; and
  - pyrazinamide (35 mg/kg) for the first 2 months.

Steroid treatment

In some hospitals in industrially developed countries, parenteral dexamethasone is used in the treatment of meningitis. There is *not* sufficient evidence to recommend routine use of dexamethasone in all children with bacterial meningitis in developing countries.

Do *not* use steroids in:

- newborns
- suspected cerebral malaria
- suspected viral encephalitis
- areas with a high prevalence of penicillin-resistant pneumococcal invasive disease.

Dexamethasone (0.6 mg/kg/day for 2–3 weeks, tailing the dose over a further 2–3 weeks) should be given to all cases of tuberculous meningitis.

Antimalarial treatment

In malarious areas, take a blood smear to check for malaria since cerebral malaria should be considered as a differential diagnosis or co-existing condition. Treat with an antimalarial if malaria is diagnosed. If for any reason a blood smear is not possible, treat presumptively with an antimalarial.

Supportive care

Examine all children with convulsions for hyperpyrexia and hypoglycaemia. Treat the hypoglycaemia (see page 143). Control high fever (≥39 °C or ≥102.2 °F) with paracetamol.

In an *unconscious* child:

- Maintain a clear airway.
- Nurse the child on the side to avoid aspiration of fluids.
- Turn the patient every 2 hours.
- Do not allow the child to lie in a wet bed.
- Pay attention to pressure points.

Oxygen treatment

Oxygen is not indicated unless the child has convulsions or associated severe pneumonia with hypoxia (SaO_2 <90%), or, if you cannot do pulse oximetry, cyanosis, severe lower chest wall indrawing, respiratory rate of >70/minute. If available, give oxygen to these children (see section 10.7, page 281).

High fever

➤ If fever (≥39 °C or ≥102.2 °F) is causing distress or discomfort, give paracetamol.

Fluid and nutritional management

There is no good evidence to support fluid restriction in children with bacterial meningitis. Give them their daily fluid requirement, but not more (see page 273) because of the risk of cerebral oedema. Monitor IV fluids very carefully and examine frequently for signs of fluid overload.

Give due attention to acute nutritional support and nutritional rehabilitation (see page 261). Feed the child as soon as it is safe. Breastfeed every 3 hours, if possible, or give milk feeds of 15 ml/kg if the child can swallow. If there is a risk of aspiration, give the sugar solution by nasogastric tube (see Chart 10, page 15). Continue to monitor the blood glucose level and treat accordingly (as above), if found to be <2.5 mmol/ litre or <45 mg/dl.

Monitoring

Nurses should monitor the child's state of consciousness, respiratory rate and pupil size every 3 hours during the first 24 hours (thereafter, every 6 hours), and a doctor should monitor the child at least twice daily.

On discharge, assess all children for neurological problems, especially hearing loss. Measure and record the head circumference of infants. If there is neurological damage, refer the child for physiotherapy, if possible, and give simple suggestions to the mother for passive exercises.

Complications

Convulsions

➤ If convulsions occur, give anticonvulsant treatment with rectal diazepam or paraldehyde (see Chart 9, page 14) or IM paraldehyde (see page 342).

Hypoglycaemia

➤ Give 5 ml/kg of 10% glucose (dextrose) solution IV rapidly (see Chart 10, page 15). Recheck the blood glucose in 30 minutes and if the level is low (<2.5 mmol/litre or <45 mg/dl), repeat the glucose (5 ml/kg)

➤ Prevent further hypoglycaemia by feeding, where possible (see above). If you give IV fluids, prevent hypoglycaemia by adding 10 ml of 50% glucose to 90 ml of Ringer's lactate or normal saline. Do not exceed maintenance fluid requirements for the child's weight (see section 10.2, page 273). If the child develops signs of fluid overload, stop the infusion and repeat the 10% glucose bolus (5 ml/kg) at regular intervals.

Follow-up

Sensorineural deafness is common after meningitis. Arrange a hearing assessment on all children one month after discharge from hospital.

Public health measures

In meningococcal meningitis epidemics, advise families of the possibility of secondary cases within the household so that they report for treatment promptly.

6.4 Measles

Measles is a highly contagious viral disease with serious complications (such as blindness in children with pre-existing vitamin A deficiency) and high mortality. It is rare in infants under 3 months of age.

Diagnosis

Diagnose measles if the mother clearly reports that the child has had a typical measles rash, or if the child has:

- fever; *and*
- a generalized maculopapular rash; *and*
- *one* of the following—cough, runny nose, or red eyes.

In children with HIV infection, these signs may not be present and the diagnosis of measles may be difficult.

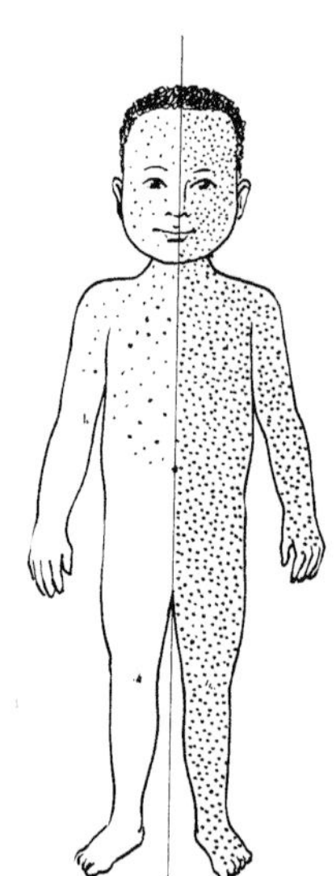

Distribution of measles rash. The left side of the drawing shows the early rash covering the head and upper part of the trunk, the right side shows the later rash covering the whole body.

6.4.1 Severe complicated measles

Diagnosis

In a child with evidence of measles (as above), any one of the following symptoms and signs indicate the presence of severe complicated measles:

- inability to drink or breastfeed
- vomits everything
- convulsions.

On *examination*, look for signs of *late complications* after the rash has disappeared, such as:

- lethargy or unconsciousness
- corneal clouding
- deep or extensive mouth ulcers.
- pneumonia (see section 4.2, page 72)
- dehydration from diarrhoea (see section 5.2, page 111)
- stridor due to measles croup
- severe malnutrition.

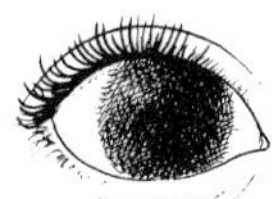 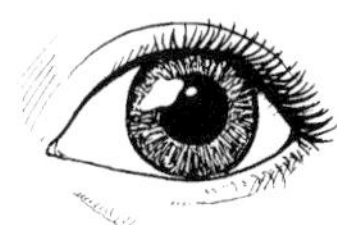

Corneal clouding—sign of xerophthalamia in vitamin A deficient child shown in comparison to the normal eye (right side)

Treatment

Children with severe complicated measles require treatment in hospital.

➤ *Vitamin A therapy.* Give oral vitamin A **to all** children with measles unless the child has already had adequate vitamin A treatment for this illness as an outpatient. Give oral vitamin A 50 000 IU (for a child aged <6 months), 100 000 IU (6–11 months) or 200 000 IU (12 months up to 5 years). See details on page 346. If the child shows any eye signs of vitamin A deficiency or is severely malnourished, a third dose must be given 2–4 weeks after the second dose. This should be given when the child comes for follow-up.

Supportive care

Fever

➤ If the temperature is ≥39 °C (≥102.2 °F) and this is causing the child distress, give paracetamol.

Nutritional support

Assess the nutritional status by weighing the child and plotting the weight on a growth chart (rehydrate before weighing). Encourage continued breastfeeding. Encourage the child to take frequent small meals. Check for mouth ulcers and treat them, if present (see below). Follow the guidelines on nutritional management given in Chapter 10 (page 261).

Complications

Follow the guidelines given in other sections of this manual for the management of the following complications:

- *Pneumonia*: see section 4.2, page 72.
- *Otitis media*: see page 162.

➤ *Diarrhoea*: treat dehydration, bloody diarrhoea or persistent diarrhoea: see Chapter 4, page 109.

➤ *Measles croup*: see section 4.5.1, page 93 for supportive care but do not give steroids.

➤ *Eye problems*. Conjunctivitis and corneal and retinal damage may occur due to infection, vitamin A deficiency, or harmful local remedies. In addition to giving vitamin A (as above), treat any infection that is present. If there is a clear watery discharge, no treatment is needed. If there is pus discharge, clean the eyes using cotton wool boiled in water, or a clean cloth dipped in clean water. Apply tetracycline eye ointment, 3 times a day for 7 days. *Never* use steroid ointment. Use a protective eye pad to prevent other infections. If there is no improvement, refer to an eye specialist.

➤ *Mouth ulcers*. If the child is able to drink and eat, clean the mouth with clean, salted water (a pinch of salt in a cup of water) at least 4 times a day.

- Apply 0.25% gentian violet to the sores in the mouth after cleaning.
- If the mouth ulcers are severe and/or smelly, give IM/IV benzylpenicillin (50 000 units/kg every 6 hours) and oral metronidazole (7.5 mg/kg 3 times a day) for 5 days.
- If the mouth sores result in decreased intake of food or fluids, the child may require feeding via a nasogastric tube.

➤ *Neurological complications*. Convulsions, excessive sleepiness, drowsiness or coma may be a symptom of encephalitis or severe dehydration. Assess the child for dehydration and treat accordingly (see section 5.1, page 111). See Chart 9, page 14, for treatment of convulsions and care of an unconscious child.

➤ *Severe malnutrition*. See guidelines in Chapter 7, page 173.

Monitoring

Take the child's temperature twice a day and check for the presence of the above complications once daily.

Follow-up

Recovery following acute measles is often delayed for many weeks and even months, especially in children who are malnourished. Arrange for the child to receive the third dose of vitamin A before discharge, if this has not already been given.

Public health measures

If possible, isolate children admitted to hospital with measles for at least 4 days after the onset of the rash. Ideally, they should be kept in a separate ward from other children. In malnourished and immunocompromised children, the isolation should be continued throughout the duration of the illness.

When there are measles cases in the hospital, immunize all other children above the age of 6 months (including those seen in outpatients, children admitted in the week following a measles case, and HIV-positive children). If infants aged 6–9 months receive measles vaccine, it is essential for the second dose to be given as soon as possible after 9 months of age.

Check the immunization status of hospital staff and immunize, if necessary.

6.4.2 Measles (non-severe)

Diagnosis

Diagnose non-severe measles in a child whose mother clearly reports that the child has had a measles rash, or if the child has:

- fever; *and*
- a generalized rash; *and*
- one of the following—cough, runny nose or red eyes; *but*
- none of the features of severe measles (see section 6.4.1, page 154).

Treatment

- ➤ Treat as an outpatient.
- ➤ *Vitamin A therapy.* Check whether the child has already been given adequate vitamin A for this illness. If not, give 50 000 IU (if aged <6 months), 100 000 IU (6–11 months) or 200 000 IU (12 months to 5 years). See details on page 346.

Supportive care

- ➤ *Fever.* If temperature ≥39 °C (≥102.2 °F) and this is causing distress or discomfort, give paracetamol.
- ➤ *Nutritional support.* Assess the nutritional status by weighing the child and plotting the weight on a growth chart. Encourage the mother to continue breastfeeding and to give the child frequent small meals. Check for mouth ulcers and treat, if present (see above).
- ➤ *Eye care.* For mild conjunctivitis with only a clear watery discharge, no treatment is needed. If there is pus, clean the eyes using cotton wool boiled in water, or a clean cloth dipped in clean water. Apply tetracycline eye ointment, 3 times a day for 7 days. *Never use* steroid ointment.

➤ *Mouth care.* If the child has a sore mouth, ask the mother to wash the mouth with clean, salted water (a pinch of salt in a cup of water) at least 4 times a day. Advise the mother to avoid giving salty, spicy or hot foods to the child.

Follow-up

Ask the mother to return with the child in two days to see whether the mouth or eye problems are resolving, and to exclude any severe complications of measles (see above).

6.5 Septicaemia

Consider septicaemia in a child with acute fever who is severely ill, when no cause can be found. Wherever meningococcal disease is common, a clinical diagnosis of meningococcal septicaemia must be made if petechiae or purpura (haemorrhagic skin lesions) are present. Non-typhoidal Salmonella is a common cause in malarious areas.

Diagnosis

On *examination*, look for the following:

- fever with no obvious focus of infection
- blood film for malaria is negative
- no stiff neck or other specific signs of meningitis (or a lumbar puncture for meningitis is negative)
- signs of systemic upset (e.g. inability to drink or breastfeed, convulsions, lethargy or vomiting everything)
- purpura may be present.

Always fully undress the child and examine carefully for signs of local infection before deciding that no cause can be found.

Where possible, *laboratory investigations* for bacteriology culture should be carried out on the blood and urine.

Treatment

➤ Give benzylpenicillin (50 000 units/kg every 6 hours) plus chloramphenicol (25 mg/kg every 8 hours) for 7 days.

➤ If the child's response to the above treatment is poor after 48 hours, change to ampicillin (50 mg/kg IM 6-hourly) plus gentamicin (7.5 mg/kg once per day) or, where *Staphylococcus aureus* is a possibility, flucloxacillin (50 mg/kg 6 hourly) plus gentamicin (7.5 mg/kg once per day).

Where there is known significant drug resistance to these antibiotics among Gram-negative bacteria, follow the national or local hospital guidelines for management of septicaemia. In many circumstances, the appropriate antibiotic may be a third-generation cephalosporin such as ceftriaxone (80 mg/kg IV, once daily over 30–60 minutes) for 7 days.

Supportive care

➤ If a high fever of ≥39 °C (or 102.2 °F) is causing the child distress or discomfort, give paracetamol.

Complications

Common complications of septicaemia include convulsions, confusion or coma, dehydration, shock, cardiac failure, disseminated intravascular coagulation (with bleeding episodes), pneumonia, and anaemia. Septicaemic shock is an important cause of death.

Monitoring

The child should be checked by nurses at least every 3 hours and by a doctor at least twice a day. Check for the presence of complications such as shock, reduced urine output, signs of bleeding (petechiae, purpura, bleeding from venepuncture sites), or skin ulceration.

6.6 Typhoid fever

Consider typhoid fever if a child presents with fever, plus any of the following: diarrhoea or constipation, vomiting, abdominal pain, headache or cough, particularly if the fever has persisted for 7 or more days and malaria has been excluded.

Diagnosis

On *examination*, key diagnostic features of typhoid are:

- fever with no obvious focus of infection
- no stiff neck or other specific signs of meningitis, or a lumbar puncture for meningitis is negative (*note:* children with typhoid can occasionally have a stiff neck)
- signs of systemic upset, e.g. inability to drink or breastfeed, convulsions, lethargy, disorientation/confusion, or vomiting everything

- rose spots on the abdominal wall in light-skinned children
- hepatosplenomegaly, tense and distended abdomen.

Typhoid fever can present atypically in young infants as an acute febrile illness with shock and hypothermia. In areas where typhus is common, it may be very difficult to distinguish between typhoid fever and typhus by clinical examination alone (see standard paediatrics textbook for diagnosis of typhus).

Treatment

- ➤ Treat with chloramphenicol (25 mg/kg every 8 hours) for 14 days, but see page 64 for treatment of young infants.
- ➤ If there is severe systemic upset or signs suggesting meningitis, treat with benzylpenicillin (50 thousand units/kg every 6 hours) for 14 days, *in addition* to chloramphenicol (25 mg/kg every 6 hours).
- ➤ If the response to treatment is poor after 48 hours, change to chloramphenicol (25 mg/kg every 8 hours) plus ampicillin (50 mg/kg IM every 6 hours).

Where drug resistance to chloramphenicol and ampicillin among *Salmonella typhi* isolates is known to be significant, follow the national guidelines for typhoid fever. In many circumstances, the appropriate antibiotic will be a third-generation cephalosporin such as ceftriaxone (80 mg/kg IM or IV, once daily, over 30–60 minutes). As multiple drug resistance is now common in some parts of the world, other treatment regimens such as ciprofloxacin (see page 333) may have to be used in areas where there is known resistance to these drugs.

Supportive care

- ➤ If the child has high fever (≥39 °C or ≥102.2 °F) which is causing distress or discomfort, give paracetamol.

Monitor haemoglobin or haematocrit levels and, if they are low and falling, weigh the benefits of transfusion against any risk of blood-borne infection (see section 10.6, page 277).

Monitoring

The child should be checked by nurses at least every 3 hours and by a doctor at least twice a day.

Complications

Complications of typhoid fever include convulsions, confusion or coma, diarrhoea, dehydration, shock, cardiac failure, pneumonia, osteomyelitis and anaemia. In young infants, shock and hypothermia can occur.

Acute gastrointestinal perforation with haemorrhage and peritonitis can occur, usually presenting with severe abdominal pain, vomiting, abdominal tenderness on palpation, severe pallor and shock. Abdominal examination may show an abdominal mass due to abscess formation, an enlarged liver and/or spleen.

If there are signs of gastrointestinal perforation, pass an IV line and nasogastric tube, and get surgical attention.

6.7 Ear infections

6.7.1 Mastoiditis

Mastoiditis is a bacterial infection of the mastoid bone behind the ear. Without treatment it can lead to meningitis and brain abscess.

Diagnosis

Key diagnostic features are:

- high fever
- tender swelling behind the ear.

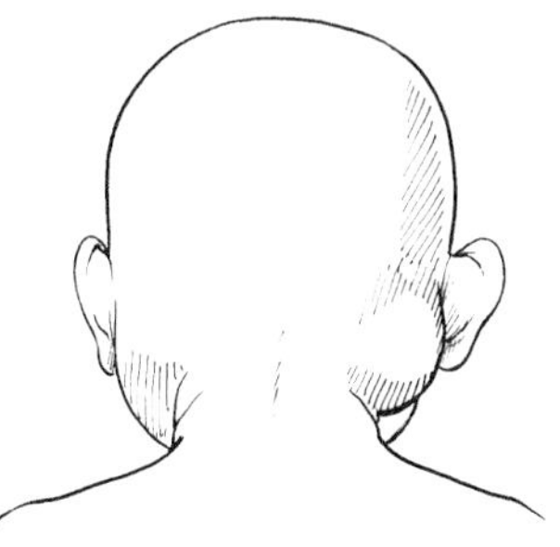

Mastoiditis—a tender swelling behind the ear which pushes the ear forward

Treatment

➤ Give chloramphenicol (25 mg/kg every 8 hours IM or IV) and benzylpenicillin (50 000 units/kg every 6 hours) until the child improves; then continue oral chloramphenicol every 8 hours for a total course of 10 days.

➤ If there is no response to treatment within 48 hours or the child's condition deteriorates, refer the child to a surgical specialist to consider incision and drainage of mastoid abscesses or mastoidectomy.

➤ If there are signs of meningitis or brain abscess, give antibiotic treatment as outlined in section 6.3 (page 148) and, if possible, refer to a specialist hospital immediately.

Supportive care

➤ If high fever (≥39 °C or ≥102.2 °F) is causing distress or discomfort to the child, give paracetamol.

Monitoring

The child should be checked by nurses at least every 6 hours and by a doctor at least once a day. If the child responds poorly to treatment, consider the possibility of meningitis or brain abscess (see section 6.3, page 148).

6.7.2 Acute otitis media

Diagnosis

This is based on a *history* of ear pain or pus draining from the ear (for a period of <2 weeks). On *examination*, confirm acute otitis media by otoscopy. The ear drum will be red, inflamed, bulging and opaque, or perforated with discharge.

Acute otitis media—bulging red eardrum (compared to normal appearance of eardrum on left)

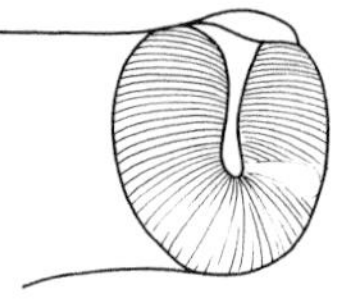

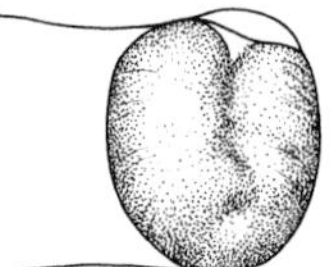

Treatment

Treat the child as an outpatient.

➤ Give oral cotrimoxazole (trimethoprim 4 mg/kg / sulfamethoxozole 20 mg/kg twice a day) or amoxicillin (15 mg/kg 3 times a day) for 5 days.

➤ If there is pus draining from the ear, show the mother how to dry the ear by wicking. Advise the mother to wick the ear 3 times daily until there is no more pus.

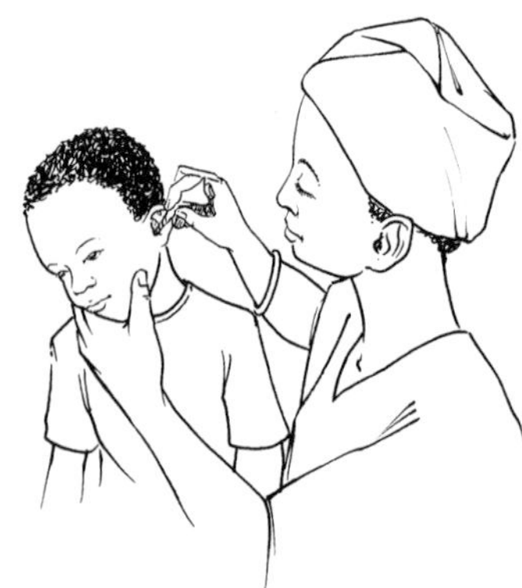

Wicking the child's ear dry in chronic otitis media

➤ Tell the mother not to place anything in the ear between wicking treatments. Do not allow the child to go swimming or get water in the ear.

➤ If the child has ear pain or high fever (≥39 °C or ≥102.2 °F) which is causing distress, give paracetamol.

Follow-up

Ask the mother to return after 5 days.

- *If ear pain or discharge persists*, treat for 5 more days with the same antibiotic and continue wicking the ear. Follow up in 5 days.

6.7.3 Chronic otitis media

If pus has been draining from the ear for 2 weeks or longer, the child has a chronic ear infection.

Diagnosis

This is based on a *history* of pus draining from the ear for more than 2 weeks. On *examination*, confirm chronic otitis media (where possible) by otoscopy.

Treatment

Treat the child as an outpatient.

➤ Keep the ear dry by wicking (see above).

➤ Instill topical antibiotic or antiseptic ear drops (with or without steroids) once daily for 2 weeks. Drops containing quinolones (norfloxacin, ofloxacin, ciprofloxacin) are more effective than other antibiotic drops.

Follow-up

Ask the mother to return after 5 days.

- *If the ear discharge persists*, check that the mother is continuing to wick the ear. Do not give repeated courses of oral antibiotics for a draining ear.
- *If the ear discharge persists*, encourage the mother to continue to wick the ear dry and consider parenteral antibiotic treatment with antibiotics that are effective against pseudomonas (such as gentamicin, azlocillin and ceftazidine.

6.8 Urinary tract infection

Urinary tract infection (UTI) is common, particularly in young female infants. As bacterial culture is usually not available in developing countries, the diagnosis is usually based on clinical signs and urine microscopy.

Diagnosis

In young children, UTI often presents with non-specific signs, on examination, such as vomiting, fever, irritability, or failure to thrive. Older children may present with more specific signs such as abdominal pain, pain on passing urine or increased frequency of passing urine.

Investigations

- Carry out microscopy of a clean, fresh, uncentrifuged specimen of urine. Cases of UTI will usually show >5 white cells per high-power field or a dipstick will show a positive result for leucocytes.
- If possible, obtain a "clean catch" urine sample for culture. In sick infants, supra-pubic aspiration may be required (see page 320).

Treatment

➤ Treat the child as an outpatient, except
  - when there is high fever and systemic upset (such as vomiting everything or inability to drink or breastfeed), or
  - where there are signs of pyelonephritis (loin pain or tenderness), or
  - in young infants.

➤ Give oral cotrimoxazole (4 mg trimethoprim/20 mg sulfamethoxazole per kg every 12 hours) for 5 days. Alternatives include ampicillin, amoxicillin and cefalexin, depending on local sensitivity patterns of *E. coli* and other Gram-negative bacilli that cause UTI, and on antibiotic availability (see page 325 for details of dosage regimens).

➤ If there is a poor response to the first-line antibiotic or the child's condition deteriorates, give gentamicin (7.5 mg/kg IM once daily) plus ampicillin (50 mg/kg IM/IV every 6 hours) or a parenteral cephalosporin (see pages 330–331). Consider complications such as pyelonephritis (tenderness in the costo-vertebral angle and high fever) or septicaemia.

➤ Treat young infants aged <2 months with gentamicin (7.5 mg/kg IM once daily) until the fever has subsided; then review, look for signs of systemic infection, and if absent, continue with oral treatment, as described above.

Supportive care

The child should be encouraged to drink or breastfeed regularly in order to maintain a good fluid intake, which will assist in clearing the infection and prevent dehydration.

Follow-up

- Investigate all episodes of UTI in >1-year-old males and in all children with more than one episode of UTI in order to identify the cause. This may require referral to a larger hospital with facilities for appropriate X-ray or ultrasound investigations.

6.9 Septic arthritis or osteomyelitis

Acute osteomyelitis is an infection of the bone, usually caused by spread of bacteria through the blood. However, some bone or joint infections result from an adjacent focus of infection or from a penetrating injury. Occasionally several bones or joints can be involved.

Diagnosis

In acute cases of bone or joint infection, the child looks ill, is febrile, and usually refuses to move the affected limb or joint, or bear weight on the affected leg. In acute osteomyelitis there is usually swelling over the bone and tenderness. In septic arthritis, the affected joint is hot, swollen and tender.

These infections sometimes present as a chronic illness, in which case the child appears less ill and may not have a fever. Local signs are less marked. Among bacterial infections, consider tuberculous osteomyelitis when the illness is chronic and there are discharging sinuses.

Laboratory investigations

X-rays are not helpful in diagnosis in the early stages of the disease. If septic arthritis is strongly suspected, introduce a sterile needle into the affected joint and aspirate the joint. The fluid may be cloudy. If there is pus in the joint, use a wide-bore needle to obtain a sample and remove the pus. Examine the fluid for white blood cells and carry out culture, if possible.

Staphylococcus aureus is the usual cause in children aged >3 years. In younger children, the commonest causes are *Haemophilus influenzae* type b, *Streptococcus pneumoniae*, or *Streptococcus pyogenes* group *A. Salmonella* is a common cause in young children in malarious areas and with sickle-cell disease.

Treatment

If culture is possible, treat according to the causative organism and the results of antibiotic sensitivity tests. Otherwise:

➤ Treat with IM/IV chloramphenicol (25 mg/kg every 8 hours) in children aged <3 years and in those with sickle-cell disease.

- ➤ Treat with IM/IV cloxacillin or flucloxacillin (50 mg/kg every 6 hours) in children aged >3 years. If this is not available, give chloramphenicol.
- ➤ Once the child's temperature returns to normal, change to oral treatment with the same antibiotic and continue this for a total of 3 weeks for septic arthritis and 5 weeks for osteomyelitis.
- ➤ In septic arthritis, remove the pus by aspirating the joint. If swelling recurs repeatedly after aspiration, or if the infection responds poorly to 3 weeks of antibiotic treatment, surgical exploration, drainage of pus, and excision of any dead bone should be carried out by a surgeon. In the case of septic arthritis, open drainage may be required. The duration of antibiotic treatment should be extended in these circumstances to 6 weeks.
- ➤ Tuberculous osteomyelitis is suggested by a history of slow onset of swelling and a chronic course, which does not respond well to the above treatment. Treat according to national tuberculosis control programme guidelines. Surgical treatment is almost never needed because the abscesses will subside with anti-tuberculosis treatment.

Supportive care

The affected limb or joint should be rested. If it is the leg, the child should not be allowed to bear weight on it until pain-free. Treat the pain or high fever (if it is causing discomfort to the child) with paracetamol.

6.10 Dengue

Dengue is caused by an arbovirus which is transmitted by Aedes mosquitoes. It is highly seasonal in many countries in Asia and South America. The illness usually starts with an acute onset of fever which remains continuously high for 2–7 days. Most children recover but a small proportion go on to develop severe disease. During the recovery period a macular or confluent blanching rash is often noted.

Diagnosis

Suspect dengue fever in an area of dengue risk if a child has fever lasting more than 2 days.

- Headache, pain behind the eyes, joint and muscle pains, abdominal pain, vomiting and/or a rash may occur but are not always present. It can be difficult to distinguish dengue from other common childhood infections.

Treatment

Most children can be managed at home provided the parents have reasonable access to the hospital.

➤ Counsel the mother to bring the child back for daily follow-up but to return immediately if any of the following occur: severe abdominal pain; persistent vomiting; cold, clammy extremities; lethargy or restlessness; bleeding e.g. black stools or coffee-ground vomit.

➤ Encourage oral fluid intake with clean water or ORS solution to replace losses from fever and vomiting.

➤ Give paracetamol for high fever if the child is uncomfortable. Do not give aspirin or ibuprofen as these drugs may aggravate bleeding.

➤ Follow up the child daily until the temperature is normal. Check the haematocrit daily where possible. Check for signs of severe disease.

➤ Admit any child with signs of severe disease (mucosal or severe skin bleeding, shock, altered mental status, convulsions or jaundice) or with a rapid or marked rise in haematocrit.

6.10.1 Severe dengue

Plasma leakage, sometimes sufficient to cause shock, is the most important complication of dengue infection in children. The patient is considered to have shock if the pulse pressure (i.e. the difference between the systolic and diastolic pressures) is ≤20 mm Hg or he/she has signs of poor capillary perfusion (cold extremities, delayed capillary refill, or rapid pulse rate). Hypotension is usually a late sign. Shock often occurs on day 4–5 of illness. Early presentation with shock (day 2 or 3 of illness), very narrow pulse pressure (≤10 mm Hg), or undetectable pulse and blood pressure suggest very severe disease.

Other complications of dengue include skin and/or mucosal bleeding and, occasionally, hepatitis and encephalopathy. However, most deaths occur in children with profound shock, particularly if the situation is complicated by fluid overload (see below).

Diagnosis

- Suspect severe dengue in an area of dengue risk if a child has fever lasting more than 2 days plus any of the following features:
- evidence of plasma leakage
  - — high or progressively rising haematocrit
  - — pleural effusions or ascites

- circulatory compromise or shock
  - cold, clammy extremities
  - prolonged capillary refill time (greater than 3 seconds)
  - weak pulse (fast pulse may be absent even with significant volume depletion)
  - narrow pulse pressure (see above)
- spontaneous bleeding
  - from the nose or gums
  - black stools or coffee-ground vomit
  - skin bruising or extensive petechiae
- altered conscious level
  - lethargy or restlessness
  - coma
  - convulsions
- severe gastrointestinal involvement
  - persistent vomiting
  - increasing abdominal pain with tenderness in the right upper quadrant
  - jaundice

Treatment

➤ Admit all patients with severe dengue to a hospital with facilities for blood pressure and haematocrit monitoring.

Fluid management – patients without shock (Pulse pressure >20 mm Hg)

➤ Give IV fluids for repeated vomiting or a high or rapidly rising haematocrit.

➤ Give only isotonic solutions such as Ringer's lactate, Hartmanns solution or 5% glucose in Ringer's lactate.

➤ Start with 6 ml/kg/hour for two hours, then reduce to 2–3 ml/kg/hour as soon as possible depending on the clinical response.

➤ Give the minimum volume required to maintain good perfusion and urine output. IV fluids are usually only needed for 24–48 hours since the capillary leak resolves spontaneously after this time.

Fluid management – patients with shock (Pulse pressure ≤20 mm Hg)

➤ Treat as an emergency. Give 20 ml/kg of an isotonic crystalloid solution such as Ringer's lactate or Hartmanns solution over one hour.

— *If the child responds* (capillary refill and peripheral perfusion start to improve, pulse pressure widens), reduce to 10 ml/kg for one hour and then gradually to 2–3 ml/kg/hr over the next 6–8 hours.

— *If the child does not respond* (continuing signs of shock), give a further 20 ml/kg of the crystalloid over one hour or consider using 10–15 ml/kg of a colloid solution such as 6% Dextran 70 or 6% HES (MW 200 000) over one hour. Revert to the crystalloid schedule described above as soon as possible.

➤ Further small boluses of extra fluid (5–10 ml/kg over 1 hour) may need to be given during the next 24–48 hours.

➤ Make fluid treatment decisions based on clinical response, i.e. review vital signs hourly and monitor urine output closely. Changes in the haematocrit can be a useful guide to treatment but must be interpreted together with the clinical response. For example, a rising haematocrit together with unstable vital signs (particularly narrowing of the pulse pressure) indicates the need for a further bolus of fluid, but extra fluid is not needed if the vital signs are stable even if the haematocrit is very high (50–55%). In these circumstances continue to monitor frequently and it is likely that the haematocrit will start to fall within the next 24 hours as the reabsorptive phase of the disease begins.

➤ In most cases, IV fluids can be stopped after 36–48 hours. Remember that many deaths result from giving too much fluid rather than too little.

Treatment of haemorrhagic complications

- Mucosal bleeding may occur in any patient with dengue but is usually minor. It is due mainly to the low platelet count, and this usually improves rapidly during the second week of illness.
- If major bleeding occurs it is usually from the gastrointestinal tract, particularly in patients with very severe or prolonged shock. Internal bleeding may not become apparent for many hours until the first black stool is passed. Consider this in children with shock who fail to improve clinically with fluid treatment, particularly if the haematocrit is stable or falling and the abdomen is distended and tender.

➤ In children with profound thrombocytopenia (<20 000 platelets/mm^3), ensure strict bed rest and protection from trauma to reduce the risk of bleeding. Do not give IM injections.

➤ Monitor clinical condition, haematocrit and, where possible, platelet count.

➤ Transfusion is very rarely necessary. When indicated it should be given with extreme care because of the problem of fluid overload. If a major bleed is suspected, give 5–10 ml/kg fresh whole blood slowly over 2–4 hours and observe the clinical response. Consider repeating if there is a good clinical response and significant bleeding is confirmed.

➤ Platelet concentrates (if available) should only be given if there is severe bleeding. They are of no value for the treatment of thrombocytopenia without bleeding and are likely to be harmful.

Treatment of fluid overload

Fluid overload is an important complication of treatment for shock. It can develop due to:

- — excess and/or too rapid IV fluids
- — incorrect use of hypotonic rather than isotonic crystalloid solutions
- — continuation of IV fluids for too long (once plasma leakage has resolved)
- — necessary use of large volumes of IV fluid in children with catastrophic leak.

■ Early signs:

- — fast breathing
- — chest indrawing
- — large pleural effusions
- — ascites
- — peri-orbital or soft tissue oedema

■ Late signs of severe overload:

- — pulmonary oedema
- — cyanosis
- — irreversible shock (often a combination of ongoing hypovolaemia and cardiac failure)

The management of fluid overload varies depending on whether the child is in or out of shock:

- Children who remain in shock and show signs of severe fluid overload are extremely difficult to manage and have a high mortality.

➤ Repeated small boluses of a colloid solution may help, together with high doses of inotropic agents to support the circulation (see standard textbooks of paediatrics).

➤ Avoid diuretics since they will lead to further intravascular fluid depletion.

➤ Aspiration of large pleural effusions or ascites may be needed to relieve respiratory symptoms but there is the risk of bleeding from the procedure.

➤ If available, consider early positive pressure ventilation before pulmonary oedema develops.

- If shock has resolved but the child has fast or difficult breathing and large effusions, give oral or IV furosemide 1 mg/kg/dose once or twice daily for 24 hours and oxygen therapy (see page 281).
- If shock has resolved and the child is stable, stop IV fluids and keep the child on strict bed rest for 24–48 hours. Excess fluid will be reabsorbed and lost through urinary diuresis.

Supportive care

➤ Treat high fever with paracetamol if the child is uncomfortable. Do not give aspirin or ibuprofen as this will aggravate the bleeding.

➤ Do not give steroids.

➤ Convulsions are not common in children with severe dengue. But if they occur, manage as outlined in Chapter 1, page 22.

➤ If the child is unconscious, follow the guidelines in Chapter 1, page 22.

➤ Children with shock or respiratory distress should receive oxygen.

➤ Hypoglycaemia (blood glucose <2.5 mmol/litre or <45 mg/dl) is unusual but if present, give IV glucose as described in Chart 10, page 15.

➤ If the child has severe hepatic involvement see standard paediatric textbook for guidelines.

Monitoring

➤ **In children with shock**, monitor the vital signs hourly (particularly the pulse pressure, if possible) until the patient is stable, and check the haematocrit 3–4 times per day. The doctor should review the patient at least four times per day and only prescribe intravenous fluids for a maximum of 6 hours at a time.

➤ **For children without shock**, nurses should check the child's vital signs (temperature, pulse and blood pressure) at least four times per day and the haematocrit once daily, and a doctor should review the patient at least once daily.

➤ Check the platelet count daily, where possible, in the acute phase.

➤ Keep a detailed record of all fluid intake and output.

Notes

CHAPTER 7

Severe malnutrition

Severe malnutrition is defined in these guidelines as the presence of oedema of both feet, or severe wasting (<70% weight-for-height/length or <-3SD[a]), or clinical signs of severe malnutrition. No distinction has been made between the clinical conditions of kwashiorkor, marasmus, and marasmic kwashiorkor because the approach to their treatment is similar.

[a] SD = standard deviation score or Z-score. A weight-for-height of -2SD indicates the child is at the lower end of the normal range, and <-3SD indicates severe wasting. A weight-for-height/length of -3SD is approximately equivalent to 70% of the weight-for-height of the average (median) child. (To calculate see pages 364–366.)

7.1 Diagnosis

Key diagnostic features are:

- weight-for-length (or height) <70% or <-3SD (marasmus) (see page 364).
- oedema of both feet (kwashiorkor or marasmic kwashiorkor).

If weight-for-height or weight-for-length cannot be measured, use the clinical signs for **visible severe wasting** (see Figure). A child with visible severe wasting appears very thin and has no fat. There is severe wasting of the shoulders, arms, buttocks and thighs, with visible rib outlines.

Children <60% weight-for-age may be stunted, and not severely wasted. Stunted children do not require hospital admission unless they have a serious illness.

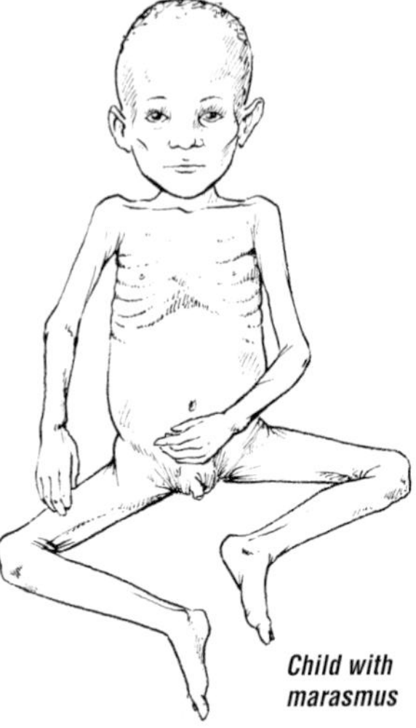

Child with marasmus

7.2 Initial assessment of the severely malnourished child

Take a *history* concerning:

- recent intake of food and fluids
- usual diet (before the current illness)
- breastfeeding
- duration and frequency of diarrhoea and vomiting
- type of diarrhoea (watery/bloody)
- loss of appetite
- family circumstances (to understand the child's social background)
- chronic cough

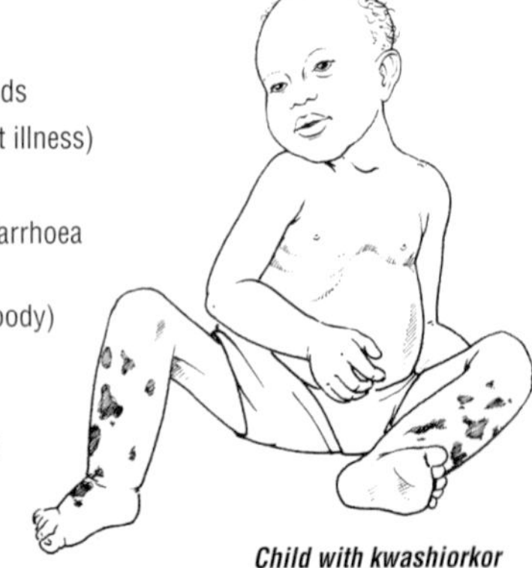

Child with kwashiorkor

- contact with tuberculosis
- recent contact with measles
- known or suspected HIV infection.

On *examination*, look for:

- signs of dehydration
- shock (cold hands, slow capillary refill, weak and rapid pulse)

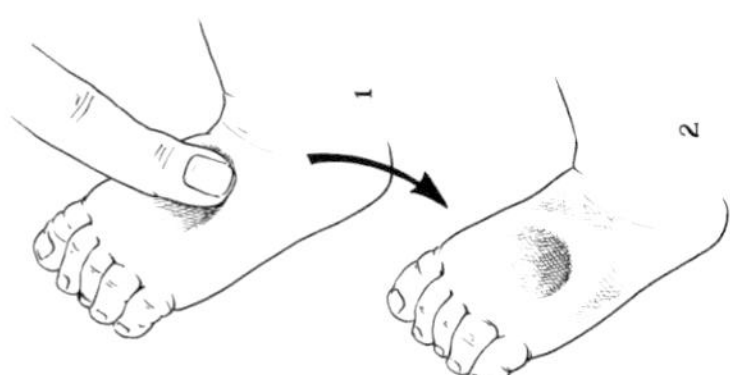

Pitting oedema on dorsum of foot. After applying pressure for a few seconds, a pit remains after the finger is removed.

- severe palmar pallor
- eye signs of vitamin A deficiency:
  - — dry conjunctiva or cornea, Bitot's spots
  - — corneal ulceration
  - — keratomalacia
- localizing signs of infection, including ear and throat infections, skin infection or pneumonia
- signs of HIV infection (see Chapter 8, page 199)
- fever (temperature ≥37.5 °C or ≥99.5 °F) or hypothermia (rectal temperature <35.5 °C or <95.9 °F)
- mouth ulcers
- skin changes of kwashiorkor:
  - — hypo- or hyperpigmentation
  - — desquamation
  - — ulceration (spreading over limbs, thighs, genitalia, groin, and behind the ears)
  - — exudative lesions (resembling severe burns) often with secondary infection (including Candida).

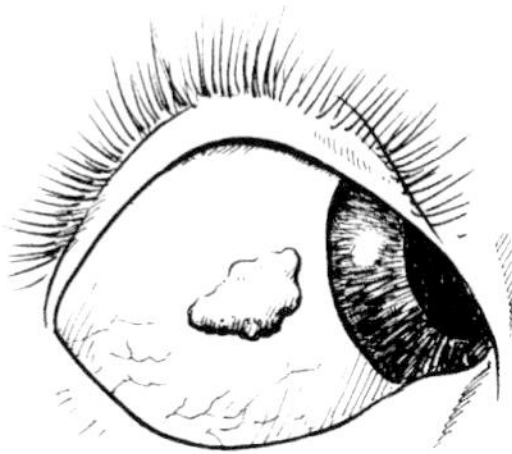

Bitot's spot (conjunctival xerosis)—sign of xerophthalmia in a vitamin A deficient child

Note: Children with vitamin A deficiency are likely to be photophobic and will keep their eyes closed. It is important to examine the eyes very gently to prevent corneal rupture.

Laboratory investigation of haemoglobin or haematocrit, if there is severe palmar pallor.

7.3 Organization of care

➤ On admission, the child with severe malnutrition should be separated from infectious children and kept in a warm area (25–30 °C, with no draughts), and constantly monitored. Washing should be kept to a minimum, after which the child should be dried immediately.

Facilities and sufficient staff should be available to ensure correct preparation of appropriate feeds, and to carry out regular feeding during the day and night. Accurate weighing machines are needed, and records should be kept of the feeds given and the child's weight so that progress can be monitored.

7.4 General treatment

Plan of treatment

For *triage assessment* of children with severe malnutrition and management of ***shock***, see Chapter 1, page 18. When there is ***corneal ulceration***, give vitamin A, instil chloramphenicol or tetracycline eye drops and atropine drops into the eye, cover with a saline soaked eye pad, and bandage (see page 190). ***Severe anaemia***, if present, will need urgent treatment (see section 7.5.2, page 191).

General treatment involves 10 steps in two phases: initial *stabilization* and *rehabilitation* (see Table 20).

Table 20. Time frame for the management of the child with severe malnutrition

	Stabilization		Rehabilitation
	Days 1–2	Days 3–7	Weeks 2–6
1. Hypoglycaemia	——————→		
2. Hypothermia	——————→		
3. Dehydration	——————→		
4. Electrolytes	——————	——————	——————→
5. Infection	——————	——————→	
6. Micronutrients	— no iron —	——————→	with iron ——→
7. Initiate feeding	——————	——————→	
8. Catch-up growth			——————→
9. Sensory stimulation	——————	——————	——————→
10. Prepare for follow-up			——————→

7.4.1 Hypoglycaemia

All severely malnourished children are at risk of hypoglycaemia and, immediately on admission, should be given a feed or 10% glucose or sucrose (see below). Frequent feeding is important.

Diagnosis

If there is any suspicion of hypoglycaemia and where blood glucose results can be obtained quickly (e.g. with dextrostix), this should be measured immediately. Hypoglycaemia is present when the blood glucose is <3 mmol/l (<54 mg/dl). If the blood glucose cannot be measured, it should be assumed that all children with severe malnutrition have hypoglycaemia.

Treatment

- ➤ Give the first feed of F-75 if it is quickly available and then continue with 2–3 hourly feeds.
- ➤ If the first feed is not quickly available give 50 ml of 10% glucose or sucrose solution (1 rounded teaspoon of sugar in 3½ tablespoons of water) orally or by nasogastric tube, followed by the first feed as soon as possible.
- ➤ Give 2–3-hourly feeds, day and night, at least for the first day.
- ➤ Give appropriate antibiotics (see page 182).
- ➤ If the child is unconscious, treat with IV 10% glucose 5 ml/kg or, if unavailable, 10% glucose or sucrose solution by nasogastric tube (see page 315).

Monitoring

If the initial blood glucose was low, repeat the measurement (using fingerprick or heelprick blood and dextrostix, where available) after 30 minutes.

- If blood glucose falls <3 mmol/1 (<54 mg/dl), repeat the 10% glucose or sugar solution.
- If the rectal temperature falls <35.5 °C or if there is deterioration in the level of consciousness, repeat the dextrostix measurement and treat accordingly.

Prevention

- ➤ Feed 2 hourly, starting immediately (see *Initial refeeding*, page 184) or, if necessary, rehydrate first. Continue feeding throughout the night.

7.4.2 Hypothermia

Diagnosis

- If the axillary temperature is <35 °C (<95 °F) or does not register on a normal thermometer, assume hypothermia. Where a low-reading thermometer is available, take the rectal temperature (<35.5 °C or <95.5 °F) to confirm the hypothermia.

Treatment

➤ Feed the child immediately (if necessary, rehydrate first).

➤ Make sure the child is clothed (including the head), cover with a warmed blanket and place a heater (not pointing directly at the child) or lamp nearby, or put the child on the mother's bare chest or abdomen (skin-to-skin) and cover them with a warmed blanket and/or warm clothing.

➤ Give appropriate antibiotics (see page 182).

Monitoring

- Take the child's rectal temperature 2-hourly until it rises to more than 36.5 °C. Take it half-hourly if a heater is being used.
- Ensure that the child is covered at all times, especially at night. Keep the head covered, preferably with a warm bonnet to reduce heat loss.
- Check for hypoglycaemia whenever hypothermia is found.

Prevention

➤ Feed the child 2-hourly, starting immediately (see *Initial refeeding*, page 184).

➤ Always give feeds through the night.

➤ Place the bed in a warm, draught-free part of the ward and keep the child covered.

➤ Change wet nappies, clothes and bedding to keep the child and the bed dry.

➤ Avoid exposing the child to cold (e.g. after bathing, or during medical examinations).

➤ Let the child sleep with the mother for warmth in the night.

7.4.3 Dehydration

Diagnosis

Dehydration tends to be overdiagnosed and its severity overestimated in severely malnourished children. This is because it is difficult to estimate dehydration status accurately in the severely malnourished child using clinical signs alone. Assume that all children with *watery diarrhoea* may have *some* dehydration.

Note: Low blood volume can co-exist with oedema.

Treatment

Do *not* use the IV route for rehydration except in cases of shock (see page 18). Standard WHO-ORS solution for general use has a high sodium and low potassium content, which is not suitable for severely malnourished children. Instead, give special rehydration solution for malnutrition, ReSoMal (see recipe below, or use commercially available ReSoMal).

➤ Give the *ReSoMal rehydration fluid*, orally or by nasogastric tube, much more slowly than you would when rehydrating a well-nourished child:

— give 5 ml/kg every 30 minutes for the first 2 hours

— then give 5–10 ml/kg/hour for the next 4–10 hours.

The exact amount depends on how much the child wants, volume of stool loss, and whether the child is vomiting.

➤ If rehydration is still occurring at 6 hours and 10 hours, give starter F-75 (see recipes on page 186) *instead* of ReSoMal at these times. Use the same volume of starter F-75 as for ReSoMal.

• Then initiate refeeding with starter F-75.

Recipe for ReSoMal

Ingredient	Amount
Water	2 litres
WHO-ORS	One 1-litre packet*
Sucrose	50 g
Electrolyte/mineral solution**	40 ml

* 2.6 g sodium chloride, 2.9 g trisodium citrate dihydrate, 1.5 g potassium chloride, 13.5 g glucose.

** See page 180 for the recipe for the electrolyte/mineral solution. If you use a commercially prepared electrolyte and mineral powder, follow the manufacturer's instructions. If these cannot be made up, use 45 ml of KCl solution (100 g KCl in 1 litre of water) instead.

ReSoMal contains approximately 37.5 mmol Na, 40 mmol K, and 3 mmol Mg per litre.

Formula for concentrated electrolyte/mineral solution

This is used in the preparation of starter and catch-up feeding formulas and ReSoMal. Electrolyte and mineral powders are produced by some manufacturers. If these are not available or affordable, prepare the solution (2500 ml) using the following ingredients:

	g	mol/20 ml
Potassium chloride: KCl	224	24 mmol
Tripotassium citrate	81	2 mmol
Magnesium chloride: $MgCl_2 . 6H_2O$	76	3 mmol
Zinc acetate: Zn acetate.$2H_2O$	8.2	300 µmol
Copper sulfate: $CuSO_4 . 5H_2O$	1.4	45 µmol
Water: make up to	2500 ml	

If available, also add selenium (0.028 g of sodium selenate, $NaSeO_4 . 10H_2O$) and iodine (0.012 g of potassium iodide, KI) per 2500 ml.

- Dissolve the ingredients in cooled boiled water.
- Store the solution in sterilized bottles in the fridge to retard deterioration. Discard if it turns cloudy. Make fresh each month.
- Add 20 ml of the concentrated electrolyte/mineral solution to each 1000 ml of milk feed.If it is not possible to prepare this electrolyte/ mineral solution and pre-mixed sachets are not available, give K, Mg and Zn separately. Make a 10% stock solution of potassium chloride (100 g in 1 litre of water) and a 1.5% solution of zinc acetate (15 g in 1 litre of water).

For the oral rehydration solution ReSoMal, use 45 ml of the stock KCl solution instead of 40 ml electrolyte/mineral solution

For milk feeds F-75 and F-100, add 22.5 ml of the stock KCl solution instead of 20 ml of the electrolyte/mineral solution to 1000 ml of feed. Give the 1.5% zinc acetate solution by mouth 1 ml/kg/day. Give 0.3 ml/kg of 50% magnesium sulfate intramuscularly once to a maximum of 2 ml.

Monitoring

During rehydration, respiration and pulse rate should fall and urine start to be passed. The return of tears, a moist mouth, less sunken eyes and fontanelle, and improved skin turgor are also signs that rehydration is proceeding, but many severely malnourished children will not show these changes even when fully rehydrated. Monitor weight gain.

Monitor the progress of rehydration half-hourly for 2 hours, then hourly for the next 4–10 hours. Be alert for signs of overhydration, which is very dangerous and may lead to heart failure. Check:

- respiratory rate
- pulse rate
- urine frequency
- frequency of stools and vomit.

If you find signs of overhydration (increasing respiratory rate by 5/min and pulse rate by 15/min), stop ReSoMal immediately and reassess after 1 hour.

Prevention

Measures to prevent dehydration from continuing watery diarrhoea are similar to those for well-nourished children (see Treatment Plan A on page 120), except that ReSoMal fluid is used instead of standard ORS.

➤ If the child is breastfed, continue breastfeeding.

➤ Initiate refeeding with starter F-75.

➤ Give ReSoMal between feeds to replace stool losses. As a guide, give 50–100 ml after each watery stool.

7.4.4 Electrolyte imbalance

All severely malnourished children have deficiencies of potassium and magnesium which may take two weeks or more to correct. Oedema is partly a result of these deficiencies. Do *not* treat oedema with a diuretic. Excess body sodium exists even though the plasma sodium may be low. *Giving high sodium loads could kill the child.*

Treatment

➤ Give extra potassium (3–4 mmol/kg daily).

➤ Give extra magnesium (0.4–0.6 mmol/kg daily).

The extra potassium and magnesium should be added to the feeds during their preparation. See page 180 for a recipe to make a combined electrolyte/mineral solution. Add 20 ml of this solution to 1 litre of feed to supply the extra potassium and magnesium required. Alternatively, use commercially available pre-mixed sachets (specially formulated for the malnourished child).

➤ When rehydrating, give low sodium rehydration fluid (ReSoMal) (see recipe, page 179).

➤ Prepare food without adding salt.

7.4.5 **Infection**

In severe malnutrition, the usual signs of infection such as fever are often absent, yet multiple infections are common. Therefore, assume that all malnourished children have an infection on their arrival in hospital and treat with antibiotics straightaway. Hypoglycaemia and hypothermia are signs of severe infection.

Treatment

Give all severely malnourished children:

➤ a broad-spectrum antibiotic

➤ measles vaccine if the child is ≥6 months and not immunized, or if the child is >9 months and had been vaccinated before the age of 9 months, but delay vaccination if the child is in shock.

Choice of broad-spectrum antibiotic

➤ *If the child appears to have no complications*, give cotrimoxazole (dosage: see page 335) for 5 days

➤ *If there are complications* (hypoglycaemia, hypothermia, or the child looks lethargic or sickly), give:

— ampicillin (50 mg/kg IM/IV 6-hourly for 2 days), then oral amoxicillin (15 mg/kg 8-hourly for 5 days) OR, if amoxicillin is not available, oral ampicillin (50 mg/kg 6-hourly for 5 days) over a total of 7 days

AND

— gentamicin (7.5 mg/kg IM/IV) once daily for 7 days.

➤ *If the child fails to improve within 48 hours*, add chloramphenicol (25 mg/kg IM/IV 8-hourly) for 5 days.

Depending on local resistance patterns, these regimens should be adapted.

If meningitis is suspected, do a lumbar puncture for confirmation, where possible, and treat with chloramphenicol (25 mg/kg 6 hourly) for 10 days (see page 150). If you identify other specific infections (such as pneumonia, dysentery, skin- or soft-tissue infections), give antibiotics as appropriate. Add antimalarial treatment if the child has a positive blood film for malaria parasites. Tuberculosis is common, but anti-tuberculosis treatment should only be given when tuberculosis is diagnosed or strongly suspected (see section 7.5.5, page 192). For HIV-exposed children, see Chapter 8.

Note: Some experienced doctors routinely give metronidazole (7.5 mg/kg 8-hourly for 7 days) in addition to broad-spectrum antibiotics. However, the efficacy of this treatment has not been established by clinical trials.

Treatment for parasitic worms

If there is evidence of worm infestation, give mebendazole (100 mg orally twice a day) for 3 days. In countries where infestation is very prevalent, also give mebendazole to children with no evidence of infestation after day 7 of admission.

Monitoring

If there is anorexia after the above antibiotic treatment, continue for a full 10-day course. If anorexia still persists, reassess the child fully.

7.4.6 Micronutrient deficiencies

All severely malnourished children have vitamin and mineral deficiencies. Although anaemia is common, do not give iron initially but wait until the child has a good appetite and starts gaining weight (usually in the second week), because iron can make the infections worse.

Treatment

Give daily (for at least 2 weeks):

- a multivitamin supplement
- folic acid (5 mg on day 1, then 1 mg/day)
- zinc (2 mg Zn/kg/day)
- copper (0.3 mg Cu/kg/day)
- *once gaining weight*, ferrous sulfate (3 mg Fe/kg/day).

➤ Give vitamin A orally (aged <6 months: 50 000 IU; aged 6–12 months: 100 000 IU; older children: 200 000 IU) on day 1.

Zinc and copper supplements can be combined with the potassium and magnesium to make an electrolyte/mineral solution, which is added to ReSoMal and to the feeds (see page 180 for recipe). As an alternative, pre-mixed sachets containing electrolytes and all appropriate micronutrients are simpler to use.

Note: When using pre-mixed sachets, give single doses of vitamin A and folic acid on day 1, and give iron only after the child gains weight.

7.4.7 **Initial refeeding**

In the initial phase, a cautious approach is required because of the child's fragile physiological state.

Treatment

Essential features of initial feeding are:

- frequent small feeds of low osmolality and low lactose
- oral or nasogastric feeds (*never* parenteral preparations)
- 100 kcal/kg/day
- protein: 1–1.5 g/kg/day
- liquid: 130 ml/kg/day (100 ml/kg/day if the child has severe oedema)
- if the child is breastfed, continue with this, but make sure the prescribed amounts of starter formula are given (see below).

Days	Frequency	Vol/kg/feed	Vol/kg/d
1–2	2-hourly	11 ml	130 ml
3–5	3-hourly	16 ml	130 ml
6 onwards	4-hourly	22 ml	130 ml

The suggested starter formula and feeding schedules (see below) are designed to meet these targets. Milk-based formulas, such as starter F-75 (with 75 kcal/100 ml and 0.9 g of protein/100 ml), will be satisfactory for most children (see page 186 for recipes). Since cereal-based F-75 partially replaces sugar with cereal flour, it has the advantage of lower osmolarity which may benefit some children with persistent diarrhoea, but it needs to be cooked.

Feed from a cup or a bowl, or use a spoon, dropper or syringe to feed very weak children.

Table 21. Volumes of F-75 per feed (approx 130 ml/kg/day)

Child's weight (kg)	2-hourly (ml/feed)	3-hourly (ml/feed)	4-hourly (ml/feed)
2.0	20	30	45
2.2	25	35	50
2.4	25	40	55
2.6	30	45	55
2.8	30	45	60
3.0	35	50	65
3.2	35	55	70
3.4	35	55	75
3.6	40	60	80
3.8	40	60	85
4.0	45	65	90
4.2	45	70	90
4.4	50	70	95
4.6	50	75	100
4.8	55	80	105
5.0	55	80	110
5.2	55	85	115
5.4	60	90	120
5.6	60	90	125
5.8	65	95	130
6.0	65	100	130
6.2	70	100	135
6.4	70	105	140
6.6	75	110	145
6.8	75	110	150
7.0	75	115	155
7.2	80	120	160
7.4	80	120	160
7.6	85	125	165
7.8	85	130	170
8.0	90	130	175
8.2	90	135	180
8.4	90	140	185
8.6	95	140	190
8.8	95	145	195
9.0	100	145	200
9.2	100	150	200
9.4	105	155	205
9.6	105	155	210
9.8	110	160	215
10.0	110	160	220

Recipes for refeeding formulas F-75 and F-100

	F-75 [a] (starter: cereal-based)	F-75 [b,c] (starter)	F-100 [d] (catch-up)
Dried skimmed milk (g)	25	25	80
Sugar (g)	70	100	50
Cereal flour (g)	35	—	—
Vegetable oil (g)	27	27	60
Electrolyte/mineral soln (ml)	20	20	20
Water: make up to (ml)	1000	1000	1000
Contents per 100 ml			
Energy (kcal)	75	75	100
Protein (g)	1.1	0.9	2.9
Lactose (g)	1.3	1.3	4.2
Potassium (mmol)	4.2	4.0	6.3
Sodium (mmol)	0.6	0.6	1.9
Magnesium (mmol)	0.46	0.43	0.73
Zinc (mg)	2.0	2.0	2.3
Copper (mg)	0.25	0.25	0.25
% energy from protein	6	5	12
% energy from fat	32	32	53
Osmolality (mOsm/l)	334	413	419

[a] Cook for 4 minutes. This may be helpful for children with dysentery or persistent diarrhoea.

[b] A comparable starter formula can be made from 35 g whole dried milk, 100 g sugar, 20 g oil, 20 ml electrolyte/mineral solution, and water to make 1000 ml. If using fresh cow's milk, take 300 ml milk, 100 g sugar, 20 ml oil, 20 ml electrolye/mineral solution, and water to make 1000 ml.

[c] This formula has a high osmolarity (413 mOsm/l) and might not be tolerated by all children, especially those with diarrhoea. Isotonic versions of F-75 (280 mOsmol/l) are available commercially, in which maltodextrins replace some of the sugar.

[d] A comparable catch-up formula can be made from 110 g whole dried milk, 50 g sugar, 30 g oil, 20 ml electrolyte/mineral solution, and water to make 1000 ml. If using fresh cow's milk, take 880 ml milk, 75 g sugar, 20 ml oil, 20 ml electrolyte/mineral solution, and water to make 1000 ml.

Recipes for refeeding formulas F-75 and F-100

Alternative for F-75 if milk is unavailable.

Use precooked corn-soya blend (CSB) or wheat-soya blend (WSB)

CSB or WSB 50 g
Sugar 85 g
Oil 25 g
20 ml electrolyte/mineral mix
Make up to 1000 ml with (boiled) water

Note: Milk-based F-75 is best. If milk is limited, prioritize it for making the milk-based F-75 and use a non-milk alternative for F-100 (see below).

Alternative for F-100 if milk is unavailable.

Use precooked corn-soya blend (CSB) or wheat-soya blend (WSB)

CSB or WSB 150 g
sugar 25 g
oil 40 g
20 ml electrolyte/mineral mix
Make up to 1000 ml with (boiled) water.

A recommended schedule, with gradual increase in the feed volume and gradual decrease in feeding frequency, is shown on page 184:

For children with a good appetite and no oedema, this schedule can be completed in 2–3 days.

Note: If staff resources are limited, give priority to 2-hourly feeds for only the most seriously ill children, and aim for at least 3-hourly feeds initially. Get mothers and other carers to help with feeding. Show them what to do and supervise them. Night feeds are essential and staff rosters may need to be adjusted. If, despite all efforts, not all the night feeds can be given, the feeds should be spaced equally through the night to avoid long periods without a feed (with the risk of increased mortality).

If the child's intake (after allowing for any vomiting) does not reach 80 kcal/kg/day, despite frequent feeds, coaxing and re-offering, give the remaining feed by nasogastric tube. *Do not exceed 100 kcal/kg/day in this initial phase.*

In very hot climates, children might need extra water as these foods may not contain enough water if children are sweating.

Monitoring

Monitor and record:

- amounts of feed offered and left over
- vomiting
- stool frequency and consistency
- daily body weight

7.4.8 Catch-up growth

Signs that a child has reached this phase are:

- return of appetite
- most/all of the oedema has gone.

Treatment

Make a gradual transition from starter to catch-up formula.

➤ Replace the starter F-75 with an equal amount of catch-up F-100 for 2 days.

Give a milk-based formula, such as catch-up F-100 which contains 100 kcal/100 ml and 2.9 g of protein per 100 ml (see recipe, page 186). Modified porridges or complementary foods can be used, provided they have comparable energy and protein concentrations (see page 186 and 268–9 for recipes).

➤ Then increase each successive feed by 10 ml until some feed remains uneaten. The point when some of the feed remains unconsumed is likely to occur when intakes reach about 200 ml/kg/day.

After a gradual transition, give:

— frequent feeds, unlimited amounts

— 150–220 kcal/kg/day

— 4–6 g of protein/kg/day.

If the child is breastfed, continue to breastfeed. However, breast milk does not have sufficient energy and protein to support rapid catch-up growth, so give F-100 as indicated.

Monitoring

Avoid causing heart failure. Monitor for early signs of heart failure (rapid pulse and fast breathing).

CALCULATING WEIGHT GAIN

This example shows how to calculate weight gain of a child. It is for a weight gain over 3 days:

- Current weight of the child in grams = 6300 g
- Weight 3 days ago in grams = 6000 g

Step 1. Calculate weight gain in g (6300–6000 = 300 g)

Step 2. Calculate average daily weight gain (300g ÷ 3 days = 100g/day)

Step 3. Divide by child's average weight in kg
(100 g/day ÷ 6.15kg = 16.3 g/kg/day).

If both pulse and breathing rates increase (breathing by 5 breaths/minute and pulse by 25 beats/minute), and the increase is sustained for two successive 4-hourly readings:

- reduce the volume fed to 100 ml/kg/day for 24 hours
- then, slowly increase as follows:
  - 115 ml/kg/day for next 24 hours
  - 130 ml/kg/day for following 48 hours
  - then, increase each feed by 10 ml as described earlier.

Assess progress. After the transition, progress is assessed by the rate of weight gain:

- Weigh the child every morning before being fed, and plot the weight.
- Calculate and record the weight gain every 3 days as g/kg/day (see box).

If the weight gain is:

- poor (<5 g/kg/day), the child requires a full re-assessment
- moderate (5–10 g/kg/day), check whether the intake targets are being met, or if infection has been overlooked
- good (>10 g/kg/day).

7.4.9 Sensory stimulation

Provide:

- tender loving care
- a cheerful stimulating environment

- structured play therapy for 15–30 minutes a day
- physical activity as soon as the child is well enough
- maternal involvement as much as possible (e.g. comforting, feeding, bathing, play).

Provide suitable toys for the child (see page 285). Ideas for the organization of play activities are also given.

7.4.10 **Malnutrition in infants <6 months**

Malnutrition in infants <6 months is less common than in older children, and an organic cause for the malnutrition or failure to thrive should be considered, and, where appropriate, be treated. For nutritional rehabilitation, the basic principles for older children apply as well. However, these young infants are less able to excrete salt and urea with their urine, especially in hot climates. Therefore, the preferred diets in the stabilization phase are (in order of preference)

- Breastmilk (if it is available in sufficient quantity)
- Commercial infant formula

Diluted F-100 (add water in formula page 186 up to 1.5 litres instead of 1 litre) is acceptable during the rehabilitation phase.

7.5 **Treatment of associated conditions**

7.5.1 **Eye problems**

If the child has any eye signs of vitamin A deficiency (see page 175):

➤ give vitamin A orally on days 1, 2 and 14 (aged <6 months, 50 000 IU; aged 6–12 months, 100 000 IU; older children, 200 000 IU). If the first dose was given in the referring centre, treat on days 1 and 14 only.

If the eyes show signs of corneal clouding or ulceration, give the following additional care to the affected eye(s) to prevent corneal rupture and extrusion of the lens:

➤ instil chloramphenicol or tetracycline eye drops, 4 times daily as required for 7–10 days

➤ instil atropine eye drops, 1 drop 3 times daily for 3–5 days

➤ cover with saline-soaked eye pads

➤ bandage the eye(s).

Note: Children with vitamin A deficiency are likely to be photophobic and have their eyes closed. It is important to examine their eyes very gently to prevent corneal rupture.

7.5.2 **Severe anaemia**

A blood transfusion is required if:

- Hb is <4 g/dl
- Hb is 4–6 g/dl *and* the child has respiratory distress.

In severe malnutrition, the transfusion must be slower and of smaller volume than for a well-nourished child. Give:

➤ whole blood, 10 ml/kg *slowly* over 3 hours

➤ furosemide, 1 mg/kg IV at the start of the transfusion.

If the child has signs of heart failure, give 10 ml/kg of packed cells because whole blood is likely to worsen this condition. Children with kwashiorkor may have redistribution of fluid leading to apparent low Hb which does not require transfusion.

Monitor the pulse and breathing rates every 15 minutes during the transfusion. If either increases (breathing by 5 breaths/minute or pulse by 25 beats/minute), transfuse more slowly.

Note: After the transfusion, if the Hb is still low, do not repeat the transfusion within 4 days. For further details on giving transfusion, see page 277.

7.5.3 **Skin lesions in kwashiorkor**

Zinc deficiency is usual in children with kwashiorkor and their skin quickly improves with zinc supplementation. In addition:

➤ Bathe or soak the affected areas for 10 minutes/day in 0.01% potassium permanganate solution.

➤ Apply barrier cream (zinc and castor oil ointment, or petroleum jelly, or tulle gras) to the raw areas, and apply gentian violet (or, if available, nystatin cream) to skin sores.

➤ Omit using nappies/diapers so that the perineum can stay dry.

7.5.4 Continuing diarrhoea

Treatment

Giardiasis

Where possible, examine the stools by microscopy.

➤ If cysts or trophozoites of *Giardia lamblia* are found, give metronidazole (7.5 mg/kg 8-hourly for 7 days).

Lactose intolerance

Diarrhoea is only rarely due to lactose intolerance. Only treat for lactose intolerance if the continuing diarrhoea is preventing general improvement. Starter F-75 is a low-lactose feed. In exceptional cases:

➤ substitute milk feeds with yoghurt or a lactose-free infant formula

➤ reintroduce milk feeds gradually in the rehabilitation phase.

Osmotic diarrhoea

This may be suspected if the diarrhoea worsens substantially with hyperosmolar F-75 and ceases when the sugar content and osmolarity are reduced. In these cases:

➤ use a lower osmolar cereal-based starter F-75 (see recipe, page 186) or, if necessary, use a commercially available isotonic starter F-75

➤ introduce catch-up F-100 gradually.

7.5.5 Tuberculosis

If tuberculosis is strongly suspected:

- perform a Mantoux test (note: *false negatives are frequent*)
- take a chest X-ray, if possible.

If these are positive or tuberculosis is highly suspected, treat according to national tuberculosis guidelines (see section 4.8, page 101).

7.6 Discharge and follow-up

A child who is 90% weight-for-length (equivalent to –1SD) can be considered to have recovered. The child is still likely to have a low weight-for-age because of stunting.

Show the parent how to:

- feed frequently with energy-rich and nutrient-dense foods

- give structured play therapy (see page 285).

Ask the parent to bring the child back for regular follow-up (at 1, 2 and 4 weeks, then monthly for 6 months) and make sure the child receives:

  — booster immunizations

  — 6-monthly vitamin A.

Discharge before full recovery

Children who have not recovered fully are still at increased risk of relapse.

The timing of discharge takes into consideration the benefit of further inpatient management of the child, especially in terms of weight gain, and the risk of acquiring infections while remaining in contact with children with infections in the ward. Social factors such as loss of earnings for the mother and care for other children are also to be taken into account. Make a careful assessment of the child and of the available community support. The child will need continuing care as an outpatient to complete rehabilitation and prevent relapse. Some considerations for the success of home treatment are given below.

The child:

- should have completed antibiotic treatment
- should have a good appetite
- should show good weight gain
- should have lost oedema or at least be losing oedema (if the child was oedematous)

The mother or carer:

- should be available for child care
- should have received specific training on appropriate feeding (types, amount, frequency)
- should have the resources to feed the child. If this is not the case, advise on available support.

It is important to prepare the parents for home treatment. This might include switching the child to a locally affordable and available food (see pages 268–9 for examples). This will require feeding the child at least 5 times per day with foods that contain approximately 100 kcal and 2–3 g protein per 100 g of food. Mothers should understand that it is essential to give frequent meals with a high energy and protein content.

Fortified spreads (ready to use therapeutic foods) can be used in children older than 6 months.

- ➤ Give appropriate meals (and the correct quantity of food) at least 5 times daily.
- ➤ Give high-energy snacks between meals (e.g. milk, banana, bread, biscuits).
- ➤ Assist and encourage the child to complete each meal.
- ➤ Give food separately to the child so that the child's intake can be checked
- ➤ Give electrolyte and micronutrient supplements.
- ➤ Breastfeed as often as the child wants to.

Organizing follow-up for children discharged before recovery

If the child is discharged early, make a plan for the follow-up of the child until recovery and contact the outpatient department, nutrition rehabilitation centre, local health clinic, or health worker who will take responsibility for continuing supervision of the child. In general, the child should be weighed weekly after discharge. If there is failure to gain weight over a 2-week period or weight loss between any two measurements, the child should be referred back to hospital.

7.7 Monitoring the quality of care

7.7.1 Mortality audit

A register of admissions, discharges and deaths should be kept. This should contain information about the children (such as weight, age, sex), day of admission, date of discharge, or date and time of death.

To identify factors which can be changed to improve care, determine whether the majority of deaths occurred:

- *within 24 hours:* consider untreated or delayed treatment of hypoglycaemia, hypothermia, septicaemia, severe anaemia, or incorrect rehydration fluid or volume of fluid, or overuse of IV fluids
- *within 72 hours:* check whether refeeding was with too high a volume per feed or with wrong formulation; potassium and antibiotics given?
- *at night:* consider hypothermia related to insufficient covering of the child or no night feeds
- *when beginning F-100:* consider too rapid a transition from starter to catch-up formula.

7.7.2 Weight gain during rehabilitation phase

Standardize the weighing on the ward. Calibrate scales every day. Weigh the child the same time of the day (e.g. morning), after removing clothes.

Weight gain is defined as follows:

— poor: <5 g/kg/day

— moderate: 5–10 g/kg/day

— good: >10 g/kg/day.

If the weight gain is <5 g/kg/day, determine:

- whether this occurred in all cases being treated (if so, a major review of case management is required)
- whether this occurred in specific cases (reassess these children as if they were new admissions).

General areas to check, if the weight gain is poor, are described below.

Inadequate feeding

Check:

- that night feeds are given.
- that target energy and protein intakes are achieved. Is the actual intake (i.e. what was offered minus what was left over) correctly recorded? Is the quantity of feed recalculated as the child gains weight? Is the child vomiting or ruminating?
- feeding technique: is the child fed frequent feeds, unlimited amounts?
- quality of care: are staff motivated/gentle/loving/patient?
- all aspects of feed preparation: scales, measurement of ingredients, mixing, taste, hygienic storage, adequate stirring if separating out.
- whether complementary foods given to the child are energy dense enough.
- adequacy of multivitamin composition and shelf-life.
- preparation of mineral mix and whether correctly prescribed and administered. If in a goitrous region, check whether potassium iodide (KI) is added to the electrolyte/mineral mix (12 mg/2500 ml), or give all children Lugol's iodine (5–10 drops/day).
- if complementary foods are given, check that they contain electrolyte/mineral solution.

Untreated infection

If feeding is adequate and there is no malabsorption, suspect a hidden infection. The following are easily overlooked: urinary tract infections, otitis media, tuberculosis and giardiasis. In such a case:

- re-examine carefully
- repeat urine microscopy for white blood cells
- examine the stool
- if possible, take a chest X-ray.

HIV/AIDS

Recovery from malnutrition is possible in children with HIV and AIDS, but it may take longer and treatment failures are more common. Initial nutritional treatment of severe malnutrition in children with HIV/AIDS should be the same as for HIV-negative children.

For other HIV-related conditions, see Chapter 8, p. 199.

Psychological problems

Check for abnormal behaviour such as stereotyped movements (rocking), rumination (i.e. self-stimulation through regurgitation), and attention-seeking. Treat by giving the child special love and attention. For the child who ruminates, firmness, with affection, can assist. Encourage the mother to spend time playing with the child (see page 285).

Notes

Notes

CHAPTER 8

Children with HIV/AIDS

HIV infection is becoming a more important child health problem in many countries. In general, the management of specific conditions in HIV-infected children is similar to that of other children (see guidelines in Chapters 3 to 7). Most infections in HIV-positive children are caused by the same pathogens as in HIV-negative children, although they may be more frequent, more severe and occur repeatedly. Some, however, are due to unusual pathogens. Many HIV-positive children actually die from common childhood illnesses. Some of these deaths are preventable by early diagnosis and correct management, or by giving routine scheduled immunizations and improving nutrition. In particular, these children have a greater risk of pneumococcal infections and pulmonary tuberculosis. Co-trimoxazole prophylaxis and antiretroviral therapy dramatically decrease the number of children dying early.

This chapter discusses the following aspects of management of children with HIV/AIDS: counselling and testing, diagnosis of HIV infection, clinical staging, antiretroviral therapy, management of HIV-related conditions, supportive care, breastfeeding, discharge and follow-up, and palliative care for the terminally ill child.

The rate of mother-to-child transmission of HIV (without antiretroviral prophylaxis) is estimated to range from 15–45%. Evidence from industrially developed countries shows that such transmission can be greatly reduced (to less than 2% in recent studies) by the use of antiretrovirals during pregnancy and at delivery and by replacement feeding and elective Cesarean section. This has more recently become available in resource poor settings as well, and is having a major impact on the transmission of HIV and thus survival of the child.

8.1 Sick child with suspected or confirmed HIV infection

8.1.1 Clinical diagnosis

The clinical expression of HIV infection in children is highly variable. Some HIV-positive children develop severe HIV-related signs and symptoms in the first year of life. Other HIV-positive children may remain asymptomatic or mildly symptomatic for more than a year and may survive for several years.

Suspect HIV if any of the following signs, which are not common in HIV-negative children, are present.

Signs that may indicate possible HIV infection.

- *Recurrent infection*: three or more severe episodes of a bacterial infection (such as pneumonia, meningitis, sepsis, cellulitis) in the past 12 months.
- Oral thrush: Erythema and white-beige pseudomembranous plaques on the palate, gums and buccal mucosa. After the neonatal period, the presence of oral thrush—without antibiotic treatment, or lasting over 30 days despite treatment, or recurring, or extending beyond the tongue—is highly suggestive of HIV infection. Also typical is extension to the back of the throat which indicates oesophageal candidiasis.
- *Chronic parotitis*: the presence of unilateral or bilateral parotid swelling (just in front of the ear) for ≥14 days, with or without associated pain or fever.
- *Generalized lymphadenopathy*: the presence of enlarged lymph nodes in two or more extra-inguinal regions without any apparent underlying cause.
- *Hepatomegaly with no apparent cause*: in the absence of concurrent viral infections such as cytomegalovirus (CMV).

- *Persistent and/or recurrent fever*: fever (>38 °C) lasting ≥7 days, or occurring more than once over a period of 7 days.
- *Neurological dysfunction*: progressive neurological impairment, microcephaly, delay in achieving developmental milestones, hypertonia, or mental confusion.
- *Herpes zoster (shingles)*: painful rash with blisters confined to one dermatome on one side.
- *HIV dermatitis*: erythematous papular rash. Typical skin rashes include extensive fungal infections of the skin, nails and scalp, and extensive molluscum contagiosum.
- Chronic suppurative lung disease.

Signs common in HIV-infected children, but also common in ill non-HIV infected children

- *Chronic otitis media*: ear discharge lasting ≥14 days.
- *Persistent diarrhoea*: diarrhoea lasting ≥14 days.
- *Moderate or severe malnutrition*: weight loss or a gradual but steady deterioration in weight gain from the expected growth, as indicated in the child's growth card. Suspect HIV particularly in breastfed infants <6 months old who fail to thrive.

Signs or conditions very specific to HIV-infected children

Strongly suspect HIV infection if the following are present: pneumocystis pneumonia (PCP), oesophageal candidiasis, lymphoid interstitial pneumonia (LIP) or Kaposi's sarcoma. These conditions are very specific to HIV-infected children. Acquired recto-vaginal fistula in girls is also very specific but rare.

8.1.2 Counselling

If there are reasons to suspect HIV infection and the child's HIV status is not known, the family should be counselled and diagnostic testing for HIV should be offered.

Pre-test counselling includes obtaining informed consent before any tests proceed. As the majority of children are infected through vertical transmission from the mother, this implies that the mother, and often the father, is also infected. They may not know this. Even in high-prevalence countries, HIV remains an extremely stigmatizing condition and the parents may feel reluctant to undergo testing.

HIV counselling should take account of the child as part of a family. This should include the psychological implications of HIV for the child, mother, father and other family members. Counselling should stress that, although cure is currently not possible, there is much that can be done to improve the quality and duration of the child's life and the mother's relationship with the child. Where antiretroviral treatment is available, this greatly improves survival and the quality of life of the child and the parents. Counselling should make it clear that the hospital staff want to help, and that the mother should not be frightened of going to a health centre or hospital early in an illness, if only to ask questions.

Counselling requires time and has to be done by trained staff. If staff at the first referral level have not been trained, assistance should be sought from other sources, such as local community AIDS support organizations.

Indications for HIV counselling

HIV counselling is indicated in the following situations.

1. **Child with unknown HIV status presenting with clinical signs of HIV infection and/or risk factors (such as a mother or sibling with HIV/AIDS)**

   — Decide if you will do the counselling or if you will refer the child.

   — If you are doing the counselling, make time for the counselling session.

   Take advice from local people experienced in counselling so that any advice given is consistent with what the mother will receive from professional counsellors at a later stage.

   — Where available, arrange an HIV test, according to national guidelines, to confirm the clinical diagnosis, alert the mother to HIV-related problems, and discuss prevention of future mother-to-child transmissions.

   Note: If HIV testing is not available, discuss the presumptive diagnosis of HIV infection in the light of the existing signs/symptoms and risk factors.

   — If counselling is not being carried out at the hospital, explain to the parent why they are being referred elsewhere for counselling.

2. **Child known to be HIV-infected but responding poorly to treatment, or needing further investigations**

   Discuss the following in the counselling sessions:

   — the parents' understanding of HIV infection

   — management of current problems

   — role of ART

— the need to refer to a higher level, if necessary

— support from community-based groups, if available.

3. **Child known to be HIV-infected who has responded well to treatment and is to be discharged (or referred to a community-based care programme for psychosocial support)**

   Discuss the following in the counselling sessions:

   — the reason for referral to a community-based care programme, if appropriate

   — follow-up care

   — risk factors for future illness

   — immunization and HIV

   — adherence and ART treatment support.

8.1.3 Testing and diagnosis of HIV infection in children

The diagnosis of HIV infection in perinatally exposed infants and young children is difficult because passively acquired maternal HIV antibodies may be present in the child's blood until the child is 18 months of age. Additional diagnostic challenges arise if the child is still breastfeeding or has been breastfed. Although HIV infection cannot be ruled out until 18 months for some children, many children will have lost HIV antibodies between 9 and 18 months.

HIV testing should be voluntary and free of coercion, and informed consent is required before HIV testing (see above 8.1.2).

All diagnostic HIV testing of children must be:

- **confidential**
- be accompanied by **counselling**
- only be conducted with informed **consent** so that it is both informed and voluntary.

For children this usually means parental or guardian's consent. For the older minor, parental consent to testing/treatment is not generally required; however it is obviously preferable for young people to have their parents' support, and consent may be required by law. Accepting or refusing HIV testing should not lead to detrimental consequences to the quality of care offered.

HIV antibody test (ELISA or rapid tests)

Rapid tests are increasingly available and are safe, effective, sensitive and reliable for diagnosing HIV infection in children from the age of 18 months. For the child

<18 months, rapid HIV antibody tests are a sensitive, reliable way of detecting the **HIV exposed infant** and to exclude HIV infection in non-breastfeeding children.

You can use rapid HIV tests to exclude HIV infection in a child presenting with malnutrition or other serious clinical events in high HIV-prevalence areas. For children <18 months, confirm all positive HIV antibody tests by virological tests as soon as possible (see below).

Where this is not possible, repeat antibody testing at 18 months.

Virological testing

Virological testing for HIV-specific RNA or DNA is the most reliable method for diagnosing HIV infection in children <18 months of age. This requires sending a blood sample to a specialized laboratory which can perform this test, but these are becoming available in many countries. It is relatively cheap, easy to standardize, and can be done using dried blood spots. If the child has had zidovudine (ZDV) prophylaxis during and after delivery, virological testing is not recommended until 4–8 weeks after delivery, as ZDV interferes with the reliability of the test. One virological test which is positive at 4–8 weeks is sufficient to diagnose infection in a young infant. If the young infant is still breastfeeding, and the RNA virological test is negative, it needs to be repeated 6 weeks after the complete cessation of breastfeeding to confirm that the child is not HIV infected.

8.1.4 Clinical staging

In a child with diagnosed or highly suspected HIV infection, the clinical staging system helps to recognize the degree of damage to the immune system and to plan treatment and care options. The stages determine the likely prognosis of HIV, and are a guide when to start, stop or substitute ARV therapy in HIV-infected children.

The clinical stages identify a progressive sequence from least to most severe, with each higher clinical stage having a poorer prognosis. For classification purposes, once a stage 3 clinical condition has occurred, the child's prognosis will likely remain that of stage 3, and will not improve to that of stage 2, even with resolution of the original condition, or appearance of a new stage 2 clinical event. Antiretroviral treatment with good adherence dramatically improves prognosis.

The clinical staging events can also be used to identify the response to ARV treatment if there is no easy or affordable access to viral load or CD4 testing.

Table 22. The WHO paediatric clinical staging system

For use in those <13 years with confirmed laboratory evidence of HIV infection (HIV AB where age >18 months, DNA or RNA virological testing for those age <18 months)

STAGE 1

Asymptomatic
Persistent generalized lymphadenopathy (PGL)

STAGE 2

Hepatosplenomegaly
Papular pruritic eruptions
Seborrhoeic dermatitis
Fungal nail infections
Angular cheilitis
Lineal gingival erythema (LGE)
Extensive human papilloma virus infection or molluscum infection (>5% body area)
Recurrent oral ulcerations (2 or more episodes in 6 months)
Parotid enlargement
Herpes zoster
Recurrent or chronic upper respiratory tract infections (otitis media, otorrhoea, sinusitis, 2 or more episodes in any 6 month period)

STAGE 3

Unexplained moderate malnutrition not responding to standard therapy
Unexplained persistent diarrhoea (>14 days)
Unexplained persistent fever (intermittent or constant, for longer than 1 month)
Oral candidiasis (outside neonatal period)
Oral hairy leukoplakia
Pulmonary tuberculosis[1]
Severe recurrent presumed bacterial pneumonia (2 or more episodes in 6 months)
Acute necrotizing ulcerative gingivitis/periodontitis
LIP (lymphoid interstitial pneumonia)
Unexplained anaemia (<8 gm/dl), neutropenia (<500/mm^3) or thrombocytopenia (<30,000/mm^3) for >1 month

(Continued)

Table 22. The WHO paediatric clinical staging system (continued)

STAGE 4

Unexplained severe wasting or severe malnutrition not responding to standard therapy
Pneumocystis pneumonia
Recurrent severe presumed bacterial infections (2 or more episodes within one year, e.g. empyema, pyomyositis, bone or joint infection, meningitis, but excluding pneumonia)
Chronic orolabial or cutaneous herpes simplex infection (of >1 month duration)
Disseminated or extrapulmonary tuberculosis
Kaposi sarcoma
Oesophageal candida
Symptomatic HIV seropositive infant <18 months with 2 or more of the following; oral thrush, +/– severe pneumonia, +/– failure to thrive, +/– severe sepsis[2]
CMV retinitis
CNS toxoplasmosis
Any disseminated endemic mycosis including cryptococcal meningitis (e.g. extra-pulmonary cryptococcosis, histoplasmosis, coccidiomycosis, penicilliosis)
Cryptosporidiosis or isosporiasis (with diarrhoea >1 month)
Cytomegalovirus infection (onset at age >1 month in an organ other than liver, spleen, or lymph nodes)
Disseminated mycobacterial disease other than tuberculous
Candida of trachea, bronchi or lungs
Acquired HIV-related recto-vesico fistula
Cerebral or B cell non-Hodgkin's lymphoma
Progressive multifocal leukoencephalopathy (PML)
HIV encephalopathy
HIV-related cardiomyopathy
HIV-related nephropathy

1 TB may occur at any CD4 count and CD4 % should be considered where available
2 Presumptive diagnosis of stage 4 disease in seropositive children <18 months requires confirmation with HIV virological tests or using HIV antibody test after 18 months of age.

8.2 Antiretroviral therapy (ART)

Antiretroviral drugs are becoming more widely available, and have revolutionized HIV/AIDs care. ARV drugs are not a cure for HIV but they have dramatically reduced mortality and morbidity, and improved the quality of life for adults and children. WHO recommends that in resource-limited settings, HIV-infected adults and children should start ARV therapy based upon clinical or immunological criteria, and using simplified standardized treatment guidelines. Resistance to single or dual agents is quick to emerge, and so single drug regimens are contraindicated; indeed at least three drugs are the recommended minimum standard for all settings. While new ARV drugs are emerging on the market, frequently these are not available for use in children, either due to lack of formulations or dosage data as well as high costs. As children with HIV are often part of a household with an adult with HIV, ideally access to treatment and ARV drugs needs to be ensured for other family members, and where possible similar drug regimens should be used. Fixed-dose combinations are increasingly available, and are preferred to promote and support treatment adherence as well as reduction in the cost of treatment. Existing tablets often cannot be divided into lower dosages for children (under 10 kg), so syrups/solutions and suspensions are needed.

The underlying principles of antiretroviral therapy (ART) and choice of first-line ART in children are largely the same as in adults. However it is also important to consider:

- availability of a suitable formulation that can be taken in appropriate doses
- simplicity of the dosage schedule
- taste/palatability and hence compliance in young children
- the ART regimen which the parent(s) or guardians are or will be taking.

Suitable formulations for children are not available for some ARVs (particularly the protease inhibitor class of drugs).

8.2.1 Antiretroviral drugs

Antiretrovirals fall into three main classes of drugs: nucleoside analogue reverse transcriptase inhibitors (NRTIs), non-nucleoside reverse transcriptase inhibitors (NNRTIs), and protease inhibitors (PIs) (see Table 23).

Triple therapy is the standard of care. WHO currently recommends that first-line regimens should be based upon two nucleoside analogue reverse transcriptase inhibitors (NRTI) plus one non-nucleoside drug (NNRTI). The use of triple NRTI as first-line therapy is currently considered a secondary alternative because of

Table 23. Classes of antiretroviral drugs recommend for use in children in resource-poor settings

Nucleoside analogue reverse transcriptase inhibitors	
— Zidovudine	ZDV (AZT)
— Lamivudine	3TC
— Stavudine	d4T
— Didanosine	ddI
— Abacavir	ABC
Non-nucleoside reverse transcriptase inhibitors	
— Nevirapine	NVP
— Efavirenz	EFV
Protease inhibitors	
— Nelfinavir	NFV
— Lopinavir/ritonavir	LPV/r
— Saquinavir	SQV

Table 24. Possible first-line treatment regimens for children

WHO-recommended first-line ARV regimen for infants and children	
First-line regimen	**Second-line regimen**
Stavudine (d4T) or Zidovudine (ZDV)	Abacavir (ABC)
plus	*plus*
Lamivudine (3TC)	Didanosine (ddI)
plus	*plus*
Nevirapine (NVP) or Efavirenz (EFV)[1]	Protease inhibitor: Lopinavir/ritonavir (LPV/r) or Nelfinavir (NFV) or Saquinavir (SQV)[2]

[1] Give Efavirenz only to children >3 years and 10 kg body weight
Efavirenz is the treatment of choice for children who receive rifampicin for tuberculosis

[2] Give Saquinavir only to children >25 kg body weight

recent research findings in adults. Protease inhibitors are usually recommended to be part of second-line regimens in most resource-limited settings.

EFV is the NNRTI of choice in children who are on rifampicin, if treatment needs to start before anti-tuberculous therapy is completed. For drug dosages and regimens see Appendix 2, page 348.

Calculation of drug dosages

Drug doses are given on pages 348–352, per kg for some drugs and per m^2 surface area of the child for others. A table giving the equivalent weights of various surface area values is also given in Appendix 2 (page 325) to help in dosage calculation. In general, children metabolize PI and NNRTI drugs faster than adults and require higher than adult equivalent doses to achieve appropriate drug levels. Drug doses have to be increased as the child grows; otherwise there is a risk of underdosage and development of resistance.

Formulations

Liquid formulations may not be easily available, are more expensive and may have reduced shelf-life. As the child gets older, the amount of syrup to take becomes quite considerable. Therefore, from 10 kg of weight, it is preferred to give parts of scored tables or combination preparations (see drug table)

8.2.2 When to start ART

About 20% of HIV-infected infants in developing countries progress to AIDS or death by 12 months of age (with a substantial contribution from PCP infections in infants under 6 months not receiving cotrimoxazole treatment). It is possible that early therapy (even for a limited period) in the primary infection of infants may improve disease outcome. Currently, US guidelines recommend early ART for infants but European guidelines are more conservative. In developing countries, the benefits of starting ART early in children are balanced by potential problems with adherence, resistance, and diagnostic difficulties. Clear clinical benefit shown by clinical trials is required before early ART can be recommended.

For infants and children with confirmed HIV infection, the indications for starting treatment are outlined in Table 25.

In children aged 12–18 months who are HIV (antibody) positive, with symptoms and in whom HIV is strongly suspected on clinical grounds, it may be reasonable to start ART.

Starting ART in *asymptomatic* children is not encouraged because of inevitable development of resistance with time. Treatment should generally be deferred until after acute infections have been treated. In the case of tuberculosis which is frequently (but generally only presumptively) diagnosed in HIV-infected children, treatment should be deferred at least until after 2 months of antituberculous therapy has been completed, and preferably until completion of all antituberculosis therapy. This is to avoid interactions with rifampicin and also possible non-adherence due to the number of medications needed to be administered. Choice of ART is similar to that in adults.

8.2.3 Side-effects of antiretroviral therapy and monitoring

The response to antiretroviral treatment and side-effects of treatment need to be monitored. Where CD4 cell count is available, this should be done every 3–6 months and can inform on the successful response to treatment or its failure and therefore guide changes in treatment. Where this is not possible, clinical parameters, including clinical staging events, need to be used (see Table 22).

Monitoring response after ARV initiation:

- After ARV initiation or ARV change:
  - See the child at 2 and 4 weeks after the start/change.
- Child should be seen if there are any problems that concern the caregiver, or intercurrent illness.

Long-term follow-up

- A clinician should see the child at least every 3 months.
- A non-clinician (ideally, the provider of ARV medication, such as pharmacist, who would assess adherence and provide adherence counselling) should see the child monthly.
- Child should be seen more frequently, preferably by a clinician, if clinically unstable.

The organization of follow-up care depends on the local expertise, and should be decentralized as far as possible.

Monitoring response

- Weight and height (monthly)
- Neurodevelopment (monthly)
- Adherence (monthly)
- CD4 (%) if available (then every 3–6 months)
- Baseline Hb or Hct (if on ZDV/AZT), ALT if available
- Symptom-related determination: Hb or Hct or full blood count, ALT

Table 25. Summary of indications for initiating ART in children, based on clinical staging

Clinical stages	ART
4	Treat
Presumptive stage 4	Treat
3	Treat all, except if the child is >18 months and CD4 >15%, or >5 years and CD4 >10% or >200/mm^3
1 and 2	Treat only where CD4 available and child Under 18 months: CD4 % <25% 18–59 months: CD4 % <15% 5 years or over: CD4 % <10% or <200/mm^3

Note:

A presumptive diagnosis of stage 4 clinical disease should be made if:

An infant is HIV-antibody positive (ELISA or rapid test), aged under 18 months and symptomatic with two or more of the following:

- +/- oral thrush;
- +/- severe pneumonia[1]
- +/- severe wasting/malnutrition
- +/- severe sepsis[2]

CD4 values, where available, may be used to guide decision-making; CD4 percentages below 25% require ART

Other factors that support the diagnosis of clinical stage 4 HIV infection in an HIV-seropositive infant are:

- — recent HIV related maternal death
- — advanced HIV disease in the mother.

Confirmation of the diagnosis of HIV infection should be sought as soon as possible.

[1] Pneumonia requiring oxygen.

[2] Requiring intravenous therapy.

SIDE-EFFECTS OF ANTIRETROVIRAL THERAPY AND MONITORING

General, long-term side-effects of antiretroviral therapy include lipodystrophy. Specific side-effects of individual antiretroviral drugs are summarized in Table 26.

Table 26. Common side-effects of antiretroviral drugs

Drug		Side-effects	Comments
Nucleoside analogue reverse transcriptase inhibitors (NRTI)			
Lamivudine	3TC	Headache, abdominal pain, pancreatitis	Well tolerated
Stavudine [a]	d4T	Headache, abdominal pain, neuropathy	Large volume of suspension, capsules can be opened
Zidovudine	ZDV (AZT)	Headache, anaemia	Do not use with d4T (antagonistic antiretroviral effect)
Abacavir	ABC	Hypersensitivity reaction: fever, mucositis, rash: stop drug	Tablets can be crushed
Didanosine	ddI	Pancreatitis, peripheral neuropathy, diarrhoea and abdominal pain	On empty stomach, give with antacid
Non-nucleoside reverse transcriptase inhibitors (NNRTI)			
Efavirenz	EFV	strange dreams, sleepiness, rash	Take at night, avoid taking with fatty food
Nevirapine	NVP	Rash, liver toxicity	With rifampicin coadministration, increase NVP dose by ~30%, or avoid use. Drug interactions
Protease inhibitors (PI)			
Lopinavir/ritonavir [a]	LPV/r	Diarrhoea, nausea	Take with food, bitter taste
Nelfinavir	NFV	Diarrhoea, vomiting, rash	Take with food
Saquinavir [a]	SQV	Diarrhoea, abdominal discomfort	Take within 2 hours of taking food

[a] Requires cold storage and cold chain for transport.

Table 27. Clinical and CD4 definition of ARV treatment failure in children (after 6 months or more of ARV)

Clinical criteria	CD4 criteria
• Lack or decline in growth among children with initial growth response to ARV • Loss of neurodevelopmental milestones or onset of encephalopathy • New or recurrent WHO clinical Stage 4 conditions	• Return of CD4% if <6 years (% or count if age ≥6 years) to pre-therapy baseline or below, without other etiology • ≥50% fall from peak CD4% if <6 yrs (% or count if age ≥6 years), without other aetiology

8.2.4 When to change treatment

When to substitute

Drugs need to be substituted for others when there is

- Treatment limiting toxicity, such as:
  - Stevens Johnson Syndrome (SJS)
  - Severe liver toxicity
  - Severe haematologic findings
- Drug interaction (e.g. tuberculosis treatment with rifampicin interfering with NVP or PI)
- Potential lack of adherence by the patient if he cannot tolerate the regimen.

When to switch

- In absence of routine CD4 or viral load assays, judgments should be made about treatment failure based on:
  - Clinical progression
  - CD4 decline as defined in table above
- Generally, patients should have received 6 months or more of ARV therapy and adherence problems should be ruled out before considering treatment failure and switching ARV regimens.
- If an apparent deterioration is due to the immune reconstitution syndrome (IRIS), then this is not the reason to switch therapy.

Second-line treatment regimens

ABC plus ddI plus Protease inhibitor: LPV/r or NFV or SQV/r if wt ≥25 kg

8.3 Other treatment for the HIV-positive child

8.3.1 Immunization

- Children who have, or are suspected to have, HIV infection but are not yet symptomatic should be given all appropriate vaccines (according to the national EPI programme schedule), including BCG and, where relevant, yellow fever vaccine. Because most HIV-positive children have an effective immune response in the first year of life, immunization should be given as early as possible after the recommended age of vaccination.
- *Do **not** give BCG and yellow fever vaccines to children with symptomatic HIV infection.*
- Give all children with HIV infection (regardless of whether they are symptomatic or not) an extra dose of the measles vaccine at the age of 6 months, as well as the standard dose at 9 months.

8.3.2 Cotrimoxazole prophylaxis

Cotrimoxazole prophylaxis has been shown to be very effective in HIV-infected infants and children in reducing mortality and the rate of PCP as a cause of severe pneumonia. PCP is now very unusual in countries where prophylaxis is routine.

Who should get cotrimoxazole

- All HIV exposed children (children born to HIV infected mothers) from 4–6 weeks of age (whether or not part of a prevention of mother-to-child transmission [PMTCT] programme)
- Any child identified as HIV-infected with any clinical signs or symptoms suggestive of HIV, regardless of age or CD4 count.

How long should cotrimoxazole be given

Cotrimoxazole is required to be taken as follows:

- HIV exposed children—until HIV infection has been definitively ruled out and the mother is no longer breastfeeding
- HIV-infected children—indefinitely where ARV treatment is not yet available.
- Where ARV treatment is being given—cotrimoxazole may only be stopped only once clinical or immunological indicators confirm restoration of the immune system for 6 months or more (also see below). With current evidence it is not yet clear if cotrimoxazole continues to provide protection after immune restoration is achieved.

Under what circumstances should cotrimoxazole be discontinued

- Occurrence of severe cutaneous reactions such as Stevens Johnson syndrome, renal and/or hepatic insufficiency or severe haematological toxicity.
- In an HIV-exposed child, **only** after HIV infection has confidently been excluded:
  - — For a non-breastfeeding child <18 months—this is by negative DNA or RNA virological HIV testing
  - — For a breastfed HIV-exposed child <18 months—negative virological testing is only reliable if conducted 6 weeks after cessation of breastfeeding,
  - — For a breastfed HIV-exposed child >18 months—negative HIV antibody testing 6 weeks after stopping breastfeeding.
- In an HIV- infected child:
  - — If the child is on ARV therapy, cotrimoxazole can be stopped only when evidence of immune restoration has occurred. Continuing cotrimoxazole may continue to provide benefit even after the child has clinically improved.
  - — If ARV therapy is not available, cotrimoxazole should not be discontinued.

What doses of cotrimoxazole should be used?

➤ Recommended dosages of 6–8 mg/kg TMP once daily should be used. For children <6 months, give 1 paediatric tablet (or 1/4 adult tablet, 20 mg TMP/100 mg SMX); for children 6 months to 5 years, 2 paediatric tablets (or 1/2 adult tablet); and for children >5 years, 1 adult tablet. Use weight-band dosages rather than body-surface-area doses.

➤ If the child is allergic to cotrimoxazole, dapsone is the best alternative.

What follow-up is required?

- Assessment of tolerance and adherence: Cotrimoxazole prophylaxis should be a routine part of care of HIV-infected children, and be assessed at all regular clinic visits or follow-up visits by health workers and/or other members of multidisciplinary care teams. Initial clinic follow-up in children is suggested monthly, and then every three months, if cotrimoxazole is well tolerated.

8.3.3 Nutrition

- Children should eat energy-rich food and increase their energy intake
- HIV-infected adults and children should be encouraged to eat varied food which ensures micronutrient intakes.

8.4 Management of HIV-related conditions

The treatment of most infections (such as pneumonia, diarrhoea, meningitis) in HIV-infected children is the same as for other children. In cases of failed treatment, consider using a second-line antibiotic. Treatment of recurrent infections is the same, regardless of the number of recurrences.

Some HIV-related conditions require specific management. These are described below.

8.4.1 Tuberculosis

In a child with suspected or proven HIV infection, it is important always to consider the diagnosis of tuberculosis.

The diagnosis of tuberculosis in children with HIV infection is often difficult. Early in HIV infection, when immunity is not impaired, the signs of tuberculosis are similar to those in a child without HIV infection. Pulmonary tuberculosis is still the commonest form of tuberculosis, even in HIV-infected children. As HIV infection progresses and immunity declines, dissemination of tuberculosis becomes more common. Tuberculous meningitis, miliary tuberculosis, and widespread tuberculous lymphadenopathy occur.

➤ Treat tuberculosis in HIV-infected children with the same anti-tuberculosis drug regimen as for non-HIV-infected children with tuberculosis, but replace thioacetazone with an alternative antibiotic (refer to national tuberculosis guidelines or see section 4.8, page 101).

Note: Thioacetazone is associated with a high risk of severe, and sometimes fatal, skin reactions in HIV-infected children. These reactions can start with itching, but progress to severe reactions. If thioacetazone must be given, warn the parents about the risk of severe skin reactions and advise them to stop thioacetazone at once, if there is itching or skin reactions occur.

8.4.2 *Pneumocystis jiroveci* (formerly *carinii*) pneumonia (PCP)

Make a presumptive diagnosis of pneumocystis pneumonia in a child who has severe or very severe pneumonia and bilateral interstitial infiltrates on chest X-ray. Consider the possibility of pneumocystis pneumonia in children, known or suspected to have HIV, whose ordinary pneumonia does not respond to treatment. Pneumocystis pneumonia occurs most frequently in infants and is often associated with hypoxia. Fast breathing is the most common presenting sign, respiratory distress is out of proportion with chest findings, fever is often mild. Peak age is 4–6 months.

➤ Promptly give oral or preferably IV high-dose cotrimoxazole (trimethoprim (TMP) 8 mg/kg/dose, sulfamethoxazole (SMX) 40 mg/kg/dose) 3 times a day for 3 weeks.

➤ If the child has a severe drug reaction, change to pentamidine (4 mg/kg once per day) by IV infusion for 3 weeks. For the management of the child presenting with clinical pneumonia in settings with high HIV prevalence, see page 78.

➤ Continue prophylaxis on recovery, and start ART as indicated.

8.4.3 Lymphoid interstitial pneumonitis (LIP)

Suspect LIP if the chest X-ray shows a bilateral reticulo-nodular interstitial pattern, which has to be distinguished from pulmonary tuberculosis, and bilateral hilar adenopathy (see figure). The child is often asymptomatic in the early stages but may later have a persistent cough, with or without difficulty in breathing, bilateral parotid swelling, persistent generalized lymphadenopathy, hepatomegaly and other signs of heart failure, and finger-clubbing.

➤ Give a trial of antibiotic treatment for bacterial pneumonia (see section 4.2, page 72) before starting treatment with prednisolone.

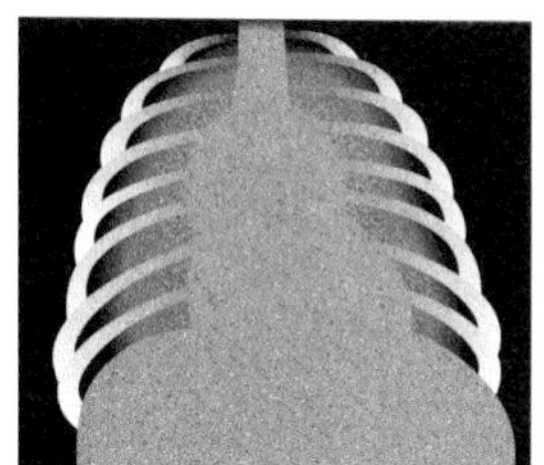

Lymphocytic insterstitial pneumonia (LIP): typical is hilar lymphadenopathy and lacelike infiltrates.

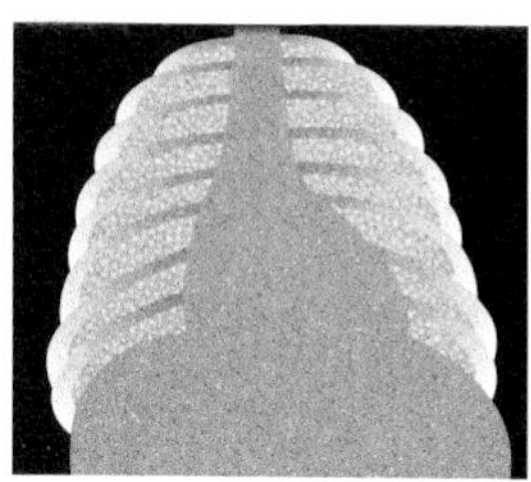

Pneumocystis jiroveci pneumonia (PCP): typical is a ground glass appearance

Start treatment with steroids, **only** if there are chest X-ray findings of lymphoid interstitial pneumonitis plus any of the following signs:

— fast or difficult breathing

— cyanosis

— pulse oximetry reading of oxygen saturation less than 90%.

➤ Give oral prednisone, 1–2 mg/kg daily for 2 weeks. Then decrease the dose over 2–4 weeks depending on treatment response.

Only start treatment if it is possible to complete the full treatment course (which may take several months depending on the resolution of signs of hypoxia), since partial treatment is not effective and could be harmful. Beware of reactivation of TB.

8.4.4 Fungal infections

Oral and oesophageal candidiasis

➤ Treat oral thrush with nystatin (100 000 units/ml) suspension. Give 1–2 ml into the mouth 4 times a day for 7 days. If this is not available, apply 1% gentian violet solution. If these are ineffective, give 2% miconazole gel, 5 ml two times a day, if available.

Suspect oesophageal candidiasis if there is difficulty or pain while vomiting or swallowing, reluctance to take food, excessive salivation, or crying during feeding. The condition may occur with or without evidence of oral thrush. If oral thrush is not found, give a trial of treatment with fluconazole (3–6 mg/kg once per day). Exclude other causes of painful swallowing (such as cytomegalovirus, herpes simplex, lymphoma and, rarely, Kaposi sarcoma), if necessary by referral to a larger hospital where appropriate testing is possible.

➤ Give oral fluconazole (3–6 mg/kg once per day) for 7 days, except if the child has active liver disease. Give amphotericin B (0.5 mg/kg/dose once per day) by IV infusion for 10–14 days to these children and in cases where there is lack of response to oral therapy, inability to tolerate oral medications, or the risk of disseminated candidiasis (e.g. in a child with leukopenia).

Cryptococcal meningitis

Suspect cryptococcus as a cause in any HIV infected child with signs of meningitis; presentation is often subacute with chronic headache or only mental status changes. India ink stain of CSF confirms the diagnosis. Treat with ampohotericin 0.5–1.5 mg/kg/day for 14 days, then with fluconazole for 8 weeks. Start fluconazole prophylaxis after treatment.

8.4.5 Kaposi sarcoma

Consider Kaposi sarcoma in children presenting with nodular skin lesions, diffuse lymphadenopathy and lesions on the palate and conjunctiva with periorbital bruising. Diagnosis is usually clinical but can be confirmed by a needle biopsy of skin lesions or lymph node biopsy. Suspect also in children with persistent diarrhoea, weight loss, intestinal obstruction, abdominal pain or large pleural effusion.

Consider referral to a larger hospital for management.

8.5 HIV transmission and breastfeeding

HIV transmission may occur during pregnancy, labour and delivery, or through breastfeeding. The best way to prevent transmission is to prevent HIV infection in general, especially in pregnant women, and to prevent unintended pregnancies in HIV-positive women. If an HIV-infected woman becomes pregnant, she should be provided with services including prophylactic antiretroviral drugs (and ART where clinically indicated), safer obstetric practices, and infant feeding counseling and support.

There is evidence that the additional risk of HIV transmission through breastfeeding is about 5–20%. HIV can be transmitted through breast milk at any point during lactation, and thus the rate of infection in breastfed infants increases with duration of breastfeeding.

Defer counselling on HIV transmission until the child's condition has stabilized. Where a decision has been made to continue breastfeeding because the child is already infected, infant feeding options should be discussed for future pregnancies. This should be carried out by a trained and experienced counsellor.

- If a child is known to be HIV-infected and is being breastfed, encourage the mother to continue breastfeeding.
- If the mother is known to be HIV-positive and the child's HIV status is unknown, the mother should be counselled about the benefits of breastfeeding as well as the risk of HIV transmission through breastfeeding. If replacement feeding is acceptable, feasible, affordable, sustainable and safe, avoidance of further breastfeeding is recommended. Otherwise, exclusive breastfeeding should be practised if the child is less than 6 months of age, and breastfeeding should be discontinued as soon as these conditions are in place.

Infants born to HIV-positive mothers who have escaped perinatal infection have a lower risk of acquiring HIV if they are not breastfed. However, their risk of death may be increased if they are not breastfed in situations where there is no regular access to nutritionally adequate, safely prepared breast milk substitutes.

The counselling should be carried out by a trained and experienced counsellor. Take advice from local people experienced in counselling so that any advice given is consistent with what the mother will receive from professional counsellors at a later stage.

If the mother decides to use breast milk substitutes, counsel the mother about their correct use and demonstrate safe preparation.

8.6 Follow-up

8.6.1 Discharge from hospital

HIV-infected children may respond slowly or incompletely to the usual treatment. They may have persistent fever, persistent diarrhoea and chronic cough. If the general condition of these children is good, they do not need to remain in the hospital, but can be seen regularly as outpatients.

8.6.2 Referral

If facilities are not available in your hospital, consider referring a child suspected to have HIV infection:

- for HIV testing with pre- and post-test counselling
- to another centre or hospital for further investigations or second-line treatment if there has been little or no response to treatment
- to a trained counsellor for HIV and infant feeding counselling, if the local health worker cannot do this
- to a community/home-based care programme, or a community/institution-based voluntary counselling and testing centre, or a community-based social support programme for further counselling and continuing psychosocial support.

A special effort should be made to refer orphans to essential services including health care education and birth registration.

8.6.3 Clinical follow-up

Children who are known or suspected to be HIV-infected should, when not ill, attend well-baby clinics like other children. In addition, they need regular clinical follow-up at first-level facilities at least twice a year to monitor:

— their clinical condition

— growth
— nutritional intake
— immunization status
— psychosocial support (where possible, this should be given through community-based programmes).

8.7 Palliative and end-of-life care

An HIV-infected child often has considerable discomfort, so good palliative care is essential. Take all decisions together with the mother, and communicate them clearly to other staff (including night staff). Consider palliative care at home as an alternative to hospital care. Some treatments for pain control and relief of distressing conditions (such as oesophageal candidiasis or convulsions) can significantly improve the quality of the child's remaining life.

Give end-of-life (terminal) care if:

— the child has had a progressively worsening illness
— everything possible has been done to treat the presenting illness.

Ensuring that the family has appropriate support to cope with the impending death of the child is an important part of care in the terminal stages of HIV/AIDS. Parents should be supported in their efforts to give palliative care at home so that the child is not kept in hospital unnecessarily.

8.7.1 Pain control

The management of pain in HIV-infected children follows the same principles as for other chronic diseases such as cancer or sickle-cell disease. Particular attention should be paid to ensuring that care is culturally appropriate and sensitive. The underlying principles should be:

— give analgesia *by mouth*, where possible (IM treatment is painful)
— give it *regularly*, so that the child does not have to experience the recurrence of severe pain in order to get the next dose of analgesia
— give it in *increasing doses*, or start with mild analgesics and progress to strong analgesics as the requirement for pain relief rises or tolerance develops
— set the *dose for each child*, because children will have different dose requirements for the same effect.

Use the following drugs for effective pain control:

1. ***Local anaesthetics:*** for painful lesions in the skin or mucosa or during painful procedures.
   — Lidocaine: apply on a gauze to painful mouth ulcers before feeds (apply with gloves, unless the family member or health worker is HIV-positive and does not need protection from infection); it acts in 2–5 minutes.
   — TAC (tetracaine, adrenaline, cocaine): apply to a gauze pad and place over open wounds; it is particularly useful when suturing.
2. ***Analgesics:*** for mild and moderate pain (such as headaches, post-traumatic pain, and pain from spasticity).
   — paracetamol
   — nonsteroidal anti-inflammatory drugs, such as ibuprofen.
3. ***Potent analgesics such as opiates:*** for moderate and severe pain not responding to treatment with analgesics.
   — morphine, an inexpensive and potent analgesic: give orally or IV every 4–6 hours, or by continuous IV infusion.
   — pethidine: give orally every 4–6 hours
   — codeine: give orally every 6–12 hours, combined with non-opioids to achieve additive analgesia.

   Note: Monitor carefully for respiratory depression. If tolerance develops, the dose will need to be increased to maintain the same degree of pain relief.
4. ***Other drugs:*** for specific pain problems. These include diazepam for muscle spasm, carbamazepine or amitryptiline for neuralgic pain, and corticosteroids (such as dexamethasone) for pain due to an inflammatory swelling pressing on a nerve.

8.7.2 Management of anorexia, nausea and vomiting

Loss of appetite in a terminal illness is difficult to treat. Encourage carers to continue providing meals and to try:

— small feeds given more frequently, particularly in the morning when the child's appetite may be better
— cool foods rather than hot foods
— avoiding salty or spicy foods.

If there is very distressing nausea and vomiting, give oral metoclopramide (1–2 mg/kg) every 2–4 hours, as required.

8.7.3 Prevention and treatment of pressure sores

Teach the carers to turn the child at least once every 2 hours. If pressure sores develop, keep them clean and dry. Use local anaesthetics such as TAC to relieve pain.

8.7.4 Care of the mouth

Teach the carers to wash out the mouth after every meal. If mouth ulcers develop, clean the mouth at least 4 times a day, using clean water or salt solution and a clean cloth rolled into a wick. Apply 0.25% or 0.5% gentian violet to any sores. Give paracetamol if the child has a high fever, or is irritable or in pain. Crushed ice wrapped in gauze and given to the child to suck may give some relief. If the child is bottle-fed, advise the carer to use a spoon and cup instead. If a bottle continues to be used, advise the carer to clean the teat with water before each feed.

If oral thrush develops, apply miconazole gel to the affected areas at least 3 times daily for 5 days, *or* give 1 ml nystatin suspension 4 times daily for 7 days, pouring slowly into the corner of the mouth so that it reaches the affected parts.

If there is pus due to a secondary bacterial infection, apply tetracycline or chloramphenicol ointment. If there is a foul smell in the mouth, give IM benzylpenicillin (50 000 units/kg every 6 hours), plus oral metronidazole suspension (7.5 mg/kg every 8 hours) for 7 days.

8.7.5 Airway management

If the parents want the child to die at home, show them how to nurse an unconscious child and how to keep the airway clear

If respiratory distress develops as the child nears death, put the child in a comfortable sitting position and manage the airway, as required. Give priority to keeping the child comfortable rather than prolonging life.

8.7.6 Psychosocial support

Helping parents and siblings through their emotional reaction towards the dying child is one of the most important aspects of care in the terminal stage of HIV disease. How this is done depends on whether care is being given at home, in hospital or in a hospice. At home, much of the support can be given by close family members, relatives and friends.

Keep up to date on how to contact local community-based home care programmes and HIV/AIDS counselling groups. Find out if the carers are receiving support from these groups. If not, discuss the family's attitude towards these groups and the possibility of linking the family with them.

Notes

Notes

CHAPTER 9

Common surgical problems

Infants and children develop distinct surgical diseases and have special perioperative needs. This chapter provides guidelines for the supportive care of children with surgical problems and briefly describes the management of the most common surgical conditions.

9.1 Care before, during and after surgery

Good surgical care neither begins nor ends with the procedure. In most instances it is the preparation for surgery, the anaesthetic and the postoperative care that ensures a good outcome.

9.1.1 Preoperative care

Both the child and the parents need to be prepared for the procedure and need to consent.

- Explain why the procedure is needed, the anticipated outcome and the potential risks and benefits.
- Ensure that the child is medically fit for an operation.
  - — Correct fluid deficits prior to emergency procedures (intravenous normal saline bolus, 10–20 ml/kg—repeat as needed). Restoration of urine output implies adequate volume resuscitation.
  - — Correct anaemia. Severe anaemia interferes with oxygen transport. As a consequence the heart must pump more blood. Surgery may cause blood loss and the anaesthetic may affect oxygen transport in the blood. Ideally, the child's haemoglobin should be checked to see if it is normal for the age and population.
    - Reserve blood transfusions for situations where the anaemia must be corrected quickly, e.g. emergency surgery.
    - Correct anaemia in elective surgical children with oral medications (page 339).
    - Children with haemoglobinopathies (HbSS, HbAS, HbSC and thalass-aemias) who need surgery and anaesthesia require special care. Please refer to standard texts of paediatrics for details.
  - — Check that the child is in the best nutritional state possible. Good nutrition is needed to heal wounds.
- Check that the child has an empty stomach prior to a general anaesthetic.
  - — Infants under 12 months: the child should be given no solids orally for 8 hrs, no formula for 6 hrs, no clear liquids for 4 hours or no breast milk for 4 hrs before the operation.
  - — If prolonged periods of fasting are anticipated (>6 hrs) give intravenous fluids that contain glucose.
- Preoperative lab screening is generally not essential. However, carry out the following if this is possible:
  - — Infants less than 6 months: check haemoglobin or haematocrit
  - — Children 6 months–12 years:
    - minor surgery (e.g. hernia repair)—no investigations
    - major surgery—check haemoglobin or haematocrit.

— Other investigations may be indicated after full clinical examination of the child.

- Preoperative antibiotics should be given for:
  — Infected and contaminated cases (e.g. those requiring bowel or bladder surgery):
    - Bowel: give ampicillin (25–50 mg/kg IM or IV four times a day), gentamicin (7.5 mg/kg IM or IV once a day) and metronidazole (7.5 mg/kg three times a day) before and for 3–5 days after the operation.
    - Urinary tract: give ampicillin (25–50 mg/kg IM or IV four times a day), and gentamicin (7.5 mg/kg IM or IV once a day) before and for 3–5 days after the operation.

  — Children at risk for endocarditis (children with congenital heart disease or valvular heart disease) undergoing dental, oral, respiratory and oesophageal procedures.
    - Give amoxicillin 50 mg/kg orally before the operation or, if unable to take oral medications, ampicillin 50 mg/kg IV within 30 minutes before the surgery

9.1.2 Intraoperative care

Successful procedures require teamwork and careful planning. The operating room should function as a team. This includes surgeons, anaesthesia staff, nurses, scrub technicians and others. Ensure that essential supplies are readily available before the start of the operation.

Anaesthesia

Infants and children experience pain just like adults, but may express it differently.

- Make the procedure as painless as possible.

➤ For minor procedures in co-operative children—give a local anaesthetic such as lidocaine 4–5 mg/kg or bupivacaine 0.25% (dose not to exceed 1 mg/kg).

- For major procedures— give general anaesthesia
  — Ketamine is an excellent anaesthetic when muscle relaxation is not required.
    - Insert an intravenous cannula (it may be more convenient to delay this until after ketamine has been given IM).

➤ Give ketamine 5–8 mg/kg IM or 1–2 mg/kg IV; following IV ketamine, the child should be ready for surgery in 2–3 minutes, if given IM in 3–5 minutes.

➤ Give a further dose of ketamine (1–2 mg/kg IM or 0.5–1 mg/kg IV) if the child responds to a painful stimulus.

- At the end of the procedure turn the child into the lateral position and closely supervise the recovery in a quiet place.

Special considerations

- ***Airway***

— The smaller diameter airway in children makes them especially susceptible to airway obstruction so they often need intubation to protect their airway during surgical procedures.

— Small children also have difficulty in moving heavy columns of air making adult vaporiser units unacceptable.

— Endotracheal tube sizes for children are given in Table 28.

Table 28. Endotracheal tube size, by age

Age (years)	Tube size (mm)
Premature infant	2.5–3.0
Newborn	3.5
1	4.0
2	4.5
2–4	5.0
5	5.5
6	6
6–8	6.5
8	Cuffed 5.5
10	Cuffed 6.0

Alternatively, as a rough guide for normally nourished children more than 2 years old, use the following formula:

$$\text{Internal diameter of the tube (mm)} = \frac{\text{Age (years)}}{4} + 4$$

Another rough indicator of the correct tube size is the diameter of the child's little finger. Always have tubes one size bigger and smaller available. With a non-cuffed tube there should be a small air leak. Listen to the lungs with a stethoscope following intubation to ensure the breath sounds are equal on both sides.

- ***Hypothermia***

Children lose heat more rapidly than adults because they have a greater relative surface area and are poorly insulated. This is important as hypothermia can affect drug metabolism, anaesthesia, and blood coagulation.

— Prevent hypothermia in the operating room by turning off the air conditioner, warming the room (aim for a temperature of >28 °C when operating on an infant or small child) and covering exposed parts of child.

— Use warmed fluids (but not too hot),

— Avoid long procedures (>1 hour) unless the child can be kept warm.

— Monitor the child's temperature as frequently as possible and at the completion of the operation.

- ***Hypoglycaemia***

Infants and children are at risk for developing hypoglycaemia because of a limited ability to utilize fat and protein to synthesize glucose.

— Use glucose infusions during anaesthesia to help maintain blood sugar level. For most paediatric operations, other than minor ones, give Ringer's lactate plus glucose 5% (or glucose 4% with saline 0.18%) at a rate of 5 ml/kg of body weight per hour in addition to replacing the measured fluid losses.

- ***Blood loss***

Children have smaller blood volumes than adults. Even small amounts of blood loss can be life threatening.

— Measure blood loss during operations as accurately as possible.

— Consider blood transfusion if blood loss exceeds 10% of blood volume (see Table 29).

— Have blood readily available in the operating room if blood loss is anticipated.

Table 29. Blood volume of children by age

	ml/kg body weight
Neonate	85–90
Children	80
Adults	70

9.1.3 Postoperative care

Communicate to the family the outcome of the operation, problems encountered during the procedure, and the expected postoperative course.

Immediately following surgery

- Ensure that the child recovers safely from the anaesthetic.
  - — Monitor the vital signs—respiratory rate, pulse (see Table 30) and, if necessary, blood pressure every 15–30 minutes until stable.
- Avoid settings where high-risk children cannot be adequately monitored.
- Investigate and treat abnormal vital signs.

Table 30. Normal pulse rate and blood pressure in children

Age	Pulse rate (normal range)	Systolic blood pressure (normal)
0–1 year	100–160	Above 60
1–3 years	90–150	Above 70
3–6 years	80–140	Above 75

Note: normal pulse rates are 10% slower in sleeping children.

Note: In infants and children a presence or absence of a strong central pulse is often a more useful guide to the presence or absence of shock than a blood pressure reading.

Fluid management

- Postoperatively, children commonly require more than maintenance fluid. Children with abdominal operations typically require 150% of baseline requirements (see page 273) and even larger amounts if peritonitis is present. Preferred IV fluids are Ringer's lactate with 5% glucose or normal saline with 5% glucose or half-normal saline with 5% glucose. Note that normal saline and Ringer's lactate do not contain glucose and risk hypoglycaemia, and large amounts of 5% glucose contain no sodium and risk hyponatraemia (see Appendix 4, page 357).

- Monitor fluid status closely.
  - Record inputs and outputs (intravenous fluids, nasogastric drainage, urine drain outputs) every 4–6 hours.
  - Urine output is the most sensitive indicator of fluid status in a child.
    - Normal urine output: Infants 1–2 ml/kg/hour, children 1 ml/kg/hour.
    - If urinary retention is suspected, pass a urinary catheter. This also allows for hourly measurements of urine output to be made, which can be invaluable in severely ill children. Suspect urinary retention if bladder is palpable or the child is unable to void urine.

Pain control

Have a plan for postoperative pain management.

- Mild pain
  - ➤ Give paracetamol (10–15 mg/kg every 4–6 hours) administered by mouth or rectally. Oral paracetamol can be given several hours prior to operation or rectally at the completion of surgery.
- Severe pain
  - ➤ Give intravenous narcotic analgesics (IM injections are painful)
    - Morphine sulfate 0.05–0.1 mg/kg IV every 2–4 hours

Nutrition

- Many surgical conditions increase caloric needs or prevent adequate nutritional intake. Many children with surgical problems present in a debilitated state. Poor nutrition adversely affects their response to injury and delays wound healing.
  - Feed children as soon as possible after surgery.
  - Provide a high calorie diet containing adequate protein and vitamin supplements.
  - Consider feeding by nasogastric tube for children whose oral intake is poor.
  - Monitor the child's weight.

Common postoperative problems

- Tachycardia (raised pulse rate—see Table 30)

  May be caused by pain, hypovolaemia, anaemia, fever, hypoglycaemia, and infection.

  - Examine the child!
  - Review the child's preoperative and intraoperative care.
  - Monitor the response to pain medication, boluses of IV fluids, oxygen, and IV transfusions, where appropriate.
  - Bradycardia in a child should be considered as a sign of hypoxia until proven otherwise.

- Fever
  May be due to tissue injury, wound infections, atelectasis, urinary tract infections (from indwelling catheters), phlebitis (from an intravenous catheter site), or other concomitant infections (e.g. malaria).
  - See Sections 3.4 (page 46) and 9.3.2 which contain information on the diagnosis and treatment of wound infections (see page 243).
- Low urine output
  May be due to hypovolaemia, urinary retention or renal failure. Low urine output is almost always due to inadequate fluid resuscitation.
  - Examine the child!
  - Review the child's fluid record.
  - If hypovolaemia is suspected—give normal saline (10–20 ml/kg) and repeat as needed
  - If urinary retention is suspected (the child is uncomfortable and has a full bladder on physical examination)—pass a urinary catheter.

9.2 Newborn and neonatal problems

There are many types of congenital anomalies. Only a few of them are common. Some require urgent surgical attention. Others should be left alone until the child is older. Early recognition makes for better outcomes and allows the parents to be informed about treatment options.

9.2.1 Cleft lip and palate

These may occur together or separately (see figure). Reassure the parents that the problem can be dealt with, as there may be concern about the unattractive appearance.

Treatment

Babies with isolated cleft lip can feed normally.

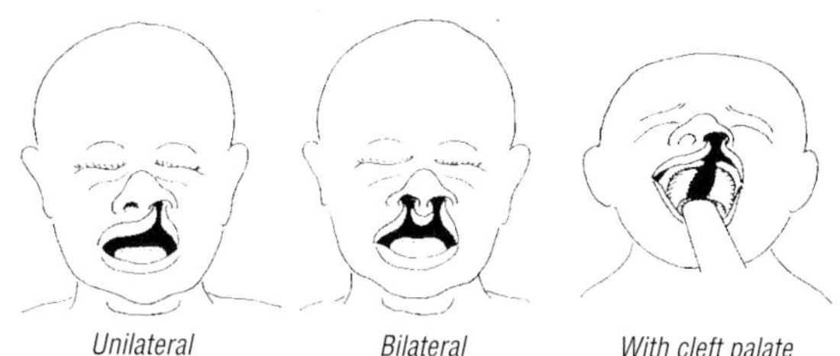

Cleft lip and palate

Cleft palate is associated with feeding difficulties. The baby is able to swallow normally but unable to suck adequately and milk regurgitates through the nose and may be aspirated into the lungs.

➤ Feed using expressed breast milk via a cup and spoon, or if available AND adequate sterility of bottles can be ensured, a special teat may be used. The technique of feeding is to deliver a bolus of milk over the back of the tongue into the pharynx by means of a spoon, pipette, or some other pouring device. The baby will then swallow normally.

- Close follow-up in infancy is required to monitor feeding and growth.
- Surgical closure of the lip at 6 months of age, of the palate at one year of age. The lip may be repaired earlier if it is safe to give an anaesthetic and the repair is technically possible.
- Follow-up after surgery to monitor hearing (middle-ear infections are common) and speech development.

9.2.2 Bowel obstruction in the newborn

May be due to hypertrophic pyloric stenosis, bowel atresia, malrotation with volvulus, meconium plug syndrome, Hirschsprung's disease (colonic aganglionosis), or imperforate anus.

Diagnosis

■ The level of obstruction determines the clinical presentation. Proximal obstruction—vomiting with minimal distension. Distal obstruction—distension with vomiting occurring late.

- Bile-stained (green) vomiting in an infant is due to a bowel obstruction until proven otherwise and is a surgical emergency.
- Pyloric stenosis presents as projectile (forceful) non-bilious vomiting, typically between 3 and 6 weeks of age.
  - Dehydration and electrolyte abnormalities are common.
  - An olive like mass (the enlarged pylorus) may be palpated in the upper abdomen.
- Consider other causes of abdominal distension (such as ileus related to sepsis, necrotizing enterocolitis and congenital syphilis, ascites)

Treatment

- ➤ Prompt resuscitation and URGENT REVIEW by a surgeon experienced in paediatric surgery.
- ➤ Give nothing orally. Pass a nasogastric tube if there is vomiting or abdominal distension.
- ➤ Intravenous fluid: use half-strength Darrow's solution or normal saline + glucose (dextrose):
  - Give 10–20 ml/kg to correct dehydration.
  - Then give maintenance fluid volume (page 273) plus the same volume that comes out of the nasogastric tube
- ➤ Give benzyl penicillin (IM 50,000 units/kg four times a day) or ampicillin (25–50 mg/kg IM or IV four times a day); plus gentamicin (7.5 mg/kg once per day)

9.2.3 Abdominal wall defects

The abdominal wall does not fully develop and remains open.

Diagnosis

- There may be exposed bowel (gastroschisis) or a thin layer covering the bowel (omphalocele) (see figure).

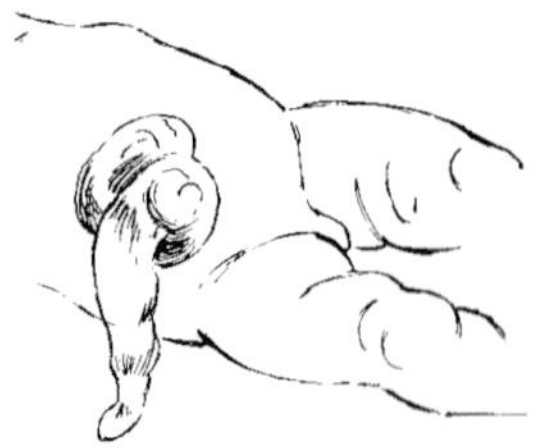

Newborn with an omphalocele

Treatment

- Apply a sterile dressing and cover with a plastic bag (to prevent fluid loss). Exposed bowel can lead to rapid fluid loss and hypothermia.
- Give nothing orally. Pass a nasogastric tube for free drainage.
- Give intravenous fluids: use normal saline + glucose (dextrose) or half-strength Darrow's solution:
  - Give 10–20 ml/kg to correct dehydration.
  - Then give maintenance fluid requirements (page 273) plus the same volume that comes out of the nasogastric tube.
- Benzyl penicillin (IM 50,000 units/kg four times a day) or ampicillin (25–50 mg/kg IM or IV four times a day); plus gentamicin (7.5 mg/kg once per day)

URGENT REVIEW by a surgeon experienced in paediatric surgery.

9.2.4 Myelomeningocele

Diagnosis

- Small sac that protrudes through a bony defect in the skull or vertebrae. The most common site is the lumbar region.
- Maybe associated with neurological problems (bowel, bladder and motor deficits in the lower extremities) and hydrocephalus.

Treatment

- Apply a sterile dressing.
- If ruptured, give benzyl penicillin (IM 50,000 units/kg four times a day) or ampicillin (25–50 mg/kg IM or IV four times a day); plus gentamicin (7.5 mg/kg once per day) for five days.

REVIEW by a surgeon experienced in paediatric surgery.

9.2.5 Congenital dislocation of the hip

Diagnosis

- Severe cases should be detected by routine physical examination at birth.
- When unilateral, the limb is short, there is limited abduction when the hip is flexed, and the skin crease at the back of the hip appears asymmetrical. When the flexed hip is abducted, a click can often be felt as the dislocated femoral head enters the acetabulum (Ortolani's sign).
- In the older infant confirm the diagnosis with X-ray. X-rays in neonates are difficult to interpret as the epiphysis of the femur and the femoral head do

not appear until 3–4 months of age (see figure). Positioning the lower limb in 45° abduction demonstrates a break in the continuity of a line drawn along the upper margin of the obturator foramen and lower aspect of the femoral neck. A) Normal Shenton's line, B) The line is broken in dislocation of the hip.

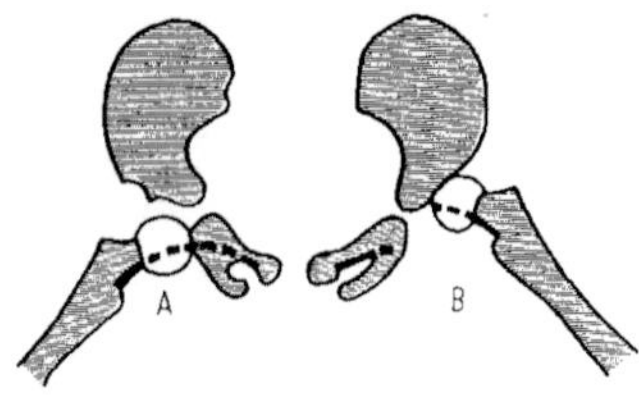

Radiological diagnosis of congenital dislocation of the hip

Treatment

- In milder cases, keep the hip in flexion and abduction through double nappies or an abduction brace in an abducted position for 2–3 months. The traditional way in many cultures of carrying the child on the back with the hip flexed and abducted will serve the same purpose.
- In more severe cases, keep the hip abducted and flexed in a splint.

REVIEW by a surgeon experienced in paediatric surgery.

9.2.6 Talipes equinovarus (club foot)

Diagnosis

- The foot cannot be placed into the normal position.
- The commonest form includes three deformities—plantar flexion of the foot, inversion (inturning of the heel) and inturning of the forefoot.

Treatment

- Mild positional deformity (the foot can be passively corrected): simple stretching of foot beginning shortly after birth.
- Moderate deformity: serial manipulations beginning shortly after birth.
  - Maintain position with either tape strapping or well-padded plaster of Paris casts. Apply this in the sequence 1 then 2 then 3 as in figure on page 239.

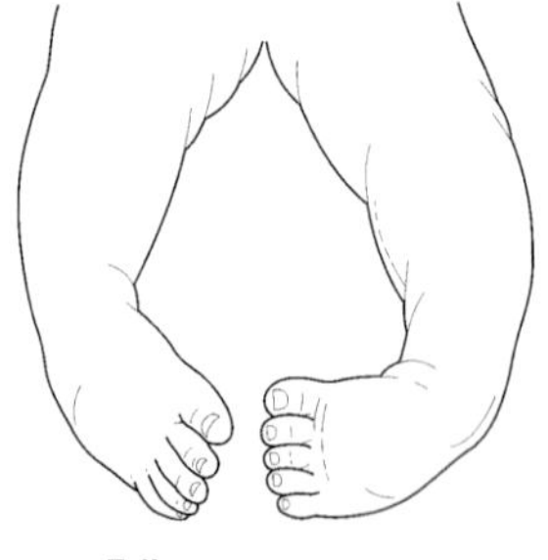

Talipes

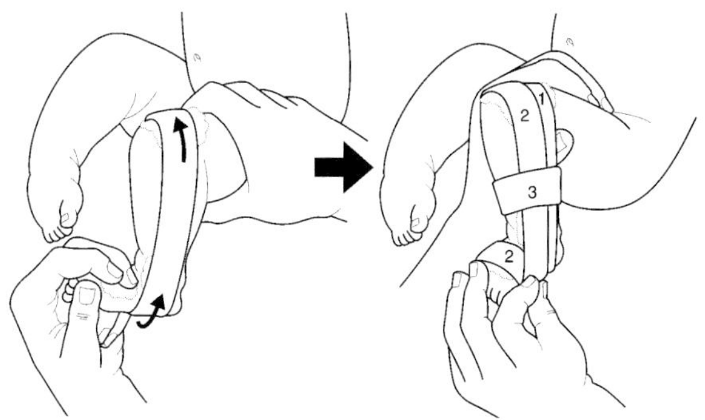

Treating talipes with tape strapping

— These manipulations need to be repeated every two weeks or until the deformity is corrected.

— Special splints may need to be worn until the child begins to walk.

➤ Severe deformity or those that present late: surgical repair.

9.3 Injuries

Injuries are the most common surgical problems affecting children. Proper treatment can prevent death and lifelong disability. Whenever possible, try to prevent childhood injuries from occurring.

- See Chapter 1 for guidelines for assessing children with severe injuries. More detailed surgical guidance is given in the WHO manual *Surgical care in the district hospital*.

9.3.1 Burns

Burns and scalds are associated with a high risk of mortality in children. Those who survive may suffer from disfigurement and psychological trauma as a result of a painful and prolonged stay in the hospital.

Assessment

Burns may be partial or full thickness. A full thickness burn means the entire thickness of the skin is destroyed, and the skin will not regenerate.

- Ask two questions:
  - — How deep is the burn?
  - — Full thickness burns are black or white, usually dry, have no feeling and do not blanch on pressure.
  - — Partial thickness burns are pink or red, blistering or weeping, and painful.
  - — How much of the body is burnt?
  - — Use a body surface area chart according to age (page 241).
  - — Alternatively, use the child's palm to estimate the burn area. A child's palm is approximately 1% of the total body surface area.

Treatment

➤ Admit all children with burns >10% of their body surface; those involving the face, hands, feet, perineum, across joints; burns that are circumferential and those that cannot be managed as outpatients.

➤ Consider whether the child has a respiratory injury due to smoke inhalation.

- — If there is evidence of respiratory distress, then provide supplemental oxygen (see page 281)
- — Severe facial burns and inhalational injuries may require early intubation or tracheostomy to prevent or treat airway obstruction.

➤ Fluid resuscitation (required for >20% total body surface burn). Use Ringer's lactate with 5% glucose, normal saline with 5% glucose or half-normal saline with 5% glucose.

- — 1st 24 hours: Calculate fluid requirements by adding maintenance fluid requirements (see page 273) and additional resuscitation fluid requirements (volume equal to 4 ml/kg for every 1% of surface burned)

  ➤ Administer 1/2 of total fluid in first 8 hours, and remaining in next 16 hours.

  Example: 20 kg child with a 25% burn.

  Total fluid in 1st 24 hrs = (60 ml/hr x 24 hours) + 4 ml x 20kg x 25% burn
  = 1440 ml + 2000 ml
  = 3440 ml (1720 ml over 1st 8 hours)

- — 2nd 24 hours: give 1/2 to 3/4 of fluid required during the first day.
- — Monitor the child closely during resuscitation (pulse, respiratory rate, blood pressure and urine output).

Chart for estimating the percentage of body surface burned

Estimate the total area burned by adding the percentage of body surface area affected as shown in the figure (refer to the table for areas A–F which change according to the age of the child).

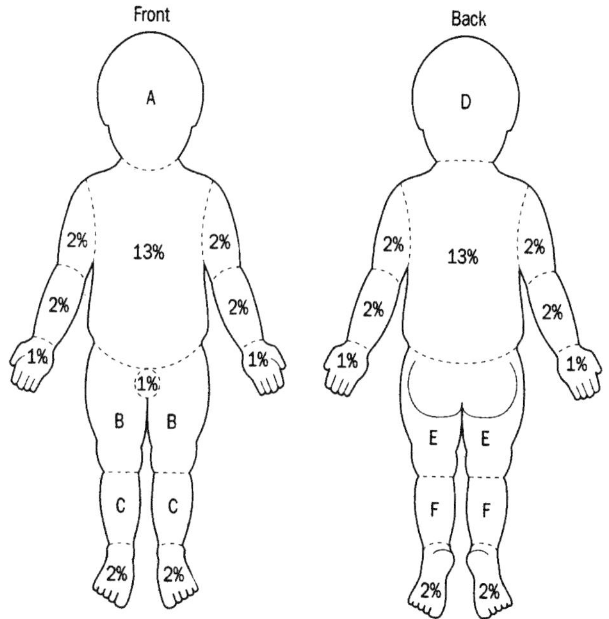

Area	By age in years			
	0	1	5	10
Head (A/D)	10%	9%	7%	6%
Thigh (B/E)	3%	3%	4%	5%
Leg (C/F)	2%	3%	3%	3%

— Blood may be given to correct anaemia or for deep burns to replace blood loss.

➤ Prevent infection

— If skin is intact, clean with antiseptic solution gently without breaking the skin.

— If skin is not intact, carefully debride the burn. Blisters should be pricked and dead skin removed.

— Give topical antibiotics/antiseptics (there are several options depending on resources available and these include: silver nitrate, silver sulfadiazine, gentian violet, betadine and even mashed papaya). Clean and dress the wound daily.

— Small burns or those in areas that are difficult to cover can be managed by leaving them open to the air and keeping them clean and dry.

➤ Treat secondary infection if present.

— If there is evidence of local infection (pus, foul odour or presence of cellulitis), treat with oral amoxicillin (15 mg/kg orally three times a day), and cloxacillin (25 mg/kg orally four times a day). If septicaemia is suspected, use gentamicin (7.5 mg/kg IM or IV once a day) plus cloxacillin (25–50 mg/kg IM or IV four times a day). If infection is suspected beneath an eschar, remove the eschar.

➤ Pain control

Make sure that pain control is adequate including before procedures such as changing dressings.

— Give paracetamol (10–15 mg/kg every 6 hours) by mouth or give intravenous narcotic analgesics (IM injections are painful), such as morphine sulfate (0.05–0.1 mg/kg IV every 2–4 hours) if pain is severe.

➤ Check tetanus vaccination status.

— If not immunized give tetanus immune globulin.

— If immunized, give tetanus toxoid booster if this is due.

➤ Nutrition.

— Begin feeding as soon as practical in the first 24 hours.

— Children should receive a high calorie diet containing adequate protein, and vitamin and iron supplements.

— Children with extensive burns require about 1.5 times the normal calorie and 2–3 times the normal protein requirements.

- Burn contractures. Burn scars across flexor surfaces contract. This happens even with the best treatment (nearly always happens with poor treatment).
  - Prevent contractures by passive mobilization of the involved areas and by splinting flexor surfaces. Splints can be made of plaster of Paris. Splints should be worn at night.
- Physiotherapy and rehabilitation.
  - Should begin early and continue throughout the course of the burn care.
  - If the child is admitted for a prolonged period, ensure the child has access to toys and is encouraged to play.

9.3.2 Principles of wound care

The goal of caring for any wound is to stop bleeding, prevent infection, assess damage to underlying structures and promote wound healing.

➤ Stop bleeding

- Direct pressure will control any bleeding (see figure on page 244).
- Bleeding from extremities can be controlled for short periods of time (<10 minutes) using a sphygmomanometer cuff inflated above the arterial pressure.
- Prolonged use of tourniquets can damage the extremity. Never use a tourniquet in a child with sickle-cell anaemia.

➤ Prevent infection

- Cleaning the wound is the most important factor in preventing a wound infection. Most wounds are contaminated when first seen. They may contain blood clots, dirt, dead or dying tissue and perhaps foreign bodies.
- Clean the skin around the wound thoroughly with soap and water or antiseptic. Water and antiseptic should be poured into the wound.
- After giving a local anaesthetic such as bupivacaine 0.25% (not to exceed 1ml/kg), search carefully for foreign bodies and carefully excise any dead tissue. Determine what damage may have been done. Major wounds require a general anaesthetic.
- Antibiotics are usually not necessary when wounds are carefully cleaned. However, there are some wounds that should be treated with antibiotics (see below).
  - Wounds older than 12 hours (these are likely to be already infected).
  - Wounds penetrating deep into tissue (e.g. a dirty stick or knife wound).

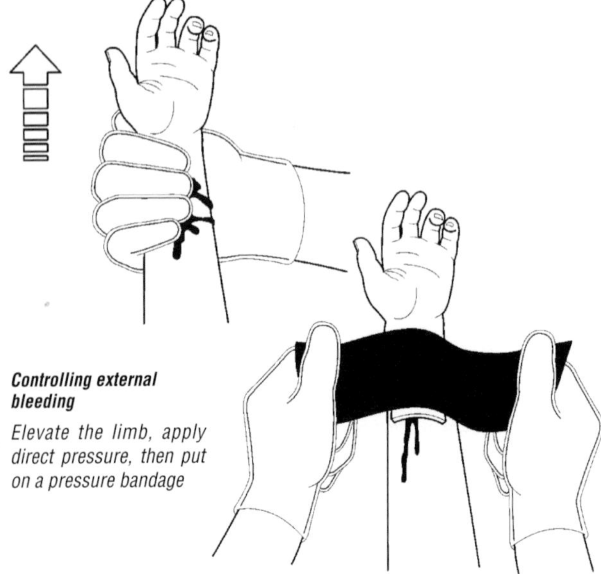

Controlling external bleeding

Elevate the limb, apply direct pressure, then put on a pressure bandage

- Tetanus prophylaxis
  - If not vaccinated, give anti-tetanus serum, if available, and start a course of tetanus toxoid vaccine.
  - If the child has had active immunization, give a booster if vaccination status is not current.
- Wound closure
  - If the wound is less than a day old and has been cleaned satisfactorily, the wound can be closed (called primary closure).
  - The wound should not be closed if it is more than 24 hours old, there has been a lot of dirt and foreign material in the wound, or if the wound has been caused by an animal bite.
  - Wounds not treated with primary closure should be packed lightly with damp gauze. If the wound is clean 48 hours later, the wound can then be closed (delayed primary closure).

— If the wound is infected, pack the wound lightly and let it heal on its own.

➤ Wound infections.

— Clinical signs: pain, swelling, redness, warmth and pus drainage from the wound.

— Treatment.

- Open wound if pus suspected
- Clean the wound with disinfectant.
- Pack the wound lightly with damp gauze. Change the dressing everyday, more frequently if needed.
- Antibiotics until surrounding cellulitis has resolved (usually 5 days).
  - ➤ Give cloxacillin (25–50 mg/kg orally four times a day) for most wounds to deal with *Staphylococcus*.
  - ➤ Give ampicillin (25–50 mg/kg orally four times a day), gentamicin (7.5 mg/kg IM or IV once a day) and metronidazole (7.5 mg/kg three times a day) if bowel flora is suspected.

9.3.3 Fractures

Children have a remarkable ability to heal fractures if the bones are aligned properly.

Diagnosis

- Pain, swelling, deformity, crepitus, unnatural movement, and loss of function.
- Fractures can be closed (where the skin is intact) or open (where there is a wound of the skin). Open fractures may lead to serious bone infection. Suspect an open fracture if there is an associated wound. A child's bones are different from adults; instead of breaking they often bend like a stick

Treatment

- Ask two questions:
  - — Is there a fracture?
  - — Which bone is broken (either by clinical exam or X-ray)?
- Consider referral for REVIEW by a surgeon experienced in paediatric surgery for complicated fractures such as those that are displaced or involve growth plates or are open.

- Open fractures require antibiotics: cloxacillin (25–50 mg/kg orally four times a day), and gentamicin (7.5 mg/kg IM or IV once a day) and meticulous cleaning to prevent osteomyelitis (see Section 9.3.2, page 243, for principles of wound care).
- Figures shown below describe simple methods for treating some of the most common childhood fractures. For further details of how to manage these fractures, consult the WHO manual *Surgical care at the district hospital* or a standard textbook of (surgical) paediatrics.

A posterior splint can be used for upper and lower extremity injuries. The extremity is first wrapped with soft padding (e.g. cotton), then a plaster of Paris splint is placed to maintain the extremity in a neutral position. The posterior splint is held in place with an elastic bandage. Monitor the fingers (capillary refill and temperature) to ensure the splint has not been placed too tightly.

The treatment of a supracondylar fracture is shown on the next page. An important complication of this fracture is constriction of the artery at the elbow—where it can become entrapped. Assess the blood flow to the hand. If the artery is obstructed the hand will be cool, capillary refill will be slow and the radial pulse will be absent. If the artery is obstructed, reduction needs to be done urgently.

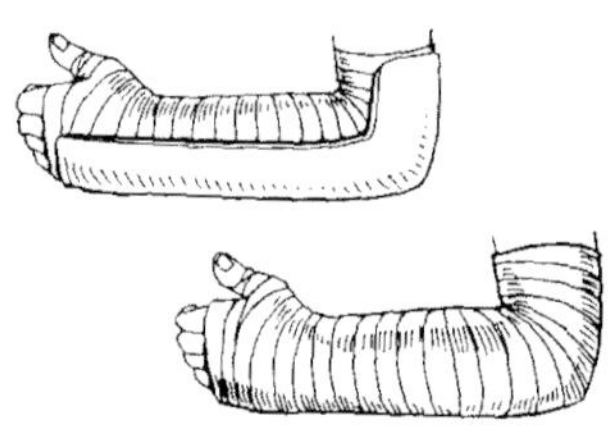

Posterior splint

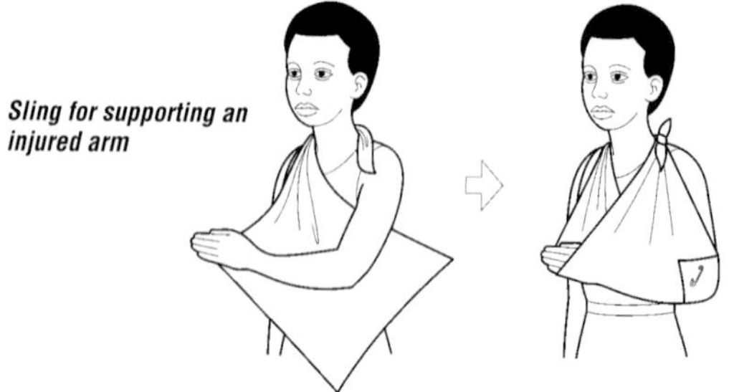

Sling for supporting an injured arm

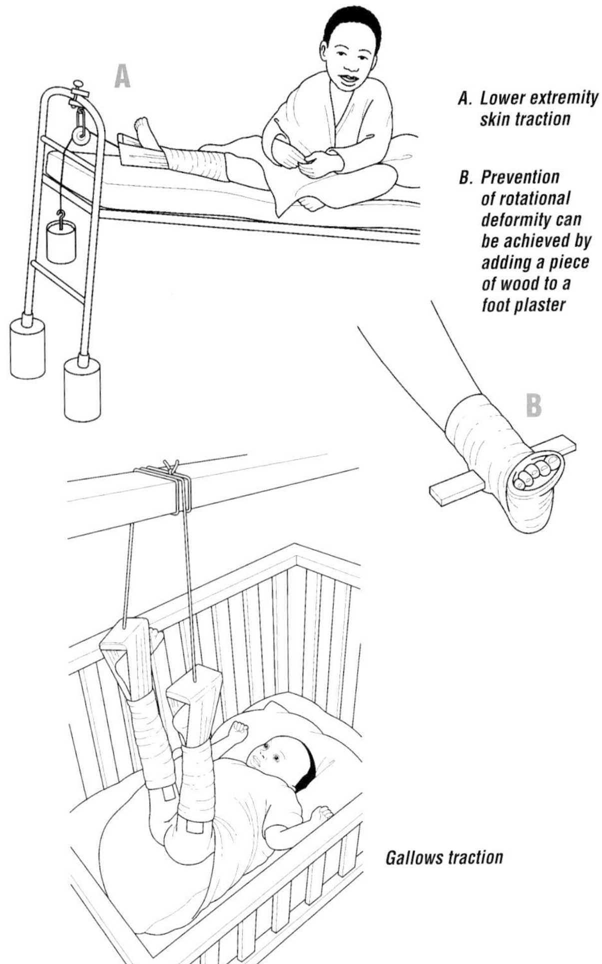

A. Lower extremity skin traction

B. Prevention of rotational deformity can be achieved by adding a piece of wood to a foot plaster

Gallows traction

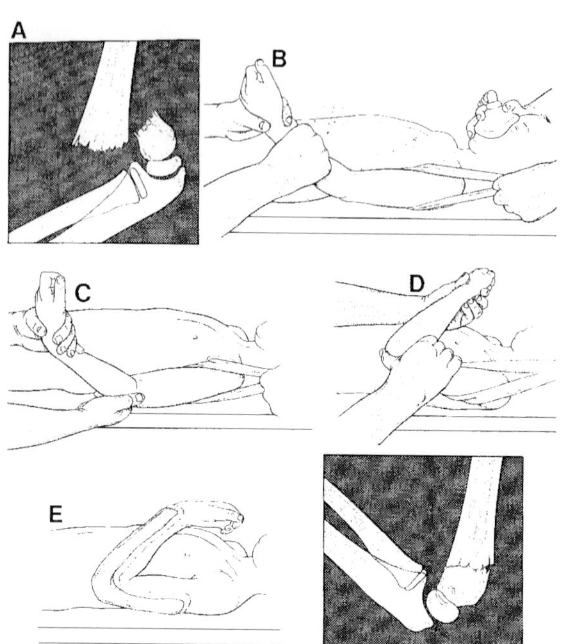

Treatment of a supracondylar fracture

A: X-ray of displaced supracondylar fracture;

B: pull as shown to reduce the fracture displacement;

C: carefully bend the elbow maintaining traction;

D: hold the elbow flexed and keep the fracture in position as shown;

E: apply a back slab;

F: check the position of the fracture on X-ray.

The treatment of a mid-shaft femoral fracture in a child under 3 years of age is by gallows splint and is shown in the figure on page 247. It is important that every few hours the attendant should check that the circulation of the feet is good and the toes are warm.

The treatment of a mid-shaft femoral fracture in an older child is by skin traction and is shown in the figure (page 247). This is a simple and effective method for treating femur fractures in children aged 3–15 years. If the child can raise his leg off the bed the fracture has united and the child is ready for ambulation on crutches (usually about 3 weeks).

9.3.4 Head injuries

There may be a skull fracture (closed, open, or depressed) and/or a brain injury. Brain injuries fall into three categories (3 C's).

- Concussion: the mildest injury where loss of brain function is temporary.
- Contusion: the brain is bruised—function may be affected for hours to days, or even weeks.
- Compression: may result from swelling or a growing blood clot (epidural or subdural haematoma). If compression is due to a blood clot, urgent operation may be required.

Diagnosis

- History of head trauma.
- Diminished level of consciousness, confusion, seizure and signs of increased intracranial pressure (unequal pupils, rigid posture, focal paralysis and irregular breathing).

Treatment

- ➤ Give nothing orally
- ➤ Protect the child's airway (see Chapter 1).
- ➤ Limit fluid intake (to $^2/_3$ of maintenance fluid requirements, see above for recommended fluids, and page 273 for fluid volumes).
- ➤ Elevate the head of the bed to 30 degrees.
- ➤ Diagnose and treat other injuries.

URGENT REVIEW by a surgeon experienced in paediatric surgery.

9.3.5 Chest and abdominal injuries

These can be life threatening and may result from blunt or penetrating injuries.

Types of injuries

- Chest injuries include rib fractures, pulmonary contusions, pneumothorax and haemothorax. Because the ribcage of children is more pliable than that of adults, there may be extensive chest injuries without rib fractures.
- Blunt and penetrating trauma to the abdomen may injure a variety of organs. Splenic injuries from blunt trauma are especially common.
  — Assume that a penetrating wound to the abdominal wall has entered the abdominal cavity and that there may be injuries to the intra-abdominal organs.
  — Be especially cautious with injuries around the anus—as penetrating rectal injuries can be easily missed.

Treatment

- Suspected chest or abdominal injuries require URGENT REVIEW by a surgeon experienced in paediatric surgery.
- See guidelines given in Chapter 1.

9.4 Abdominal problems

9.4.1 Abdominal pain

Children commonly complain of abdominal pain. Not all abdominal pain is caused by gastrointestinal infections. Abdominal pain lasting longer than four hours should be regarded as a potential abdominal emergency.

Assessment

■ Ask three questions:

  — Are there associated symptoms? The presence of nausea, vomiting, diarrhoea, constipation, fever, cough, headache, sore throat or dysuria (pain on passing urine) helps determine the severity of the problem and can help narrow the diagnosis.
  — Where does it hurt? Ask the child to point to where it hurts most. This can also help narrow the diagnosis. Periumbilical pain is a nonspecific finding.

— Does the child have peritonitis—inflammation of the lining of the peritoneal cavity? This is a critical question, as most causes of peritonitis in children require operation.

- Signs of peritonitis include tenderness during palpation, pain in the abdomen when the child jumps or has his pelvis shaken and involuntary guarding (spasm of the abdominal musculature following palpation). A rigid abdomen that does not move with respiration is another sign of peritonitis.

Treatment

- ➤ Give the child nothing orally.
- ➤ If vomiting or abdominal distension, place a nasogastric tube.
- ➤ Give intravenous fluids (most children presenting with abdominal pain are dehydrated) to correct fluid deficits (normal saline 10–20 ml/kg repeated as needed) followed by 150% maintenance fluid requirements (see page 273).
- ➤ Give analgesics if the pain is severe (this will not mask a serious intra-abdominal problem, and may even facilitate a better examination).
- ➤ Repeat the examinations if the diagnosis is in question.
- ➤ Give antibiotics if there are signs of peritonitis. To deal with enteric flora (Gram-negative rods, *Enterococcus*, and anaerobes): give ampicillin (25–50 mg/kg IM or IV four times a day), gentamicin (7.5 mg/kg IM or IV once a day) and metronidazole (7.5 mg/kg three times a day).

URGENT REVIEW by a surgeon experienced in paediatric surgery.

9.4.2 Appendicitis

This is caused by obstruction of the lumen of the appendix. Fecoliths, lymphoid hyperplasia and gastrointestinal parasites can cause obstruction. If not recognized the appendix ruptures leading to peritonitis and abscess formation.

Diagnosis

- Fever, anorexia, vomiting (variable)
- May begin as periumbilical pain, but the most important clinical finding is persistent pain and tenderness in the right lower quadrant.
- May be confused with urinary tract infections, kidney stones, ovarian problems, mesenteric adenitis, ileitis.

Treatment

- Give the child nothing orally.
- Give intravenous fluids.
  - Correct fluid deficits by giving normal saline as a 10–20 ml/kg fluid bolus, repeated as needed, followed by 150% maintenance fluid requirements.
- Give antibiotics once diagnosis established: give ampicillin (25–50 mg/kg IM or IV four times a day), gentamicin (7.5 mg/kg IM or IV once a day) and metronidazole (7.5 mg/kg three times a day).

URGENT REVIEW by a surgeon experienced in paediatric surgery. Appendectomy should be done as soon as possible to prevent perforation, peritonitis and abscess formation.

9.4.3 Bowel obstruction beyond the newborn period

This may be caused by incarcerated hernias, adhesions (scarring from previous surgery), *Ascaris* infection, and intussusception (see next section).

Diagnosis

- Clinical presentation is determined by the level of obstruction. Proximal obstruction—presents with vomiting with minimal distension. Distal obstruction—presents with distension with vomiting occurring later.
- Typically there is cramping abdominal pain, distension and no flatus.
- Sometimes peristalsis waves can be seen through abdominal wall.
- Abdominal X-rays show distended loops of bowel with air fluid levels.

Treatment

- Give the child nothing orally
- Give fluid resuscitation. Most children presenting with a bowel obstruction have been vomiting and are dehydrated.
- Correct fluid deficits with a bolus of normal saline 10–20 ml/kg, repeated as needed, followed by 150% maintenance fluid requirements
- Pass a nasogastric tube—this relieves nausea and vomiting, and prevents bowel perforation by keeping the bowel decompressed.

URGENT REVIEW by a surgeon experienced in paediatric surgery.

9.4.4 Intussusception

A form of bowel obstruction in which one segment of the intestine telescopes into the next. This most commonly occurs at the ileal-caecal junction.

Diagnosis

- Usually occurs in children <2 years of age, but can occur in older children.
- Clinical presentation:
  - — Early: colicky abdominal pain with vomiting. The child cries with pain, doubles over, and pulls the legs up.
  - — Late: pallor, abdominal distension, tenderness, bloody diarrhoea ("red currant jelly stool") and dehydration.
- Palpable abdominal mass (begins in right lower quadrant and may extend along line of colon.

Treatment

- ➤ Give an air or barium enema (this can both diagnose and reduce the intussusception). An unlubricated 35 ml Foley catheter is passed into the rectum; the bag is inflated and the buttocks strapped together. A warm solution of barium in normal saline is allowed to flow in under gravity from a height of 1 meter and its entrance into the colon is observed using an abdominal X-ray. The diagnosis is confirmed when the barium outlines a concave 'meniscus'. The pressure of the column of barium slowly reduces the intussusception, the reduction is only complete when several loops of small bowel are seen to fill with barium.
- ➤ Pass a nasogastric tube.
- ➤ Give fluid resuscitation.
- ➤ Give antibiotics if there are signs of infection (fever, peritonitis)—give ampicillin (25–50 mg/kg IM or IV four times a day), gentamicin (7.5 mg/kg IM or IV once a day) and metronidazole (7.5 mg/kg three times a day). The duration of the post-operative antibiotics depends on the severity of the disease: in an uncomplicated intussusception reduced with an air enema, give for 24–48 hours postoperatively; in a child with a perforated bowel with resection, continue antibiotics for one week.

Arrange URGENT REVIEW by a surgeon experienced in paediatric surgery. Proceed to an operation if air or barium enema is unable to reduce the intussusception. If the bowel is ischaemic or dead, then a bowel resection will be required.

9.4.5 Umbilical hernia

Diagnosis

- Soft reducible swelling at umbilicus.

Treatment

- Most close spontaneously.
- ➤ Repair if not closed by age 6 years, or if there is a history of the hernia being difficult to reduce.

Protuberant umbilicus

Umbilical hernia

9.4.6 Inguinal hernia

Diagnosis

- Intermittent reducible swelling in the groin that is observed when the child is crying or straining.
- Occurs where the spermatic cord exits the abdomen (inguinal canal).
- Distinguish from a hydrocele (fluid that collects around testicle due to a patent processus vaginalis). Hydroceles transilluminate and usually do not extend up into the inguinal canal.
- Can also occur rarely in girls.

Treatment

- Uncomplicated inguinal hernia: elective surgical repair to prevent incarceration.
- Hydrocele: repair if not resolved by age 1 year. Unrepaired hydroceles will turn into inguinal hernias.

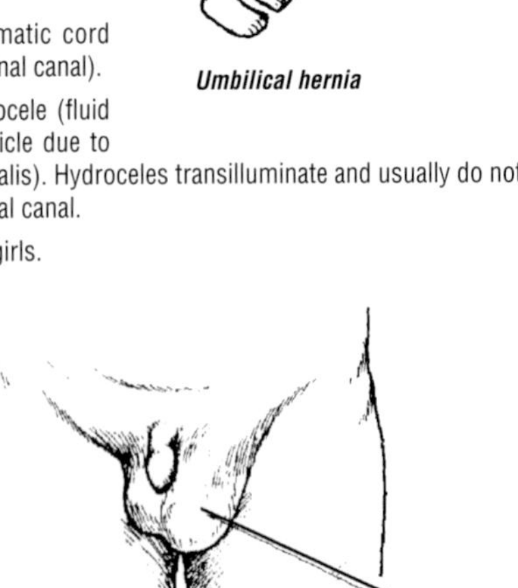

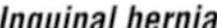

Inguinal hernia

9.4.7 Incarcerated hernias

These occur when the bowel or other intra-abdominal structure (e.g., omentum) is trapped in the hernia.

Diagnosis

- Non-reducible tender swelling at the site of an inguinal or umbilical hernia.
- There may be signs of intestinal obstruction (vomiting and abdominal distension) if the bowel is trapped in the hernia.

Treatment

- ➤ Attempt to reduce by steady constant pressure. If the hernia does not reduce easily, an operation will be required.
- ➤ Give the child nothing orally.
- ➤ Give intravenous fluids.
- ➤ Pass a nasogastric tube if there is vomiting or abdominal distension.
- ➤ Give antibiotics if compromised bowel is suspected: give ampicillin (25–50 mg/kg IM or IV four times a day), gentamicin (7.5 mg/kg IM or IV once a day) and metronidazole (7.5 mg/kg three times a day).

URGENT REVIEW by a surgeon experienced in paediatric surgery.

9.4.8 Rectal prolapse

This is caused by straining during a bowel motion and is associated with chronic diarrhoea and poor nutrition. Causative factors include gastrointestinal parasites (such as *Trichuris*) and cystic fibrosis.

Diagnosis

- The prolapse occurs on defecation. Initially the prolapsed section reduces spontaneously, but later may require manual reduction.
- May be complicated by bleeding or even strangulation with gangrene.

Treatment

- ➤ Providing the prolapsed rectum is not dead (it is pink or red and bleeds), reduce with gentle constant pressure.
- ➤ Firm strapping across buttocks to maintain the reduction.
- ➤ Correct underlying cause of diarrhoea and malnutrition.

➤ Treat for a helminth infection (such as mebendazole 100 mg orally twice a day for 3 days or 500 mg once only).

REVIEW by a surgeon experienced in paediatric surgery. Recurrent prolapse may require a Thirsch stitch.

9.5 Infections requiring surgery

9.5.1 Abscess

Infection can cause a collection of pus in almost any area of the body.

Diagnosis

- Fever, swelling, tenderness, and fluctuant mass.
- Question what might be the cause of the abscess (e.g., injection, foreign body or underlying bone infection). Injection abscesses usually develop 2–3 weeks after injection.

Treatment

➤ Incision and drainage (see figure, page 257).

- Large abscesses may require general anaesthesia.

➤ Antibiotics: cloxacillin (25–50 mg/kg four times a day) for 5 days or until surrounding cellulitis resolved. If bowel flora is suspected (e.g., perirectal abscess): give ampicillin (25–50 mg/kg IM or IV four times a day), gentamicin (7.5 mg/kg IM or IV once a day) and metronidazole (7.5 mg/kg three times a day).

9.5.2 Osteomyelitis (see page 165)

Infection of a bone usually results from blood spread. It may be caused by open fractures. The most common organisms include *Staphylococcus*, *Salmonella* (sickle-cell children) and *Mycobacterium tuberculosis*.

Diagnosis

- Acute osteomyelitis
  - Pain and tenderness of the involved bone (± fever).
  - Refusal to move the affected limb.
  - Refusal to bear weight on leg.
  - In early osteomyelitis the X-ray may be normal (it usually takes 12–14 days for X-ray changes to appear).

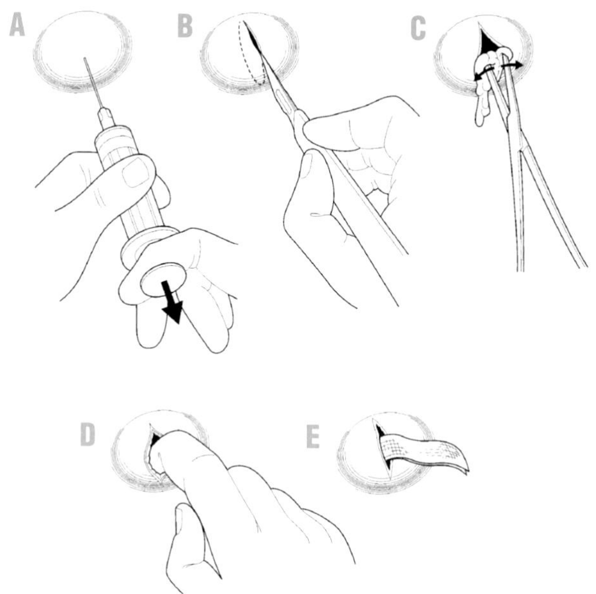

Incision and drainage of an abscess

A. Aspirating to identify site of pus; B. Elliptical incision; C–D. Breaking up loculations; E. Loose packing in place.

- Chronic osteomyelitis
  - — Chronic draining sinuses over the involved bone.
  - — X-ray: elevated periosteum and sequestrum (collection of dead bone).

Treatment

➤ REVIEW by a surgeon experienced in paediatric surgery

➤ In early osteomyelitis with fever and toxaemia, give chloramphenicol (25 mg/kg three times a day) in children <3 years and in those with sickle-cell disease;

or give cloxacillin (50 mg/kg IM or IV four times a day) in children aged >3 years for at least 5 weeks. Give parenteral antibiotics until child has clinically improved, then orally to complete the duration of the course.

➤ Chronic osteomyelitis: sequestrectomy (removal of dead bone) is usually necessary as well as antibiotic treatment, as above.

9.5.3 Septic arthritis (see page 165)

This condition is similar to osteomyelitis, but involves the joint.

Diagnosis

- Pain and swelling of the joint (± fever).
- Examination of the joint shows two important physical signs.
  - Swelling and tenderness over the joint.
  - Decreased range of movement.

Treatment

➤ Aspiration of the joint to confirm the diagnosis (see figure, page 259). The most common organism is *Staphylococcus aureus*. The aspiration should be done under sterile conditions.

- URGENT REVIEW by a surgeon experienced in paediatric surgery for washout of the joint. Pus under pressure in a joint destroys the joint.

➤ Give chloramphenicol (25 mg/kg three times a day) in children <3 years and in those with sickle cell disease; or give cloxacillin (50 mg/kg IM or IV four times a day) in children aged >3 years for at least 3 weeks. Give parenteral antibiotics until the child has clinically improved, then orally to complete the duration of the course

9.5.4 Pyomyositis

This is a condition where there is pus within the substance of a muscle.

Diagnosis

- Fever, tenderness and swelling of the involved muscle. A fluctuant mass may not be a sign as the inflammation is deep in the muscle.
- Commonly occurs in the thigh.

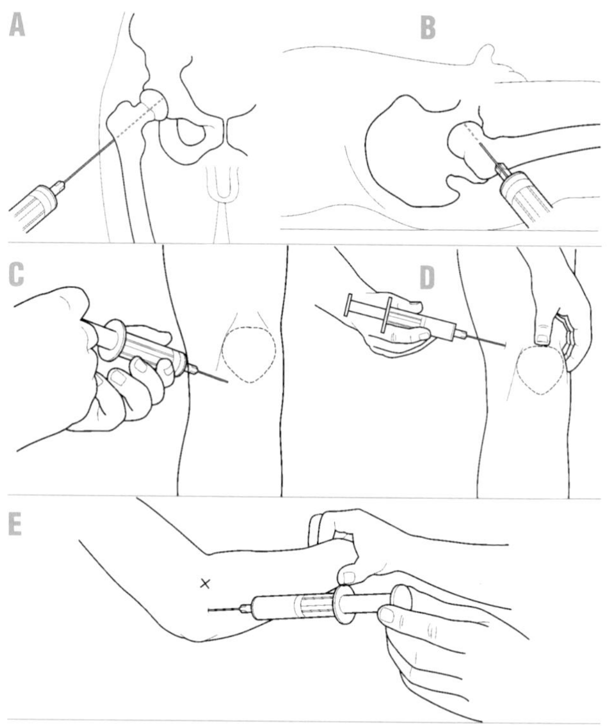

Technique for aspirating hip (A,B), knee (C,D) and elbow (E) joints.

Treatment

- Incision and drainage (usually requires a general anaesthetic).
- Leave a drain in the abscess cavity for 2–3 days.
- X-ray to exclude underlying osteomyelitis.
- Give cloxacillin (50 mg/kg IM or IV four times a day) for 5–10 days as the most common organism is *Staphylococcus aureus*.

Notes

CHAPTER 10

Supportive care

In order to provide good inpatient care, hospital policies and working practices should promote the basic principles of child care, such as:

- communicating with the parents
- arranging the paediatric ward so that the most seriously ill children get the closest attention and are close to oxygen and other emergency treatments
- keeping the child comfortable
- preventing the spread of nosocomial infection by encouraging staff to hand-wash regularly, and other measures
- keeping warm the area in which young infants or children with severe malnutrition are being looked after, in order to prevent complications like hypothermia.

10.1 Nutritional management

The health worker should follow the counselling process outlined in sections 12.3 and 12.4 (pages 295–296). A mother's card containing a pictorial representation of the advice should be given to the mother to take home as a reminder (see page 294 and Appendix 6, page 369).

10.1.1 **Supporting breastfeeding**

Breastfeeding is most important for the protection of infants from illness and for their recovery from illness. It provides the nutrients needed for a return to good health.

- Exclusive breastfeeding is recommended from birth until 6 months of age.
- Continued breastfeeding, together with adequate complementary foods, is recommended from 6 months up to 2 years of age or older.

Health workers treating sick young children have a responsibility to encourage mothers to breastfeed and to help them overcome any difficulties.

Assessing a breastfeed

Take a breastfeeding history by asking about the baby's feeding and behaviour. Observe the mother while breastfeeding to decide whether she needs help. Observe:

- How the baby is attached to the breast (see page 263).

Signs of good attachment are:

  — more areola visible above baby's mouth
  — mouth wide open
  — lower lip turned out
  — baby's chin touching the breast.

- How the mother holds her baby (see page 263).
  — baby should be held close to the mother
  — baby should face the breast
  — baby's body should be in a straight line with the head
  — baby's whole body should be supported.
- How the mother holds her breast.

Overcoming difficulties

1. 'Not enough milk'

Almost all mothers can produce enough breast milk for one or even two babies. However, sometimes the baby is not getting enough breast milk. The signs are:

- poor weight gain (<500 g a month, or <125 g a week, or less than the birth weight after 2 weeks)

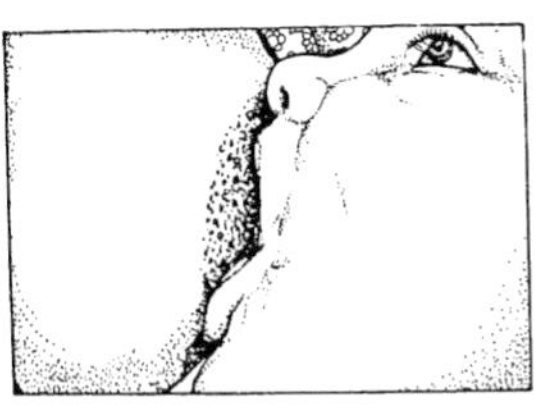
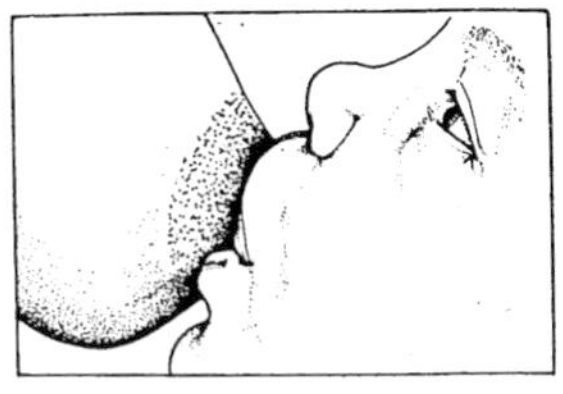

Good (left) and poor (right) attachment of infant to the mother's breast

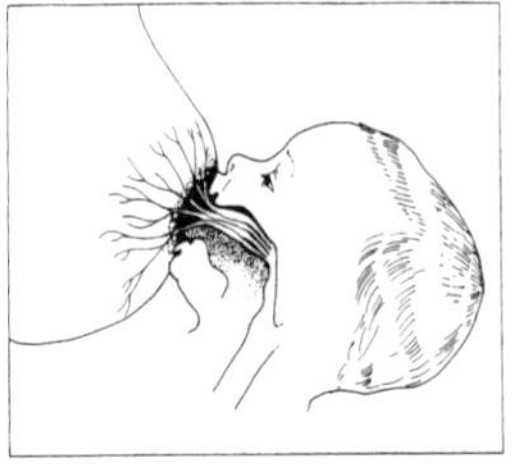
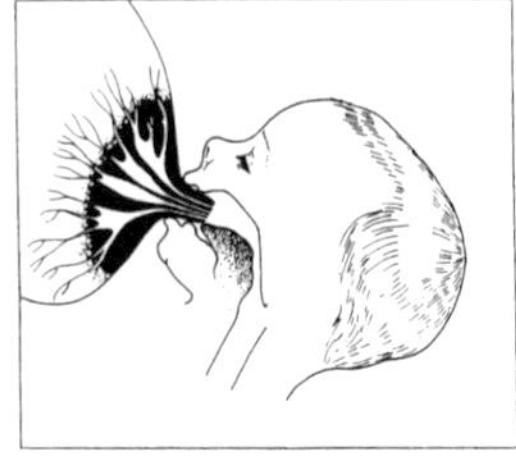

Good (left) and poor (right) attachment—cross-sectional view of the breast and baby

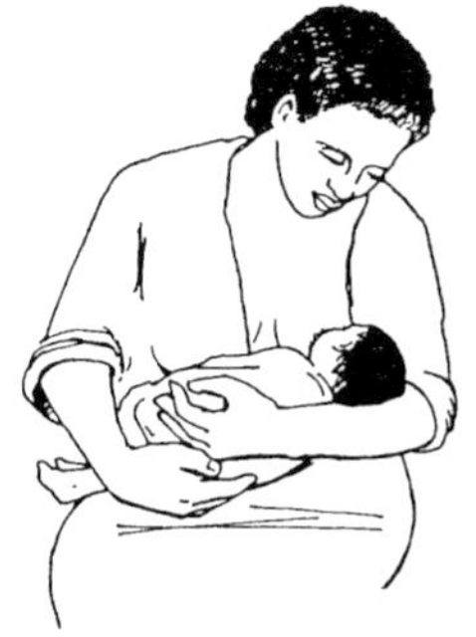
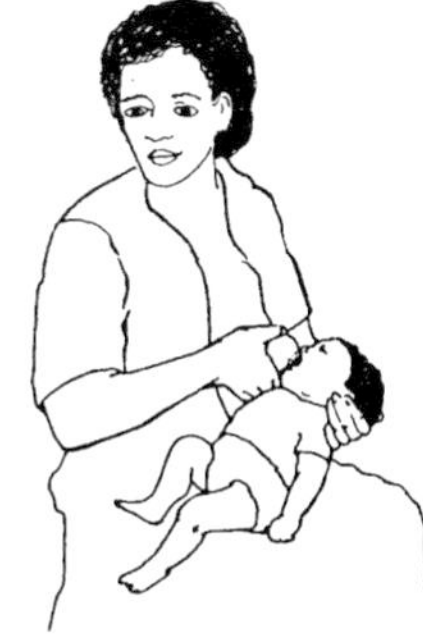

Good (left) and poor (right) positioning of infant for breastfeeding

- passing a small amount of concentrated urine (less than 6 times a day, yellow and strong-smelling).

Common reasons why a baby may not be getting enough breast milk are:

- *Poor breastfeeding practices:* poor attachment (very common cause), delayed start of breastfeeding, feeding at fixed times, no night feeds, short feeds, use of bottles, pacifiers, other foods and other fluids.
- *Psychological factors in the mother:* lack of confidence, worry, stress, depression, dislike of breastfeeding, rejection of baby, tiredness.
- *Mother's physical condition:* chronic illness (e.g. tuberculosis, severe anaemia or rheumatic heart disease), contraceptive pill, diuretics, pregnancy, severe malnutrition, alcohol, smoking, retained piece of placenta (rare).
- *Baby's condition:* illness, or congenital anomaly (such as cleft palate or congenital heart disease) which interferes with feeding.

A mother whose breast milk supply is reduced will need to increase it, while a mother who has stopped breastfeeding may need to **relactate** (see page 118).

Help a mother to breastfeed again by:

- keeping the baby close to her and not giving him/her to other carers
- having plenty of skin-to-skin contact at all times
- offering the baby her breast whenever the baby is willing to suckle
- helping the baby to take the breast by expressing breast milk into the baby's mouth, and positioning the baby so that the baby can easily attach to the breast
- avoiding use of bottles, teats and pacifiers. If necessary, express the breast milk and give it by cup. If this cannot be done, artificial feeds may be needed until an adequate milk supply is established.

2. How to increase the milk supply

The main way to increase or restart the supply of breast milk is for the baby to suckle often in order to stimulate the breast.

- Give other feeds from a cup while waiting for breast milk to come. Do not use bottles or pacifiers. Reduce the other milk by 30–60 ml per day as her breast milk starts to increase. Monitor the baby's weight gain.

3. Refusal or reluctance to breastfeed

The main reasons why a baby might refuse to breastfeed are:

- *The baby is ill, in pain or sedated*

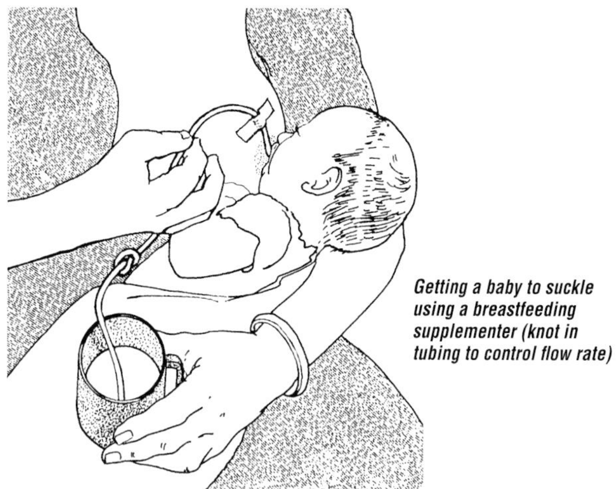

Getting a baby to suckle using a breastfeeding supplementer (knot in tubing to control flow rate)

— If the baby is able to suckle, encourage the mother to breastfeed more often. If the baby is very ill, the mother may need to express breast milk and feed by cup or tube until the baby is able to breastfeed again.

— If the baby is in hospital, arrange for the mother to stay with the baby in order to breastfeed.

— Help the mother to find a way to hold her baby without pressing on a painful place.

— Explain to the mother how to clear a blocked nose. Suggest short feeds, more often than usual, for a few days.

— A sore mouth may be due to *Candida* infection (thrush) or teething. Treat the infection with nystatin (100 000 units/ml) suspension. Give 1–2 ml dropped into the mouth, 4 times a day for 7 days. If this is not available, apply 1% gentian violet solution. Encourage the mother of a teething baby to be patient and keep offering the baby the breast.

— If the mother is on regular sedation, reduce the dose or try a less sedating alternative.

- *There is difficulty with the breastfeeding technique*
  - *Help the mother with her technique:* ensure that the baby is positioned and attached well without pressing on the baby's head, or shaking the breast.
  - *Advise her not to use a feeding bottle or pacifier:* if necessary, use a cup.
  - *Treat engorgement* by removing milk from the breast; otherwise mastitis or an abscess may develop. If the baby is not able to suckle, help the mother to express her milk.
  - *Help reduce oversupply.* If a baby is poorly attached and suckles ineffectively, the baby may breastfeed more frequently or for a longer time, stimulating the breast so that more milk is produced than required. Oversupply may also occur if a mother tries to make her baby feed from both breasts at each feed, when this is not necessary.
- *A change has upset the baby*

Changes such as separation from the mother, a new carer, illness of the mother, or in the family routine or the mother's smell (due to a different soap, food or menstruation) can upset the baby and cause refusal to breastfeed.

Low-birth-weight and sick babies

Babies with a birth weight below 2.5 kg need breast milk even more than larger babies; often, however, they cannot breastfeed immediately after birth especially if they are very small.

For the first few days, a baby may not be able to take oral feeds and may need to be fed intravenously. Begin oral feeds as soon as the baby can tolerate them.

Babies at 30–32 (or fewer) weeks gestational age usually need to be fed by nasogastric tube. Give expressed breast milk by tube. The mother can let the baby suck on her finger while being tube fed. This may stimulate the baby's digestive tract and help weight gain. Babies around 30–32 weeks may take feeds from a cup or spoon.

Babies at 32 (or more) weeks gestational age are able to start suckling on the breast. Let the mother put her baby to the breast as soon as the baby is well enough. Continue giving expressed breast milk by cup or tube to make sure that the baby gets all the nutrition needed.

Babies at 34–36 (or more) weeks gestational age can usually take all that they need directly from the breast.

Babies who cannot breastfeed

Non-breastfed babies should receive either:

- expressed breast milk (preferably from their own mothers)
- formula milk prepared with clean water according to instructions or, if possible, ready-made liquid formula
- animal milk (dilute cow's milk by adding 50 ml of water to 100 ml of milk, then add 10g of sugar to it, with an approved micronutrient supplement. If possible, do not use for premature babies).

Expressed breast milk (EBM) is the best choice—in the following amounts:

Babies ≥2.5 kg: give 150 ml/kg body weight daily, divided into 8 feeds, at 3-hour intervals.

Babies <2.5 kg: see page 53 for detailed guidance.

If the child is too weak to suck, feeding can be done with a cup. Feed by nasogastric tube if the child is lethargic or severely anorexic.

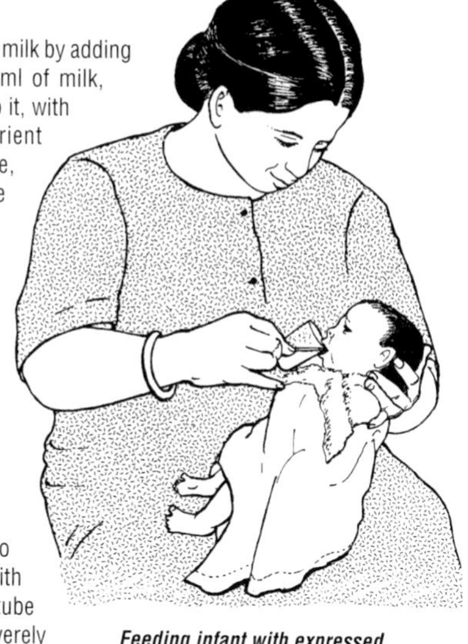

Feeding infant with expressed breast milk using a cup

10.1.2 Nutritional management of sick children

The principles for feeding sick infants and young children are:

- continue breastfeeding
- do not withhold food
- give frequent small feeds, every 2–3 hours
- coax, encourage, and be patient
- feed by nasogastric tube if the child is severely anorexic
- promote catch-up growth after the appetite returns.

Catch-up meals

The recipes provide 100 kcal and 3 g protein/100 ml. The individual servings contain approx 200 kcal and 6 g protein. A child needs to eat 7 meals in 24 hours.

Recipe 1 (Porridge without milk)

Ingredient	To make 1 litre	For one serving
Cereal flour	100 g	20 g
Groundnut/oilseed paste	100 g	20 g
Sugar	50 g	10 g

Make a thick porridge and then stir in the paste and sugar. Make up to 1 litre.

Recipe 2 (Porridge with milk/rice pudding)

Ingredient	To make 1 litre	For one serving
Cereal flour	125 g	25 g
Milk (fresh, or long-life whole milk)	600 ml	120 ml
Sugar	75 g	15 g
Oil/margarine	25 g	5 g

Make a thick porridge with milk and just a little water (or use 75 g whole milk powder instead of the 600 ml liquid milk), then add sugar and oil. Make up to 1 litre.

For rice pudding, replace cereal flour with the same amount of rice.

These recipes may need to be supplemented with vitamins and minerals.

Recipe 3 (Rice-based meal)

Ingredient	To make 600g	For one serving
Rice	75 g	25 g
Lentils (dhal)	50 g	20 g
Pumpkin	75 g	25 g
Green leaves	75 g	25 g
Oil/margarine	25 g	10 g
Water	800 ml	

Put rice, lentils, pumpkin, oil, spices and water in a pot and cook with lid on. Just before rice is cooked, add chopped leaves. Cook for a few more minutes.

Recipe 4 (Rice-based meal using cooked family foods)

Ingredient	Amount for one serving
Cooked rice	90 g (4½ big spoons)*
Cooked mashed beans, peas or lentils	30 g (1½ big spoons)
Cooked mashed pumpkin	30 g (1½ big spoons)
Margarine/oil	10 g (2 teaspoons)**

Soften the mashed foods with the oil or margarine.

Recipe 5 (Maize-based meal using family foods)

Ingredient	Amount for one serving
Thick maize porridge (cooked)	140 g (6 big spoons)*
Groundnut paste	15 g (3 teaspoons)**
Egg	30 g (1 egg)
Green leaves	20 g (handful)

Stir groundnut paste and raw egg into cooked porridge. Cook for a few minutes. Fry onion and tomato for flavour and add leaves. Stir into

* Big = 10 ml spoon, rounded; ** Teaspoon = 5 ml

The food provided should be:

- palatable (to the child)
- easily eaten (soft or liquid consistency)
- easily digested
- nutritious, and rich in energy and nutrients.

The basic principle of nutritional management is to provide a diet with sufficient energy-producing foods and high-quality proteins. Foods with a high oil or fat content are recommended. Up to 30–40% of the total calories can be given as fat. In addition, feeding at frequent intervals is necessary to achieve high energy intakes. If there is concern about the nutritional content of the food, provide multivitamin and mineral supplements.

The child should be encouraged to eat relatively small amounts frequently. If young children are left to feed by themselves, or have to compete with siblings for food, they may not get enough to eat.

A blocked nose, with dry or thick mucus, may interfere with feeding. Put drops of salted water or saline into the nose with a moistened wick to help soften the mucus.

In a minority of children who are unable to eat for a number of days (e.g. due to impaired consciousness in meningitis or respiratory distress in severe pneumonia), it may be necessary to feed by nasogastric tube. The risk of aspiration can be reduced if small volumes are given frequently.

To supplement the child's nutritional management in the hospital, feeding should be increased during convalescence to make up for any lost weight. It is important that the mother or carer should offer food to the child more frequently than normal (at least one additional meal a day) after the child's appetite increases.

CHART 16. Feeding recommendations during sickness and health*

Up to 6 months of age

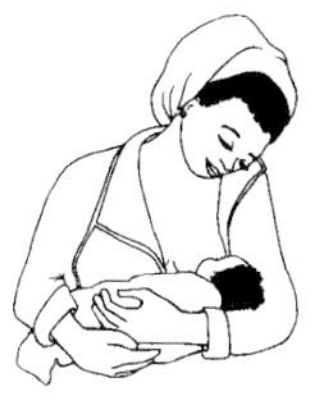

- ➤ Breastfeed as often as the child wants, day and night, at least 8 times in 24 hours.
- ➤ Do not give other foods or fluids.
- ➤ Only if the child is older than 4 months and appears hungry after breastfeeding, and is not gaining weight adequately:

  Add complementary foods (see below).

  Give 2–3 tablespoons of these foods 1 or 2 times per day after breastfeeding.

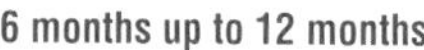

6 months up to 12 months

- ➤ Breastfeed as often as the child wants day and night, at least 8 times in 24 hours.
- ➤ Give adequate servings of locally appropriate nutrient-dense foods (see Table 31 for examples):
  - — 3 times per day if breastfed;
  - — 5 times per day if not breastfed, plus 1–2 cups of milk.

---

12 months up to 2 years

- ➤ Breastfeed as often as the child wants.
- ➤ Give adequate servings of locally appropriate nutrient-dense foods (see Table 31 for examples) or family foods 5 times per day.

---

2 years and older

- ➤ Give family foods at 3 meals each day. Also, twice daily, give nutritious food between meals (see Table 31 for examples)

---

* A good daily diet should be adequate in quantity and include an energy-rich food (for example, thick cereal with added oil); meat, fish, eggs, or pulses; and fruits and vegetables.

Table 31. Examples of local adaptations of feeding recommendations from Bolivia, Indonesia, Nepal, South Africa and Tanzania

Country	Age group: 6 months up to 12 months	12 months up to 2 years	2 years and older
Bolivia	Cereal gruel, vegetable puree, minced meat or egg yolk, fruit. From 9 months: fish, whole egg	Family meals plus additional seasonal fruit, milk-based desserts (custard, milk rice), yoghurt, cheese, give milk twice a day	
Indonesia	Give adequate amounts of rice porridge with egg / chicken / fish / meat / tempe / tahu / carrot / spinach/ green beans / oil / coconut milk. Give also snacks 2 times a day between meals such as green beans, porridge, banana, biscuit, nagasari		Give adequate amounts of family foods in 3 meals each day consisting of rice, side dishes, vegetables and fruits. Also, twice daily, give nutritious foods between meals, such as green beans, porridge, banana, biscuit, nagasari etc
Nepal	Give adequate servings of (mashed) foods such as rice, lentils (dhal), mashed bread (roti), biscuits, milk, yoghurt, seasonal fruits (such as banana, guava, mango etc), vegetables (such as potatoes, carrots, green leafy vegetables, beans etc), meat, fish and eggs		
South Africa	Porridge with added oil, peanut butter or ground peanuts, margarine and chicken, beans, full-cream milk, fruit and vegetables, mashed avocado or family food	Porridge with added oil, peanut butter or ground peanuts, margarine and chicken, beans, full-cream milk, fruit and vegetables, mashed avocado or banana, canned fish or family food	Bread and peanut butter, fresh fruit or full cream
Tanzania	Thick gruel, mixed food containing milk, mashed foods (rice, potato, ugali). Add beans, other legumes, meat, fish, or groundnuts. Add greens or fruit such as pawpaw, mango, banana, or avocado. Add spoonful of extra oil into food.		Give twice daily such as thick enriched uji, milk fruits or other nutritious snacks.

10.2 **Fluid management**

The total daily fluid requirement of a child is calculated with the following formula: 100 ml/kg for the first 10 kg, then 50 ml/kg for the next 10 kg, thereafter 25 ml/kg for each subsequent kg. For example, an 8 kg baby receives 8 x 100 ml = 800 ml per day, a 15 kg child (10 x 100) + (5 x 50) = 1250 ml per day.

Table 32. Maintenance fluid requirements

Body weight of child	Fluid (ml/day)
2 kg	200 ml/day
4 kg	400 ml/day
6 kg	600 ml/day
8 kg	800 ml/day
10 kg	1000 ml/day
12 kg	1100 ml/day
14 kg	1200 ml/day
16 kg	1300 ml/day
18 kg	1400 ml/day
20 kg	1500 ml/day
22 kg	1550 ml/day
24 kg	1600 ml/day
26 kg	1650 ml/day

Give the sick child more than the above amounts if there is fever (increase by 10% for every 1 °C of fever).

Monitoring fluid intake

Pay careful attention to maintaining adequate hydration in very sick children, who may have had no oral fluid intake for some time. **Fluids should preferably be given orally (by mouth or nasogastric tube)**.

If fluids need to be given intravenously, it is important to monitor closely any infusion of IV fluid given to a sick child because of the risk of fluid overload leading to heart failure or cerebral oedema. If it is impossible to monitor the IV fluid infusion closely, then the IV route should be used only for the management of severe dehydration, septic shock, the delivery of IV antibiotics, and in children in whom oral fluids are contraindicated (such as in perforation of the intestine or other surgical abdominal problems). Possible IV maintenance fluids include half-normal saline plus 5% glucose. Do not give 5% glucose alone for extended periods as this can lead to hyponatraemia. See Appendix 4, page 357 for composition of IV fluids.

10.3 Management of fever

Temperatures referred to in these guidelines are **rectal temperatures**, unless otherwise stated. Oral and axillary temperatures are lower by approximately 0.5 °C and 0.8 °C respectively.

Fever is *not* an indication for antibiotic treatment, and may help the immune defences against infection. However, high fever (>39 °C or >102.2 °F) can have harmful effects such as:

- reducing the appetite
- making the child irritable
- precipitating convulsions in some children aged between 6 months and 5 years
- increasing oxygen consumption (e.g. in a child with very severe pneumonia, heart failure or meningitis).

All children with fever should be examined for signs and symptoms which will indicate the underlying cause of the fever, and should be treated accordingly (see Chapter 6, page 133).

Antipyretic treatment

Paracetamol

Treatment with oral paracetamol should be restricted to children aged ≥2 months who have a fever of ≥39 °C (≥102.2 °F), and are uncomfortable or distressed because of the high fever. Children who are alert and active are unlikely to benefit from paracetamol treatment. The dose of paracetamol is 15 mg/kg 6-hourly.

Other agents

Aspirin is not recommended as a first-line antipyretic because it has been linked with Reye's syndrome, a rare but serious condition affecting the liver and brain. Avoid giving aspirin to children with chickenpox, dengue fever and other haemorrhagic disorders.

Other agents are not recommended because of their toxicity and inefficacy (dipyrone, phenylbutazone) or expense (ibuprofen).

Supportive care

Children with fever should be lightly clothed, kept in a warm but well-ventilated room, and encouraged to increase their oral fluid intake. Sponging with tepid water lowers the temperature during the period of sponging only.

10.4 **Pain control**

The underlying principles of pain control are:

— give analgesia *by mouth*, where possible (IM treatment may be painful)

— give it *regularly*, so that the child does not have to experience the recurrence of severe pain in order to get the next dose of analgesia

— give it in *increasing doses*, or start with mild analgesics and progress to strong analgesics as the requirement for pain relief rises or tolerance develops

— set the *dose for each child*, because children will have different dose requirements for the same effect.

Use the following drugs for effective pain control:

1. ***Local anaesthetics:*** for painful lesions in the skin or mucosa or during painful procedures.

   ➤ Lidocaine: apply on a gauze to painful mouth ulcers before feeds (apply with gloves, unless the family member or health worker is HIV-positive and does not need protection from infection); it acts in 2–5 minutes.

   ➤ TAC (tetracaine, adrenaline, cocaine): apply to a gauze pad and place over open wounds; it is particularly useful when suturing.

2. **Analgesics:** for mild and moderate pain (such as headaches, post-traumatic pain, and pain from spasticity).

   ➤ paracetamol

   ➤ aspirin (see comments on use page 274)

   ➤ nonsteroidal anti-inflammatory drugs, such as ibuprofen.

3. ***Potent analgesics such as opiates:*** for moderate and severe pain not responding to treatment with analgesics.

   ➤ morphine, an inexpensive and potent analgesic: give orally or IV every 4–6 hours, or by continuous IV infusion.

   ➤ pethidine: give orally or IM every 4–6 hours

   ➤ codeine: give orally every 6–12 hours, combined with non-opioids to achieve additive analgesia.

   Note: Monitor carefully for respiratory depression. If tolerance develops, the dose will need to be increased to maintain the same degree of pain relief.

4. ***Other drugs:*** for specific pain problems. These include diazepam for muscle spasm, carbamazepine for neuralgic pain, and corticosteroids (such as dexamethasone) for pain due to an inflammatory swelling pressing on a nerve.

10.5 Management of anaemia

Anaemia (non-severe)

Young children (aged <6 years) are anaemic if their haemoglobin is <9.3 g/dl (approximately equivalent to a haematocrit of <27%). If anaemia is present, begin treatment—except if the child is severely malnourished, in which case see page 183.

➤ Give (home) treatment with iron (daily dose of iron/folate tablet or iron syrup) for 14 days.

Note: If the child is taking sulfadoxine-pyrimethamine for malaria, do not give iron tablets that contain folate until a follow-up visit after 2 weeks. The folate may interfere with the action of the antimalarial. See section 7.4.6 (page 183) for use of iron in severely malnourished children.

- Ask the parent to return with the child after 14 days. Treatment should be given for 3 months, where possible. It takes 2–4 weeks to correct the anaemia and 1–3 months after the haemoglobin reverts to normal to build up iron stores.
- If the child is ≥2 years and has not had mebendazole in the previous 6 months, give one dose of mebendazole (500 mg) for possible hookworm or whipworm (see page 147).
- Advise the mother about good feeding practices.

Severe anaemia

➤ Give a *blood transfusion* as soon as possible (see below) to:

— all children with a haematocrit of ≤12% or Hb of ≤4 g/dl

— less severely anaemic children (haematocrit 13–18%; Hb 4–6 g/dl) with any of the following clinical features:

- clinically detectable dehydration
- shock
- impaired consciousness
- heart failure
- deep and laboured breathing
- very high malaria parasitaemia (>10% of red cells with parasites).

- If packed cells are available, give 10 ml/kg body weight over 3–4 hours in preference to whole blood. If not available, give fresh whole blood (20 ml/kg body weight) over 3–4 hours.
- Check the respiratory rate and pulse rate every 15 minutes. If either shows a rise, transfuse more slowly. If there is any evidence of fluid overload due to the blood transfusion, give IV furosemide, 1–2 mg/kg body weight, up to a maximum total of 20 mg.
- After the transfusion, if the haemoglobin remains as before, repeat the transfusion.
- In severely malnourished children, fluid overload is a common and serious complication. Give packed cells where available or whole blood, 10 ml/kg body weight (rather than 20 ml/kg), once only and do not repeat the transfusion (see page 191 for details).

10.6 **Blood transfusion**

10.6.1 **Storage of blood**

Use blood that has been screened and found negative for transfusion-transmissible infections. Do *not* use blood that has passed its expiry date or has been out of the refrigerator for more than 2 hours.

Large volume rapid transfusion at a rate >15 ml/kg/hour of blood stored at 4 °C may cause hypothermia, especially in small babies.

10.6.2 **Problems with blood transfusion**

Blood can be the vehicle for transmitting infections (e.g. malaria, syphilis, hepatitis B and C, HIV). Therefore, screen donors for as many of these infections as possible. To minimize the risk, only give blood transfusions when ***essential***.

10.6.3 **Indications for blood transfusion**

There are five general indications for blood transfusion:

- acute blood loss, when 20–30% of the total blood volume has been lost and bleeding is continuing
- severe anaemia
- septic shock (if IV fluids are insufficient to maintain adequate circulation and in addition to antibiotic therapy)
- to provide plasma and platelets for clotting factors, if specific blood components are not available
- exchange transfusion in neonates with severe jaundice.

10.6.4 **Giving a blood transfusion**

Before transfusion, check the following:

- the blood is the correct group and the patient's name and number are on both the label and the form (in an emergency, reduce the risk of incompatibility or transfusion reactions by cross-matching group-specific blood or giving O-negative blood if available)
- the blood transfusion bag has no leaks
- the blood pack has not been out of the refrigerator for more than 2 hours, the plasma is not pink or has large clots, and the red cells do not look purple or black

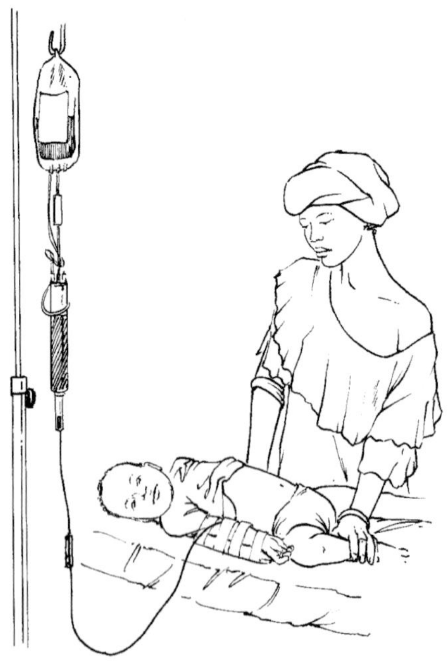

Giving a blood transfusion. Note: A burette is used to measure the blood volume, and the arm is splinted to prevent flexion of the elbow.

- any signs of heart failure. If present, give 1mg/kg of furosemide IV at the start of the transfusion in children whose circulating blood volume is normal. Do not inject into the blood pack.

Do a baseline recording of the child's temperature, respiratory rate and pulse rate.

The volume transfused should initially be 20 ml/kg body weight of whole blood, given over 3–4 hours.

During transfusion:

- if available, use an infusion device to control the rate of the transfusion
- check that the blood is flowing at the correct speed
- look for signs of a transfusion reaction (see below), particularly carefully in the first 15 minutes of the transfusion
- record the child's general appearance, temperature, pulse and respiratory rate every 30 minutes
- record the time the transfusion was started and ended, the volume of blood transfused, and the presence of any reactions.

After transfusion:

- reassess the child. If more blood is needed, a similar quantity should be transfused and the dose of furosemide (if given) repeated.

10.6.5 **Transfusion reactions**

If a transfusion reaction occurs, first check the blood pack labels and patient's identity. If there is any discrepancy, stop the transfusion immediately and notify the blood bank.

Mild reactions (due to mild hypersensitivity)

Signs and symptoms:

- itchy rash

Management:

- ➤ slow the transfusion
- ➤ give chlorphenamine 0.1 mg/kg IM, if available
- ➤ continue the transfusion at the normal rate if there is no progression of symptoms after 30 minutes
- ➤ if symptoms persist, treat as moderate reaction (see below).

Moderately severe reactions (due to moderate hypersensitivity, non-haemolytic reactions, pyrogens or bacterial contamination)

Signs and symptoms:

- severe itchy rash (urticaria)
- flushing
- fever >38 °C or >100.4 °F (*Note:* fever may have been present before the transfusion)
- rigors
- restlessness
- raised heart rate.

Management:

- ➤ stop the transfusion, but keep the IV line open with normal saline
- ➤ give IV 200 mg hydrocortisone, or chlorphenamine 0.25 mg/kg IM, if available
- ➤ give a bronchodilator, if wheezing (see pages 88–90)
- ➤ send the following to the Blood Bank: the blood-giving set that was used, blood sample from another site, and urine samples collected over 24 hours.
- ➤ if there is improvement, restart the transfusion slowly with new blood and observe carefully
- ➤ if no improvement in 15 minutes, treat as life-threatening reaction (see below), and report to doctor in charge and to the Blood Bank.

Life-threatening reactions (due to haemolysis, bacterial contamination and septic shock, fluid overload or anaphylaxis)

Signs and symptoms:

- fever >38 °C or >100.4 °F (note: fever may have been present before the transfusion)
- rigors
- restlessness
- raised heart rate
- fast breathing
- black or dark red urine (haemoglobinuria)
- unexplained bleeding

- confusion
- collapse.

Note that in an unconscious child, uncontrolled bleeding or shock may be the only signs of a life-threatening reaction.

Management:

- stop the transfusion, but keep the IV line open with normal saline
- maintain airway and give oxygen (see page 4)
- give epinephrine (adrenaline) 0.01 mg/kg body weight (equal to 0.1 ml of 1 in 10 000 solution
- treat shock (see page 4)
- give IV 200 mg hydrocortisone, or chlorpheniramine 0.1 mg/kg IM, if available
- give a bronchodilator, if wheezing (see pages 88–90)
- report to doctor in charge and to blood laboratory as soon as possible
- maintain renal blood flow with IV furosemide 1 mg/kg
- give antibiotic as for septicaemia (see page 158).

10.7 **Oxygen therapy**

Indications

Where available, oxygen therapy should be guided by pulse oximetry (see page 284). Give oxygen to children with SaO_2 <90%, and increase oxygen to achieve a SaO_2 >90%. Where pulse oximeters are not available, the need for oxygen therapy needs to be guided by clinical signs, which are less reliable.

Where the oxygen supply is *limited*, priority should be given to children with very severe pneumonia, bronchiolitis, or asthma who:

- have central cyanosis, *or*
- are unable to drink (where this is due to respiratory distress).

Where the oxygen supply is *more plentiful*, it should be given to children with any of the following:

- severe lower chest wall indrawing
- respiratory rate of 70/min or above
- grunting with every breath (in young infants)
- head nodding (see page 70).

Sources

Oxygen supplies should be available at all times. The two main sources of oxygen are cylinders and oxygen concentrators. It is important that all equipment is checked for compatibility.

Oxygen cylinders and concentrators

See list of recommended equipment for use with oxygen cylinders and concentrators and instructions for their use in the WHO technical review paper, *Oxygen therapy in the management of a child with an acute respiratory infection* and the WHO manual *Clinical use of oxygen* (see Reference on page 301).

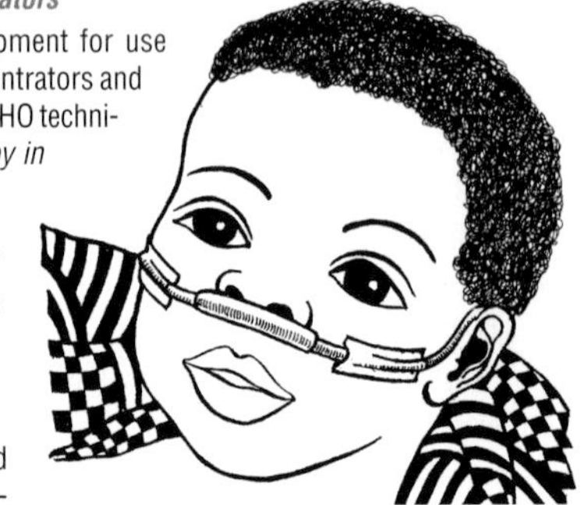

Oxygen therapy: nasal prongs correctly positioned and secured

Oxygen delivery

Three methods are recommended for the delivery of oxygen: nasal prongs, nasal catheter and nasopharyngeal catheter. Nasal prongs or a nasal catheter are preferred in most circumstances. Nasal prongs are the best method for delivering oxygen to young infants and children with severe croup or pertussis.

Use of a nasopharyngeal catheter calls for close monitoring and prompt action, in case the catheter enters the oesophagus or other serious complications develop. The use of face masks or headboxes is *not* recommended.

Nasal prongs. These are short tubes inserted into the nostrils. Place them just inside the nostrils and secure with a piece of tape on the cheeks near the nose (see figure).

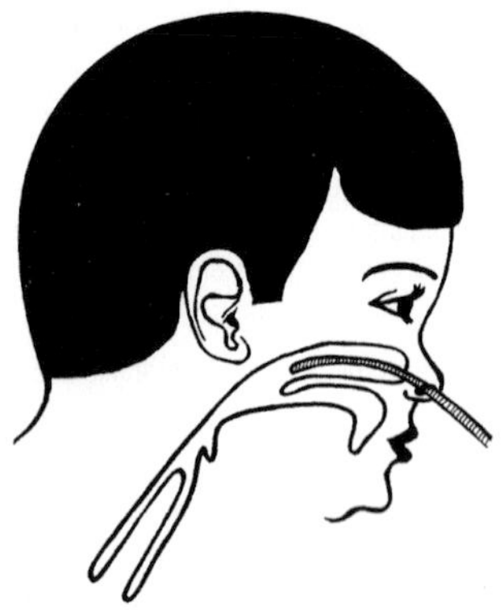

Oxygen therapy: correct position of nasal catheter (cross-sectional view)

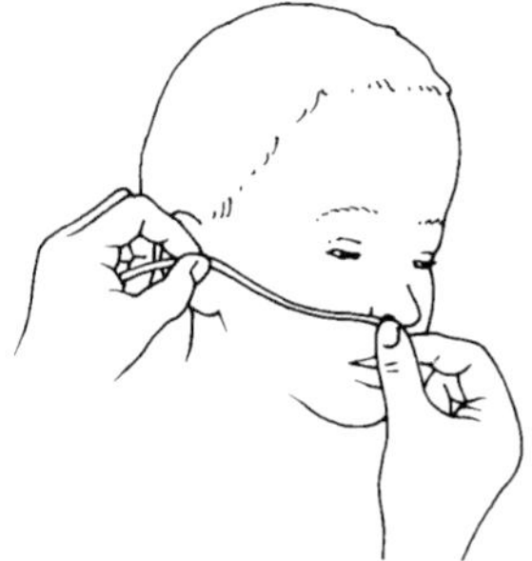

A: Measuring the distance from nose to the tragus of the ear for the insertion of a nasopharyngeal catheter

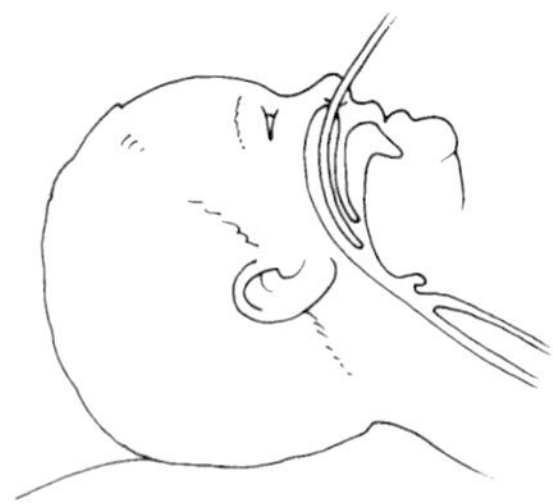

B. Cross sectional view of the position of the nasopharyngeal catheter

Care should be taken to keep the nostrils clear of mucus, which could block the flow of oxygen.

➤ Set a flow rate of 1–2 litres/min (0.5 litre/min in young infants) to deliver an inspired oxygen concentration of 30–35%. Humidification is not required with nasal prongs.

Nasal catheter. This is a 6 or 8FG catheter which is passed to the back of the nasal cavity. Place the catheter at a distance from the side of the nostril to the inner margin of the eyebrow.

➤ Set a flow rate of 1–2 litres/min. Humidification is not required with a nasal catheter.

Nasopharyngeal catheter. This is a 6 or 8FG catheter which is passed to the pharynx just below the level of the uvula. Place the catheter at a distance equal to that from the side of the nostril to the front of the ear (see figure B, above). If it is placed too far down, gagging and vomiting and, rarely, gastric distension can occur.

➤ Set a flow rate of 1–2 litres/min, which delivers an inspired oxygen concentration of 45–60%. It is important that this flow rate is not exceeded because of the risk of gastric distension. Humidification is required.

Monitoring

Train the nurses to place and secure the nasal prongs or catheter correctly. Check regularly that the equipment is working properly, and remove and clean the prongs or catheter at least twice a day.

Monitor the child at least every 3 hours to identify and correct any problems, including:

- SaO_2 by pulse oximeter
- nasal catheter or prongs out of position
- leaks in the oxygen delivery system
- oxygen flow rate not correct
- airway obstructed by mucus (clear the nose with a moist wick or by gentle suction)
- gastric distension (check the catheter's position and correct it, if necessary).

Pulse oximetry

A pulse oximeter is a machine which measures non-invasively the oxygen saturation in the blood. For this, it transmits a light beam through tissue such as a finger, a toe, or in small children the whole hand or foot. The saturation is measured in the small arteries, and is therefore referred to as the arterial oxygen saturation (SaO_2). There are reusable probes which last several months, and disposable ones.

A normal oxygen saturation at sea level in a child is 95–100%; with severe pneumonia, as oxygen uptake in the lung is impeded, it can drop. Oxygen is usually given with a saturation <90% (measured at room air). Different cut-offs might be used at altitude or if oxygen is scarce. The response to oxygen therapy can be measured with the pulse oximeter as well, as the SaO_2 should increase if the child has lung disease (with cyanotic heart disease, SaO_2 does not change when oxygen is given). The oxygen flow can be titrated with the pulse oximeter to obtain a stable SaO_2 >90% without wasting too much oxygen.

Duration of oxygen therapy

Continue giving oxygen continuously until the child is able to maintain a SaO_2 >90% in room air. When the child is stable and improving, take the child off oxygen for a few minutes. If the SaO_2 remains above 90%, discontinue oxygen, but check again ½ hour later, and 3 hourly thereafter on the first day off oxygen to ensure the child is stable. Where pulse oximetry is not available, the duration of oxygen therapy is guided by clinical signs (see p. 281), which are less reliable.

10.8 **Toys and play therapy**

Sample curriculum for play therapy

Each play session should include language and motor activities, and activities with toys.

Language activities

Teach the child local songs. Encourage the child to laugh, vocalize and describe what he or she is doing.

Motor activities

Always encourage the child to perform the next appropriate motor activity.

Activities with toys

Ring on a string (from 6 months)

Thread cotton reels and other small objects (e.g. cut from the neck of plastic bottles) on to a string. Tie the string in a ring, leaving a long piece of string hanging.

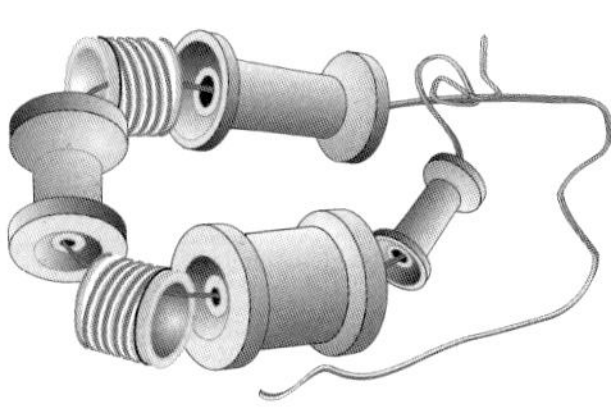

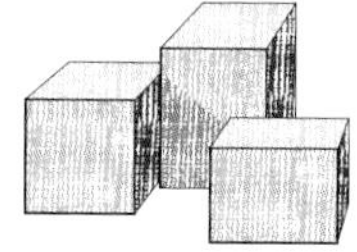

Blocks (from 9 months)

Small blocks of wood. Smooth the surfaces with sandpaper and paint in bright colours, if possible.

Nesting toys (from 9 months)

Cut off the bottom of two bottles of identical shape, but different size. The smaller bottle should be placed inside the larger bottle.

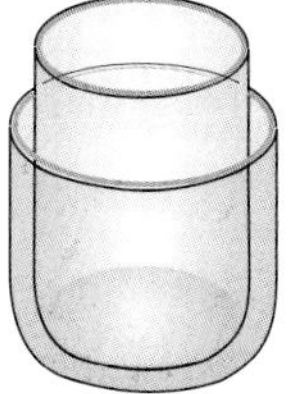

In-and-out toy (from 9 months)

Any plastic or cardboard container and small objects (not small enough to be swallowed).

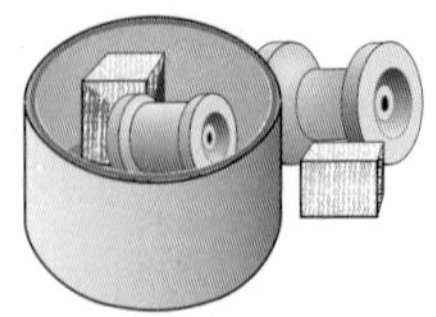

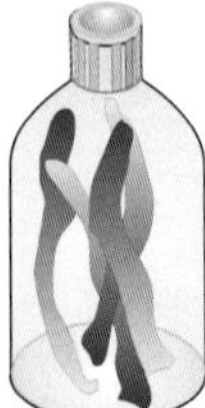

Rattle (from 12 months)

Cut long strips of plastic from coloured plastic bottles. Place them in a small transparent plastic bottle and glue the top on firmly.

Drum (from 12 months)

Any tin with a tightly fitting lid.

Doll (from 12 months)

Cut out two doll shapes from a piece of cloth and sew the edges together, leaving a small opening. Turn the doll inside-out and stuff with scraps of materials. Stitch up the opening and sew or draw a face on the doll.

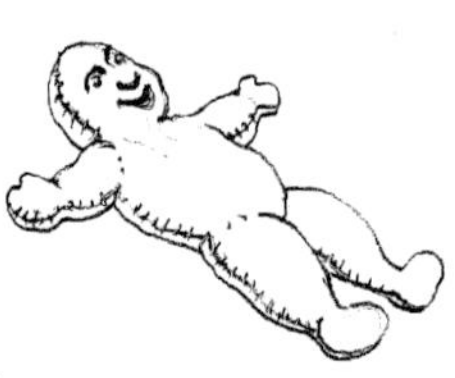

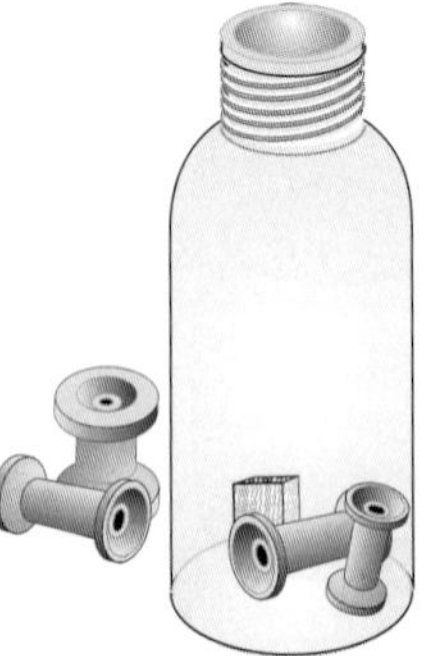

Posting bottle (from 12 months)

A large transparent plastic bottle with a small neck and small long objects that fit through the neck (not small enough to be swallowed).

Push-along toy (from 12 months)

Make a hole in the centre of the base and lid of a cylindrical-shaped tin. Thread a piece of wire (about 60 cm long) through each hole and tie the ends inside the tin. Put some metal bottle tops inside the tin and close the lid.

Pull-along toy (from 12 months)

As above, except that string is used instead of wire.

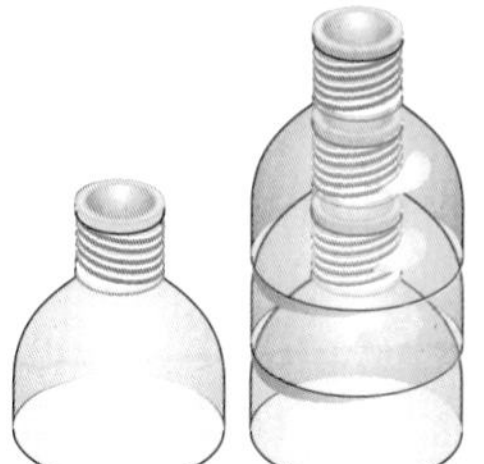

Stacking bottle tops (from 12 months)

Cut at least three identical round plastic bottles in half and stack them.

Mirror (from 18 months)

A tin lid with no sharp edges.

Puzzle (from 18 months)

Draw a figure (e.g. a doll) using a crayon on a square- or rectangular-shaped piece of cardboard. Cut the figure in half or quarters.

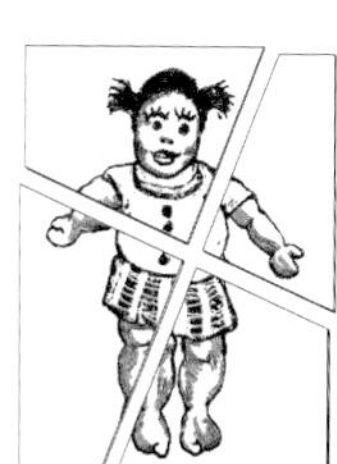

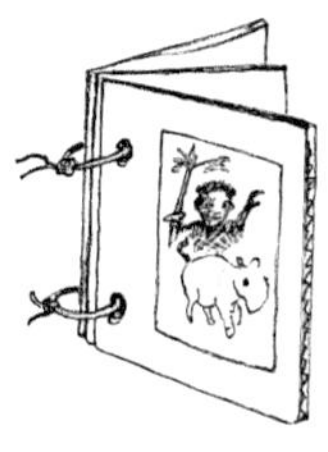

Book (from 18 months)

Cut out three rectangular-shaped pieces of the same size from a cardboard box. Glue or draw a picture on both sides of each piece. Make two holes down one side of each piece and thread string through to make a book.

Notes

CHAPTER 11

Monitoring the child's progress

11.1 **Monitoring procedures**

In order for monitoring to be effective, the health worker needs to know:

- the correct administration of the treatment
- the expected progress of the child
- the possible adverse effects of the treatment
- the complications that may arise and how these can be identified
- the possible alternative diagnoses in a child not responding to treatment.

Children treated in hospital should be checked regularly so that any deterioration in their condition, as well as complications, adverse effects of treatment, or errors in the administration of treatment can be identified promptly. The frequency of monitoring depends on the severity and nature of the illness (see relevant sections in Chapters 3 to 8).

Details of the child's condition and progress should be recorded so that they can be reviewed by other members of staff. A senior health worker who is responsible for the care of the child, and has the authority to change treatment, should supervise these records and examine the child on a regular basis.

Children who are seriously ill should be visited by a doctor (or other senior health professional) soon after the child's admission to hospital. These visits should also be seen as an opportunity to encourage communication between the families of sick children and hospital staff.

11.2 **Monitoring chart**

A monitoring chart should include the following items.

1. Patient's details
2. Vital signs (indicated by the coma score or level of consciousness, temperature, respiratory rate, pulse rate, and weight).
3. Fluid balance
4. Presence of clinical signs, complications and positive investigation findings. At each review of the child, record whether or not these signs are still present. Record any new signs or complications
5. Treatments given
6. Feeding/nutrition. Record the child's weight on admission and at appropriate intervals during treatment. There should be a daily record of the child's drinking/breastfeeding and eating. Record the amount of food taken and details of any feeding problems.
7. See Appendix 6 (page 369) for details of where to find examples of monitoring charts and critical care pathways.

11.3 **Audit of paediatric care**

The quality of care given to sick children in hospital can be improved if there is a system for reviewing the outcomes of each child admitted to the hospital. As a minimum, the system should keep records of all the children who died in the hospital. Trends in case-fatality rates over a period of time could then be compared and the treatment that was given could be discussed with all staff with the aim of identifying the problems and finding better solutions.

An audit of hospital paediatric care can be carried out by comparing the quality of care actually given with a recognized standard, such as the WHO recommendations contained in this pocket book. A successful audit calls for the full and constructive participation of all medical and nursing staff. The aim is to improve care and solve problems, without attributing blame for errors. The audit should be simple and not take up too much time, which is required for caring for the sick children. One suggestion is to ask medical and nursing staff for their views on improving the quality of care, and to give priority to these conditions or problems.

Notes

Notes

CHAPTER 12

Counselling and discharge from hospital

The discharge process for all children should include:

- correct timing of discharge from hospital
- counselling the mother on treatment and feeding of the child at home
- ensuring that the child's immunization status and record card are up-to-date
- communicating with the health worker who referred the child or who will be responsible for follow-up care
- instructions on when to return to the hospital for follow-up and on symptoms and signs indicating the need to return urgently
- assisting the family with special support (e.g. providing equipment for a child with a disability, or linking with community support organizations for children with HIV/AIDS).

12.1 Timing of discharge from hospital

In general, in the management of acute infections, the child can be considered ready for discharge after the clinical condition has improved markedly (afebrile, alert, eating and sleeping normally) and oral treatment has been started.

Decisions on when to discharge should be made on an individual basis, taking into consideration a number of factors, such as:

- the family's home circumstances and how much support is available to care for the child

- the staff's judgement of the likelihood that the treatment course will be completed at home
- the staff's judgement of the likelihood that the family will return immediately to the hospital if the child's condition should worsen.

Timing of discharge of the child with severe malnutrition is particularly important and is discussed separately in Chapter 7, page 192. In every case, the family should be given as much warning as possible of the discharge date so that appropriate arrangements can be made to support the child at home.

If the family removes the child prematurely against the advice of the hospital staff, counsel the mother on how to continue treatment at home and encourage her to bring the child for follow-up after 1–2 days, and to make contact with the local health worker for help in the follow-up care of the child.

12.2 Counselling

Mother's Card

A simple, pictorial card reminding the mother of home care instructions, when to return for follow-up care, and the signs indicating the need to return immediately to the hospital can be given to each mother. This Mother's Card will help her to remember the appropriate foods and fluids, and when to return to the health worker.

Appropriate Mother's Cards are being developed as part of local training for Integrated Management of Childhood Illness (IMCI). Check first whether one has been produced in your area and use that. If not, see Appendix 6 for details of where to find an example.

When reviewing the Mother's Card with the mother:

- Hold the card so that she can easily see the pictures, or allow her to hold it herself.
- Point to the pictures as you talk, and explain each one; this will help her to remember what the pictures represent.
- Mark the information that is relevant to the mother. For example, put a circle round the feeding advice for the child's age, and round the signs to return immediately. If the child has diarrhoea, tick the appropriate fluid(s) to be given. Record the date for the next immunization.
- Watch to see if the mother looks worried or puzzled. If so, encourage questions.
- Ask the mother to tell you in her own words what she should do at home. Encourage her to use the card to help her remember.

- Give her the card to take home. Suggest she show it to other family members. (If you do not have a large enough supply of cards to give to every mother, keep several in the clinic to show to mothers.)

12.3 Nutrition counselling

In the context of HIV counselling see page 219.

Identifying feeding problems

First, identify any feeding problems which have not been fully resolved.

Ask the following questions:

- ***Do you breastfeed your child?***
  - — How many times during the day?
  - — Do you also breastfeed during the night?
- ***Does the child take any other food or fluids?***
  - — What food or fluids?
  - — How many times a day?
  - — What do you use to feed the child?
  - — How large are the servings?
  - — Does the child receive his/her own serving?
  - — Who feeds the child and how?

Compare the child's actual feeding with the recommended guidelines for feeding a child of that age (see section 10.1.2, page 267). Identify any differences and list these as feeding problems.

In addition to the issues addressed above, consider:

- ***Difficulty in breastfeeding***
- ***Use of a feeding bottle***
- ***Lack of active feeding***
- ***Not feeding well during the illness***

Advise the mother how to overcome problems and how to feed the child.

Refer to local feeding recommendations for children of different ages. These recommendations should include details of locally appropriate energy-rich and nutrient-rich complementary foods.

Even when specific feeding problems are not found, praise the mother for what she does well. Give her advice that promotes:

- breastfeeding
- improved complementary feeding practices using locally available energy- and nutrient-rich foods
- the giving of nutritious snacks to children aged ≥2 years.

Examples of nutritionally adequate diets (see Chart 15, page 106 in the WHO manual *Management of the child with a serious infection or severe malnutrition* (see reference on page 301)) could be printed on the reverse of a locally adapted Mother's Card.

12.4 Home treatment

- Use words the mother understands.
- Use teaching aids that are familiar (e.g. common containers for mixing ORS).
- Allow the mother to practise what she must do, e.g. preparing ORS solution or giving an oral medication, and encourage her to ask questions.
- Give advice in a helpful and constructive manner, praising the mother for correct answers or good practice.

Teaching mothers is not just about giving instructions. It should include the following steps:

- ***Give information***. Explain to the mother how to give the treatment, e.g. preparing ORS, giving an oral antibiotic, or applying eye ointment.
- ***Show an example***. Show the mother how to give the treatment by demonstrating what to do.
- ***Let her practise***. Ask the mother to prepare the medicine or give the treatment while you watch her. Help her as needed, so that she does it correctly.
- ***Check her understanding***. Ask the mother to repeat the instructions in her own words, or ask her questions to see that she has understood correctly.

12.5 Checking the mother's own health

If the mother is sick, provide treatment for her and help to arrange follow-up at a first-level clinic close to her home. Check the mother's nutritional status and give any appropriate counselling. Check the mother's immunization status and, if needed, give her tetanus toxoid. Make sure the mother has access to family planning and counselling about preventing sexually-transmitted diseases and HIV. If the child has tuberculosis, the mother should have a chest X-ray and

Mantoux test. Make sure the mother knows where to have them and explain why they are needed.

12.6 Checking immunization status

Ask to see the child's immunization card, and determine whether all the immunizations recommended for the child's age have been given. Note any immunizations the child still needs and explain this to the mother; then carry them out before the child leaves hospital and record them on the card.

Recommended immunization schedule

Table 33 lists WHO's international recommendations. National recommendations will take account of local disease patterns.

Table 33. Immunization schedule for infants recommended by the Expanded Programme on Immunization

		Age				
Vaccine		**Birth**	**6 weeks**	**10 weeks**	**14 weeks**	**9 months**
BCG		x				
Oral polio		x†	x	x	x	
DPT			x	x	x	
Hepatitis B	Scheme A*	x	x		x	
	Scheme B*		x	x	x	
Haemophilus influenzae type b			x	x	x	
Yellow fever						x**
Measles						x***

† In polio-endemic countries

* Scheme A is recommended in countries where perinatal transmission of hepatitis B virus is frequent (e.g. in South-East Asia). Scheme B may be used in countries where perinatal transmission is less frequent (e.g. in sub-Saharan Africa).

** In countries where yellow fever poses a risk.

*** In exceptional situations, where measles morbidity and mortality before 9 months of age represent more than 15% of cases and deaths, give an extra dose of measles vaccine at 6 months of age. The scheduled dose should also be given as soon as possible after 9 months of age.
The extra measles dose is also recommended for groups at high risk of measles death, such as infants in refugee camps, infants admitted to hospitals, HIV-positive infants, and infants affected by disasters and during outbreaks of measles.
A second opportunity to receive a dose of measles vaccine should be provided for all children. This may be done either as part of the routine schedule or in a campaign.

Contraindications

It is important to immunize all children, including those who are sick and malnourished, unless there are contraindications. There are ***only 3 contraindications*** to immunization:

- Do not give BCG or yellow fever vaccines to a child with *symptomatic* HIV infection/AIDS, but do give the other vaccines.
- Give all immunizations, including BCG and yellow fever vaccines, to a child with *asymptomatic* HIV infection.
- Do not give DPT-2 or -3 to a child who has had convulsions or shock within 3 days of the most recent dose.
- Do not give DPT to a child with recurrent convulsions or an active neurological disease of the central nervous system.

A child with diarrhoea who is due to receive OPV should be given a dose of OPV. However, this dose should ***not*** be counted in the schedule. Make a note on the child's immunization record that it coincided with diarrhoea, so that the health worker will know this and give the child an extra dose.

12.7 Communicating with the first-level health worker

Information needed

The first-level health worker who referred the child to hospital should receive information about the child's care in hospital, which should include:

- diagnosis/diagnoses
- treatment(s) given (and duration of stay in hospital)
- response of the child to this treatment
- instructions given to the mother for follow-up treatment or other care at home
- other matters for follow-up (e.g. immunizations).

If the child has a health card, the above information can be recorded on it and the mother should be requested to show this to the health worker. Where there is no health card, these details should be recorded in a short note for the mother and health worker.

12.8 Providing follow-up care

Children who do not require hospital admission but can be treated at home

Advise all mothers who are taking their children home, after assessment in the hospital, when to go to a health worker for follow-up care. Mothers may need to return to hospital:

- for a follow-up visit in a specific number of days (e.g. when it is necessary to check progress or the response to an antibiotic)
- if signs appear that suggest the illness is worsening
- for the child's next immunization.

It is especially important to teach the mother the signs indicating the need to return to hospital immediately. Guidance on the follow-up of specific clinical conditions is given in appropriate sections of this pocket book.

Follow-up for feeding and nutritional problems

- If a child has a feeding problem and you have recommended changes in feeding, follow up in 5 days to see if the mother has made the changes, and give further counselling if needed.
- If a child has anaemia, follow up in 14 days to give more oral iron.
- If the child has a very low weight, additional follow-up is needed in 30 days. This follow-up would involve weighing the child, reassessing feeding practices, and giving further nutritional counselling.

When to return immediately

Advise the mother to return immediately if the child develops any of the following signs:

- not able to drink or breastfeed
- becomes sicker
- develops a fever
- signs of illness return again after successful treatment in hospital
- in a child with a cough or cold: fast or difficult breathing
- in a child with diarrhoea: blood in stool or drinking poorly.

Next well-child visit

Remind the mother about the child's next visit for immunization and record the date on the Mother's Card or the child's immunization record.

Notes

Further reading

The technical basis for the recommendations is regularly reviewed and updated, available under www.who.int/child-adolescent-health

Management of the child with a serious infection or severe malnutrition. WHO, Geneva, 2000. URL: http://www.who.int/child-adolescent-health/publications/CHILD_HEALTH/WHO_FCH_CAH_00.1.htm

Major Childhood Problems in Countries with limited resources. Background book on *Management of the child with a serious infection or severe malnutrition.* Geneva, World Health Organization, 2003.

TB/HIV: a clinical manual. 2nd edition. Geneva, World Health Organization, 2003.

Treatment of tuberculosis: guidelines for national programmes. 3rd edition. Geneva, World Health Organization, 2003.

Breastfeeding counselling: a training course. WHO/CDR/93.5 (WHO/UNICEF/NUT/93.3). Geneva, World Health Organization, 1993.

Management of severe malnutrition: a manual for physicians and other senior health workers. Geneva, World Health Organization, 1999.

Management of severe malaria: a practical handbook. Geneva, World Health Organization, 2000.

Surgical care at the district hospital. Geneva, World Health Organization, 2003.

Clinical use of blood. Geneva, World Health Organization, 2001.

Managing Newborn Problems: A guide for doctors, nurses and midwives. Geneva, World Health Organization, 2003.

Oxygen therapy in the management of a child with acute respiratory infection. WHO/CAR/95.3. Geneva, World Health Organization, 1995.

Clinical use of oxygen. Geneva, World Health Organization, 2005.

Emergency Triage Assessment and Treatment (ETAT) course: Manual for participants, ISBN 92 4 159687 5; *Facilitator's guide,* ISBN 92 4 159688 3. Geneva, World Health Organization, 2006.

Notes

APPENDIX 1

Practical procedures

Practical procedures should first be explained to the parents, any risks discussed with them and their consent obtained. Procedures on young infants should be carried out in warm surroundings. Good light is essential. Patients who are older children should also be told about what is to happen. Analgesia should be given, where necessary.

Sedation for procedures

For some procedures (e.g. chest tube insertion or femoral cannulation) sedation with diazepam or light anaesthesia with ketamine should be considered (see section 9.1.2, page 229).

For diazepam sedation give 0.1–0.2 mg/kg IV. For ketamine light anaesthesia give 2–4 mg/kg IM. This takes 5–10 minutes to act and lasts for about 20 minutes.

When giving any sedation, manage the child's airway, beware of respiratory depression and monitor oxygen saturation with a pulse oximeter, where possible. Ensure you have a resuscitation bag available (and if possible oxygen).

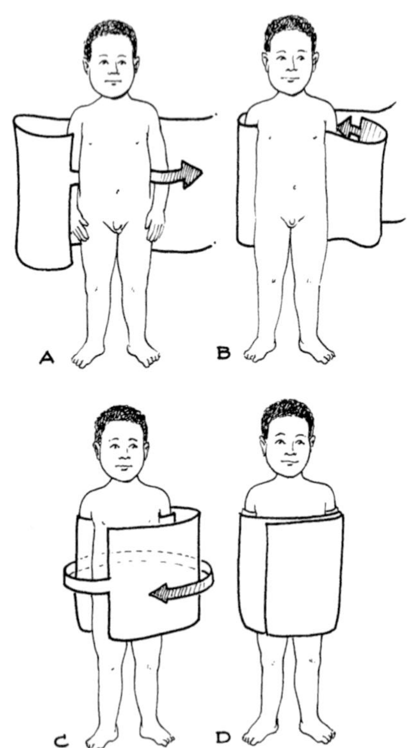

Wrapping the child to hold securely during a practical procedure

One end of a folded sheet should be pulled through under the arms on both sides (A and B). The other end is then brought across the front and wrapped around the child (C and D)

Restraining the child for examination of eyes, ears or mouth

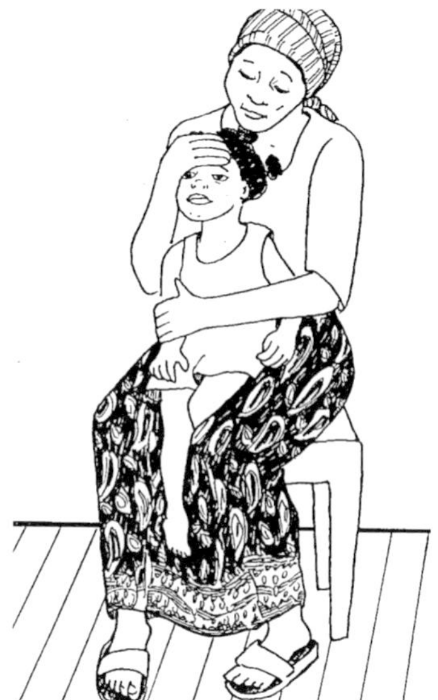

A1.1 Giving injections

First, find out whether the child has reacted adversely to drugs in the past. Wash your hands thoroughly. Where possible, use disposable needles and syringes. Or else, sterilize reusable needles and syringes.

Clean the chosen site with an antiseptic solution. Carefully check the dose of the drug to be given and draw the correct amount into the syringe. Expel the air from the syringe before injecting. Always record the name and amount of the drug given. Discard disposable syringes in a safe container.

A1.1.1 Intramuscular

In >2-year-old children, give the injection in the outer thigh or in the upper, outer quadrant of the buttock, well away from the sciatic nerve. In younger or severely malnourished children, use the outer side of the thigh midway between the hip and the knee, or over the deltoid muscle in the upper arm. Push the needle (23–25 gauge) into the muscle at a 90° angle (45° angle in the thigh). Draw back the plunger to make sure there is no blood (if there is, withdraw slightly and try again). Give the drug by pushing the plunger slowly till the end. Remove the needle and press firmly over the injection site with a small swab or cotton wool.

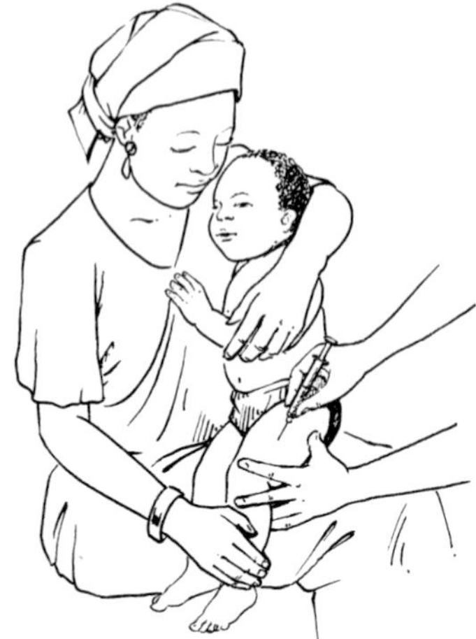

Intramuscular injection into the thigh

A1.1.2 Subcutaneous

Select the site, as described above for intramuscular injection. Push the needle (23–25 gauge) under the skin at a 45° angle into the subcutaneous fatty tissue. Do not go deep to enter the underlying muscle. Draw back the plunger to make sure there is no blood (if there is, withdraw slightly and try again). Give the drug by pushing the plunger slowly till the end. Remove the needle and press firmly over the injection site with cotton wool.

A1.1.3 Intradermal

For an intradermal injection, select an undamaged and uninfected area of skin (e.g. over the deltoid in the upper arm). Stretch the skin between the thumb and forefinger of one hand; with the other, slowly insert the needle (25 gauge), bevel upwards, for about 2 mm just under and almost parallel to the surface of the skin. Considerable resistance is felt when injecting intradermally. A raised, blanched bleb showing the surface of the hair follicles is a sign that the injection has been given correctly.

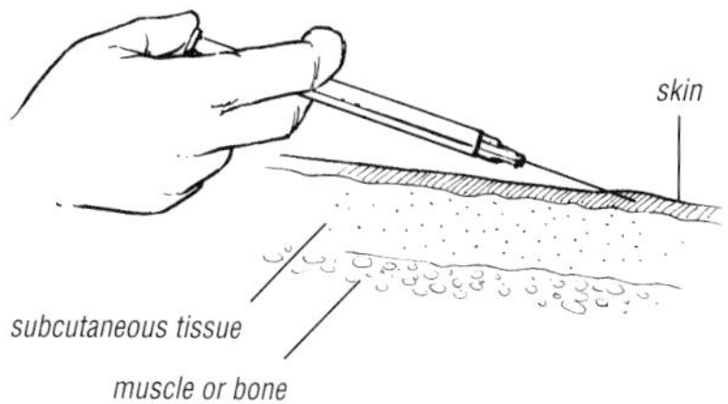

Intradermal injection (for example in Mantoux test)

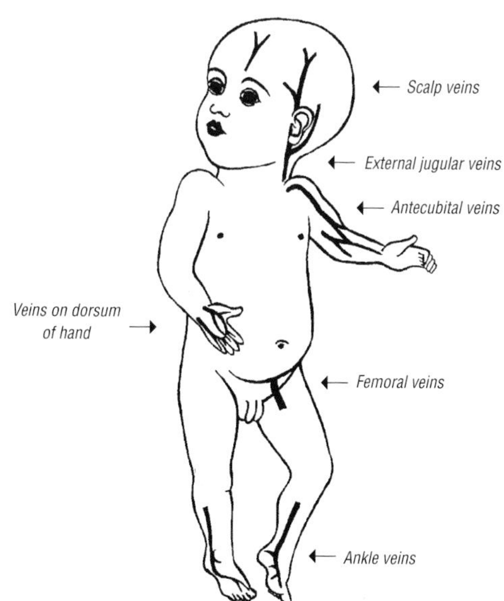

Sites for IV access in infants and young children

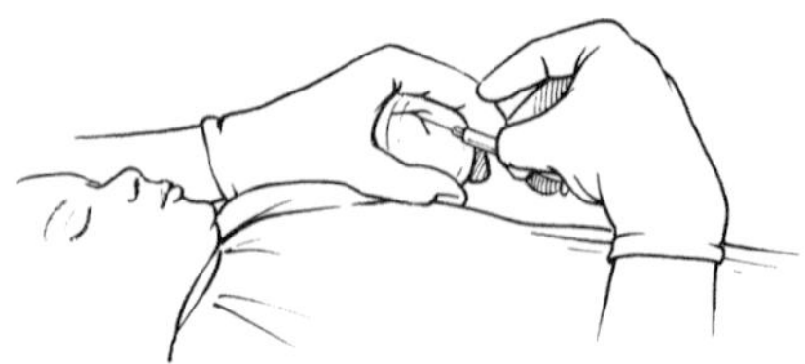

Inserting an IV cannula into a vein on the back of the hand. The hand is bent to obstruct venous return and thus make the veins visible.

A1.2 Procedures for giving parenteral fluids

A1.2.1 Insertion of an indwelling IV cannula in a peripheral vein

Select a suitable vein to place the cannula or gauge 21 or 23 butterfly needle.

Peripheral vein

- Identify an accessible peripheral vein. In young children aged >2 months, this is usually the cephalic vein in the antecubital fossa or the fourth interdigital vein on the dorsum of the hand.
- An assistant should keep the position of the limb steady and should act as a tourniquet by obstructing the venous return with his fingers lightly closed around the limb.

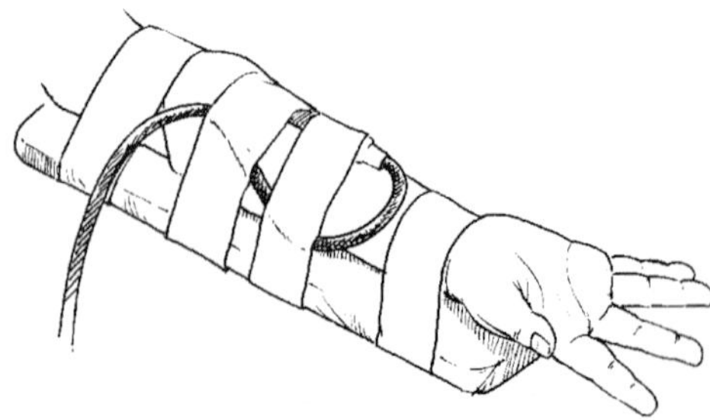

Splinted arm for IV infusion to prevent bending of the elbow

- Clean the surrounding skin with an antiseptic solution (such as spirit, iodine, isopropyl alcohol, or 70% alcohol solution), then introduce the cannula into the vein and insert most of its length. Fix the catheter securely with tape. Apply a splint with the limb in an appropriate position (e.g. elbow extended, wrist slightly flexed).

Scalp veins

These are often used in children aged <2 years but work best in young infants.

- Find a suitable scalp vein (usually in the midline of the forehead, the temporal area, or above or behind the ear).
- Shave the area if necessary and clean the skin with an antiseptic solution. The assistant should occlude the vein proximal to the site of puncture. Fill a syringe with normal saline and flush the butterfly set. Disconnect the syringe and leave the end of the tubing open. Introduce the butterfly needle as described above. Blood flowing back slowly through the tubing indicates that the needle is in the vein.
- Care should be taken not to cannulate an artery, which is recognized by palpation. If there should be a pulsatile spurting of blood, withdraw the needle and apply pressure until the bleeding stops; then look for a vein.

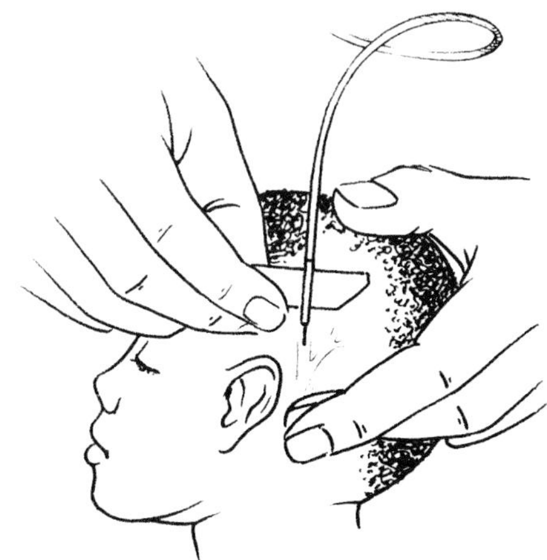

Inserting a butterfly needle into a scalp vein to set up an IV infusion in a young infant

Care of the cannula

Secure the cannula when introduced. This may require the splinting of neighbouring joints to limit the movement of the catheter. Keep the overlying skin clean and dry. Fill the cannula with heparin solution or normal saline immediately after the initial insertion and after each injection.

Common complications

Superficial *infection* of the skin at the cannula site is the commonest complication. The infection may lead to a *thrombophlebitis* which will occlude the vein and result in fever. The surrounding skin is red and tender. Remove the cannula to reduce the risk of further spread of the infection. Apply a warm moist compress to the site for 30 minutes every 6 hours. If fever persists for more than 24 hours, antibiotic treatment (effective against staphylococci) should be given, e.g. cloxacillin.

IV drug administration through an indwelling cannula

Attach the syringe containing the IV drug to the injection port of the cannula and introduce the drug. Once all the drug has been given, inject 0.5 ml heparin solution (10–100 units/ml) or normal saline into the cannula until all the blood has been expelled and the catheter is filled with the solution.

If infusion through a peripheral vein or scalp vein is not possible, and it is essential to give IV fluids to keep the child alive:

- set up an intraosseous infusion
- ***or*** use a central vein
- ***or*** perform a venous cut down.

A1.2.2 Intraosseous infusion

When carried out by a well trained and experienced health worker, intraosseous infusion is a safe, simple and reliable method of giving fluid and drugs *in an emergency*.

The first choice for the puncture is the proximal tibia. The site for needle insertion is in the middle of the antero-medial surface of the tibia, at the junction of the upper and middle third to avoid damaging the epiphyseal plate (which is higher in the tibia). An alternative site for needle insertion is the distal femur, 2 cm above the lateral condyle.

- Prepare the necessary equipment, i.e.:
  - — bone marrow aspiration or intraosseous needles (15–18 gauge or, if not

available, 21 gauge). If these are not available, large-bore hypodermic or butterfly needles can be used in young children
- — antiseptic solution and sterile gauze to clean the site
- — a sterile 5-ml syringe filled with normal saline
- — a second sterile 5-ml syringe
- — IV infusion equipment
- — sterile gloves.

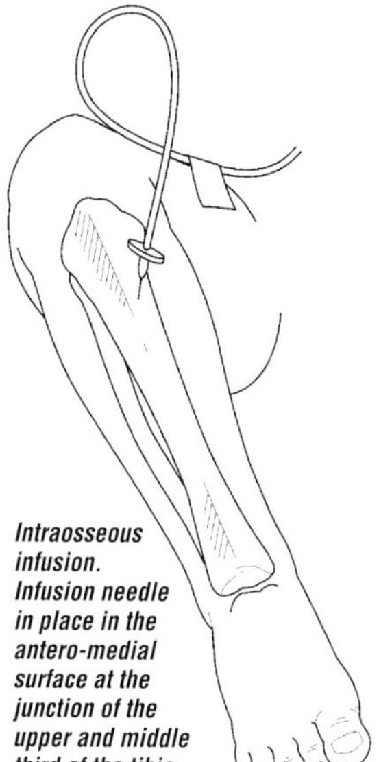

Intraosseous infusion. Infusion needle in place in the antero-medial surface at the junction of the upper and middle third of the tibia.

- Place padding under the child's knee so that it is bent 30° from the straight (180°) position, with the heel resting on the table.
- Locate the correct position (described above and shown in the illustration).
- Wash the hands and put on sterile gloves.
- Clean the skin over and surrounding the site with an antiseptic solution.
- Stabilize the proximal tibia with the left hand (this hand is now not sterile) by grasping the thigh and knee above and lateral to the cannulation site, with the fingers and thumb wrapped around the knee but not directly behind the insertion site.
- Palpate the landmarks again with the sterile glove (right hand).
- Insert the needle at a 90° angle with the bevel pointing towards the foot. Advance the needle slowly using a gentle but firm, twisting or drilling motion.
- Stop advancing the needle when you feel a sudden decrease in resistance or when you can aspirate blood. The needle should now be fixed in the bone.
- Remove the stylet.
- Aspirate 1 ml of the marrow contents (looks like blood), using the 5-ml syringe, to confirm that the needle is in the marrow cavity.
- Attach the second 5-ml syringe filled with normal saline. Stabilize the needle

and slowly inject 3 ml while palpating the area for any leakage under the skin. If no infiltration is seen, start the infusion.

- Apply dressings and secure the needle in its place.

Note: Failure to aspirate marrow contents does not mean that the needle is not correctly placed.

- Monitor the infusion by the ease with which the fluid flows and by the clinical response of the patient.
- Check that the calf does not swell during the infusion.

Stop the intraosseous infusion as soon as venous access is available. In any case, it should not continue for more than 8 hours.

Complications include:

- Incomplete penetration of the bony cortex

  Signs: The needle is not well fixed; infiltration occurs under the skin.
- Penetration of the posterior bone cortex (more common)

  Sign: Infiltration occurs, calf becomes tense.
- Infection

  Signs: Cellulitis at the site of the infusion.

A1.2.3 **Central vein cannulation**

These should not be used routinely, and only when IV access is urgent. Remove the cannula from a central vein as soon as possible (i.e. when IV fluid is no longer essential or when a peripheral vein can be cannulated successfully).

External jugular vein

- Hold the child securely, with the head turned to one side away from the puncture site and slightly lower than the body (15–30 degree head down position). Restrain the child as necessary in this position.
- After cleaning the skin with an antiseptic solution, identify the external jugular vein as it passes over the sternocleidomastoid muscle at the junction of its middle and lower thirds. An assistant should occlude the vein to keep it distended and keep its position steady by pressing over the lower end of the visible part of the vein just above the clavicle. Pierce the skin over the vein, pointing in the direction of the clavicle. A short firm thrust will push the needle into the vein. Proceed with cannulation of the vein, as described above with a peripheral vein.

Femoral vein

- Do not attempt in young infants.
- The child should be supine with buttocks 5 cm elevated on a rolled up towel so that the hip is slightly extended. Abduct and externally rotate the hip joint and flex the knee. An assistant should hold the leg in this position and keep the other leg out of the way. If the child has pain, infiltrate the area with 1% lignocaine.
- Clean the skin with an antiseptic solution. Palpate the femoral artery (below the inguinal ligament in the middle of the femoral triangle). The femoral nerve lies lateral and the femoral vein runs medial to the artery.
- Clean the skin with antiseptic. Introduce the needle at 10–20 degrees to the skin, 1–2 cm distal to the inguinal ligament, 0.5–1 cm medial to the femoral artery.
- Venous blood will flow into the syringe when the needle is in the femoral vein.
- Proceed with cannulation of the vein by advancing the cannula at an angle of 10 degrees to the skin.
- Stitch the cannula in place and put a sterile occlusive dressing on the skin under the cannula and another one over the top of the cannula. Fix firmly in place with adhesive tape. It may be necessary to splint the leg to prevent flexion of the hip.
- Monitor the site closely for as long as the cannula is in place, taking care to keep the leg immobile during the infusion. A femoral line can last for up to 5 days with correct care.
- Withdraw the cannula after the IV infusion has been given, and apply firm pressure for 2–3 minutes over the site.

A1.2.4 Venous cut-down

This is less appropriate if speed is essential.

- Immoblize the child's lower leg and clean the skin, as described above. Identify the long saphenous vein, which lies half a fingerbreadth (in the infant) or one fingerbreadth (in the older child) superior and anterior to the medial malleolus.
- Infiltrate the skin with 1% lignocaine and make an incision through the skin perpendicular to the course of the vein. Bluntly dissect the subcutaneous tissue with haemostat forceps.

- Identify and free a 1–2 cm strip of vein. Pass a proximal and distal ligature.
- Tie off the distal end of the vein, keeping the ties as long as possible.
- Make a small hole in the upper part of the exposed vein and insert the cannula into this, while holding the distal tie to stabilize the position of the vein.
- Secure the cannula in place with the upper ligature.
- Attach a syringe filled with normal saline and ensure that the fluid flows freely up the vein. If it does not, check that the cannula is in the vein or try withdrawing it slightly to improve the flow.
- Tie the distal ligature around the catheter, then close the skin incision with interrupted sutures. Fix the cannula to the skin and cover with a sterile dressing.

A1.2.5 Umbilical vein catheterization

This procedure can be used for resuscitation or exchange transfusion and is usually possible in neonates in the first few days of life. In some circumstances it might be possible up to 5 days of life.

- Attach a sterile 3-way tap and syringe to a 5 French gauge catheter and fill with sterile 0.9% saline, then close the tap to prevent air entry (which may cause an air embolus)
- Clean the umbilical cord and surrounding skin with an antiseptic solution, then tie a suture around the base of the cord.
- Cut the cord 1–2 cms from the base with a sterile scalpel. Identify the umbilical vein (larger gaping vessel) and umbilical arteries (two thicker walled vessels apart from the vein). Hold the cord (near the umbilical vein) with sterile forceps.
- Hold near end of catheter with sterile forceps and advance it into the vein (it should pass easily) for 4–6 cms
- Check that catheter is not kinked and that blood draws back easily; if there is a block pull gently on the cord, pull back the catheter partly and re-insert
- Secure with 2 sutures into the cord leaving 5 cm long suture ends. Tape suture and catheter (see diagram)
- After removal, apply pressure to the umbilical stump for 5–10 minutes.

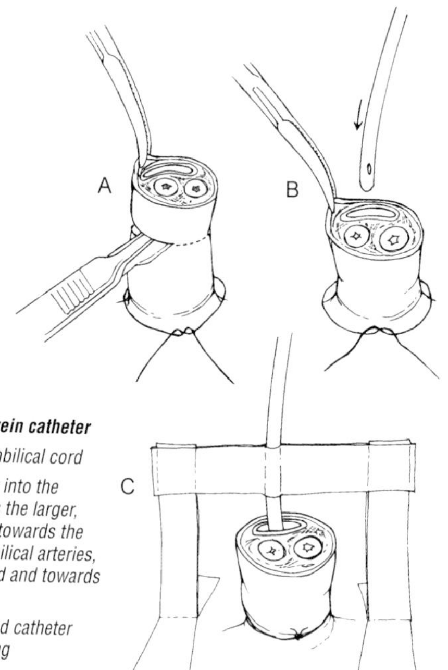

Inserting an umbilical vein catheter

A. Preparation of the umbilical cord

B. Inserting the catheter into the umbilical vein. This is the larger, thin walled structure towards the head. Note the 2 umbilical arteries, which are thick-walled and towards the legs of the baby.

C. Fixation of the inserted catheter which prevents kinking

A1.3 Insertion of a nasogastric tube

- Holding the tip of the tube against the child's nose, measure the distance from the nose to the ear lobe, then to the xiphisternum (epigastrium). Mark the tube at this point.
- Hold the child firmly. Lubricate the tip of the catheter with water and pass it directly into one nostril, pushing it slowly in. It should pass easily down into the stomach without resistance. When the measured distance is reached, fix the tube with tape at the nose.
- Aspirate a small amount of stomach contents with a syringe to confirm that the tube is in place (check that it turns blue litmus paper pink). If no aspirate

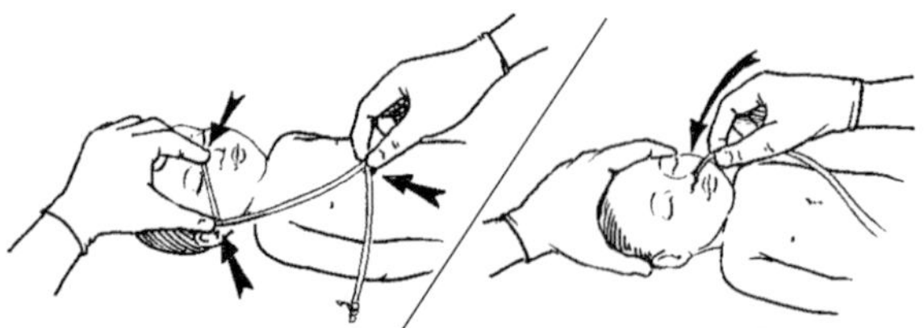

Inserting a nasogastric tube. The distance is measured from the nose to the ear and then to the epigastrium, and then the tube is inserted to the measured distance.

is obtained, inject air down the tube and listen over the abdomen with a stethoscope.

- If there is any doubt about the location of the tube, withdraw it and start again.
- When the tube is in place, fix a 20-ml syringe (without the plunger) to the end of the tube, and pour food or fluid into the syringe, allowing it to flow by gravity.

If oxygen therapy is to be given by nasopharyngeal catheter at the same time, pass both tubes down the same nostril and try to keep the other nostril patent by wiping away crusts and secretions or pass the feeding tube through the mouth.

A1.4 Lumbar puncture

The following are *contraindications*:

- signs of raised intracranial pressure (unequal pupils, rigid posture or paralysis in any of the limbs or trunk, irregular breathing)
- skin infection in the area through which the needle will have to pass.

If contraindications are present, the potential value of the information gained from a lumbar puncture should be carefully weighed against the risk of the procedure. If in doubt, it might be better to start treatment for suspected meningitis, and delay performing a lumbar puncture.

- *Position the child*

There are two possible positions:

— the child lying down on the left side (particularly for young infants)

— in the sitting position (particularly for older children).

Lumbar puncture when the child is lying on the side:

- A hard surface should be used. Place the child on the side so that the vertebral column is parallel to this surface and the transverse axis of the back is vertical (see Figure).
- The assistant should flex the back of the child, pull up the knees towards the chest, and hold the child at the upper back between the shoulders and buttocks so that the back is bent. Hold the child firmly in this position. Make sure that the airway is not obstructed and the child can breathe normally. Take particular care in holding young infants. The assistant should not hold a young infant by the neck nor flex the neck to avoid airway obstruction.
- *Check anatomical landmarks*
  - Locate the space between the third and fourth or between the fourth and fifth lumbar vertebrae. (The third lumbar vertebra is at the junction of the line between the iliac crests and the vertebral column).
- *Prepare the site*
  - Use aseptic technique. Scrub the hands and wear sterile gloves.
  - Prepare the skin around the site with an antiseptic solution.
  - Sterile towels may be used.
  - In older children who are alert, give a local anaesthetic (1% lignocaine) infiltrated in the skin over the site.

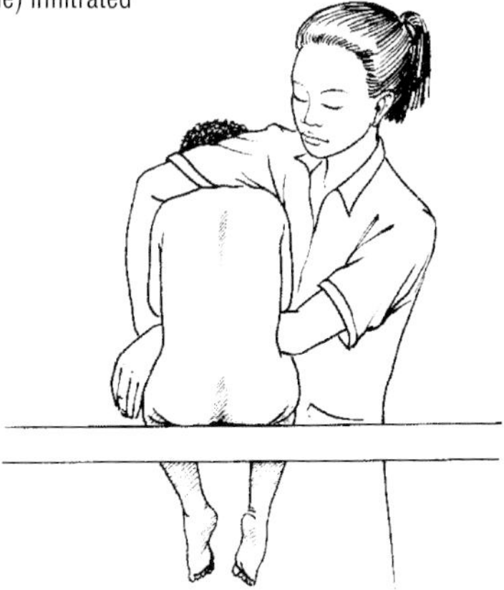

Restraining an older child in sitting position in order to carry out a lumbar puncture

- *Perform the lumbar puncture*
  - Use an LP needle with stylet (22 gauge for a young infant, 20 gauge for an older infant and child; if these are not available, hypodermic needles may be used). Insert the needle into the middle of the intervertebral space and aim the needle towards the umbilicus.
  - Advance the needle slowly. The needle will pass easily until it encounters the ligament between the vertebral processes. More pressure is needed to penetrate this ligament, less resistance is felt as the dura is penetrated. In young infants this decrease in resistance is not always felt, so advance the needle very carefully.
  - Withdraw the stylet, and drops of cerebrospinal fluid will pass out of the needle. If no CSF is obtained, the stylet can be reinserted and the needle advanced slightly.
  - Obtain a sample of 0.5–1 ml CSF and place in a sterile container.
  - Withdraw the needle and stylet completely and put pressure over the site for a few seconds. Put a sterile dressing over the needle puncture site.

If the needle is introduced too far, a lumbar vein may be punctured. This will result in a "traumatic tap" and the spinal fluid will be bloody. The needle should be withdrawn and the procedure repeated in another disc space.

A1.5 Insertion of a chest drain

Pleural effusions should be drained, except when small. It is sometimes necessary to drain both sides of the chest. You may have to drain the chest 2 or 3 times if the fluid keeps coming back.

Diagnostic procedure

- Consider giving the child sedation or light anaesthesia with ketamine.
- Wash the hands and put on sterile gloves.
- Lay the child on the back.
- Clean the skin over the chest for at least 2 minutes with an antiseptic solution (for example, 70% alcohol).
- Select a point in the mid-axillary line (at the side of the chest) just below the level of the nipple (fifth intercostal space, see Figure, page 319).
- Inject about 1ml of 1% lignocaine into the skin and subcutaneous tissue at this point.

- Insert a needle or catheter through the skin and pleura and aspirate to confirm the presence of pleural fluid. Withdraw a sample for microscopy and other tests and place in a container.

If the fluid is clear (straw-coloured or brownish), pull out the needle or catheter after withdrawing enough fluid to relieve distress and put a dressing over the puncture site. Consider a differential diagnosis of tuberculosis (see section 4.8, page 101).

If the fluid is thin pus or cloudy (like milk), leave the catheter in place so that you can draw out more pus several times a day. Make sure you seal the end of the catheter so that no air can get in.

If the fluid is thick pus which cannot pass easily through the needle or catheter, insert a chest tube (see below).

Insertion of a chest tube

- Select and prepare the site as described above.
  - Make a 2–3 cm skin incision along the line of the intercostal space, just *above* the rib below (to avoid damaging the vessels which lie under the lower edge of each rib).

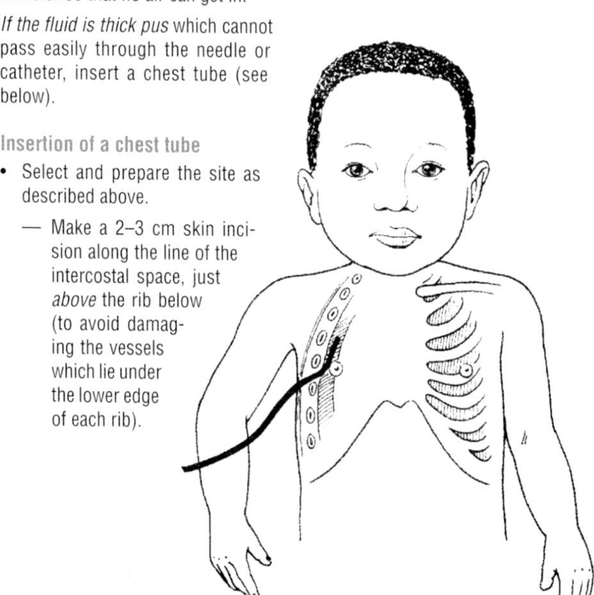

Insertion of a chest tube: the site is selected in the mid-axillary line in the 5th intercostal space (at the level of the nipple) on the superior aspect of the 6th rib.

- Use sterile forceps to push through the subcutaneous tissue just above the upper edge of the rib and puncture the pleura.
- Pass a gloved finger into the incision and clear a path to the pleura (this is not possible in infants).
- Use the forceps to hold the drainage catheter (16 gauge) and introduce it into the chest for several centimetres, pointing upwards. Ensure that all drainage holes of the catheter are inside the chest.
- Connect the catheter to a collection bottle with an underwater seal.
- Suture the catheter in place, secure with tape, and apply a gauze dressing.

A1.6 Supra-pubic aspiration

Aspirate to a depth of 3 cm in the midline at the proximal transverse crease above the pubis with a 23 G needle under sterile conditions. Do this only in a child with a full bladder, which can be demonstrated by percussion. Do not use urine bags to collect urine because the specimens may become contaminated.

Have a clean urine jar ready in case the child passes urine during the procedure.

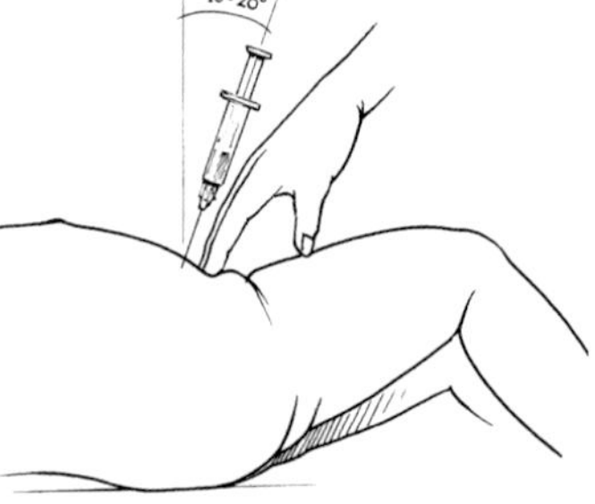

Position for carrying out suprapubic aspirate—side view. Note the angle of insertion of the needle.

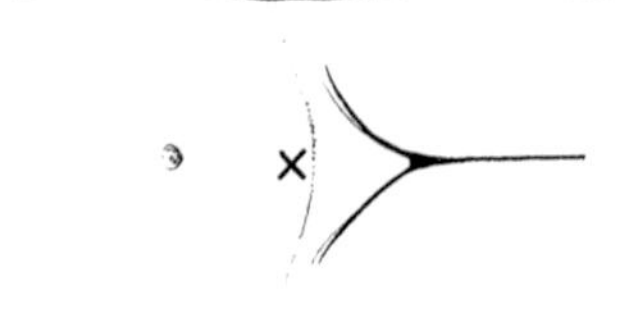

Selecting the place for a suprapubic aspirate. The bladder is punctured in the midline, just above the symphysis.

A1.7 Measuring blood glucose

Blood glucose can be measured with rapid diagnostic tests ("Dextrostix") at the bedside, which provide an estimation of blood glucose within a few minutes. There are several brands on the market, which differ slightly in how they should be used. Instructions on the box and the package leaflet must therefore be read before using them.

Generally, a drop of blood is placed on the reagent strip, and left for 30 seconds to one minute, depending on the brand of strip. The blood is then wiped off, and after another fixed period of time (e.g. one further minute), the colour change on the reagent field of the strip is read. For this, the resulting colour is compared with a colour scale printed on the box. This allows to estimate the glucose level to be within a certain range, e.g. between 2 and 5 mmol/l, but does not allow exact determinations.

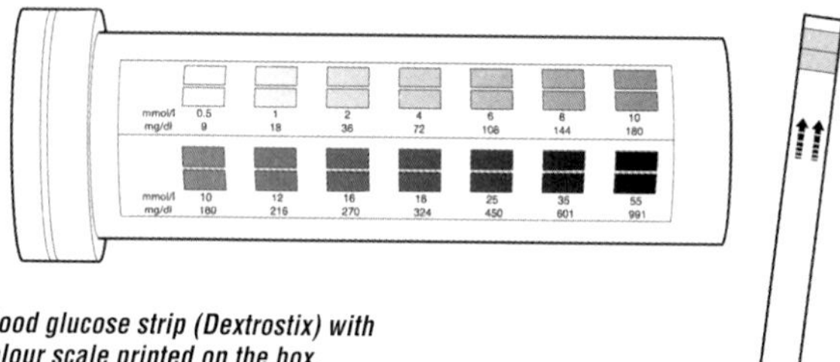

Blood glucose strip (Dextrostix) with colour scale printed on the box.

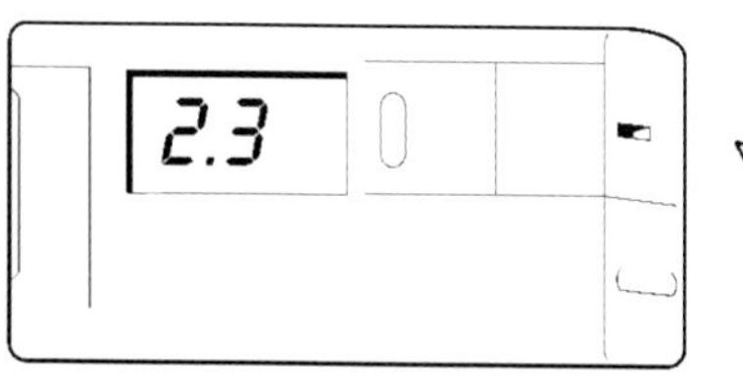

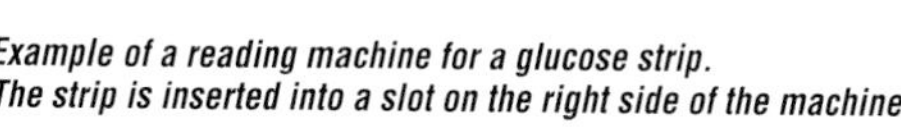

Example of a reading machine for a glucose strip. The strip is inserted into a slot on the right side of the machine.

Some strips come with an electronic reading machine, which has a battery as a power source. After the blood is wiped off, the strip is inserted into the reading machine, which provides a more accurate value.

As the reagents deteriorate with exposure to ambient humidity, it is important that they are kept in a closed box, and that the box is closed again right after a strip has been taken out.

Notes

Notes

APPENDIX 2

Drug dosages/regimens

This section gives drug doses for the drugs mentioned in these guidelines. For ease of use and to avoid the need to make calculations, doses are given according to body weight of the child. Errors in calculating drug doses are common in hospital practice worldwide, so calculations should be avoided, where possible. A number of doses are given covering a range of body weights from 3–29 kg.

A drug table for neonates in the first 2 months of life is included in Chapter 3, pages 62–66.

However for some drugs (for example, antiretrovirals), it is better to calculate the EXACT individual drug doses based on the body weight of the child, where this is possible. These drugs include those for which the exact dose is critically important to ensure a therapeutic effect or to avoid toxicity, e.g. digoxin, chloramphenicol, aminophylline and antiretroviral drugs.

For some antiretroviral drugs, recommended dosages are often given according to the surface area of the child. A table giving approximate child surface areas for different weight categories is given below to help with this calculation. The doses in the table can then be used to check that the calculated dose is approximately correct (and to check that a calculation error has not been made).

$$\text{Body surface area in m}^2 = \sqrt{\frac{\{\text{height (cm) x weight (kg)}\}}{3600}}$$

thus a child weighing 10 kg and 72 cm long has a body surface area of

$$\sqrt{(10\text{x}72/3600)} = 0.45.$$

DRUGS

Drug dosage by surface area (m^2) of the child

Age or weight of child	Surface area
Neonatal (< 1 month)	0.2–0.25 m^2
Young infant (1–<3 months)	0.25–0.35 m^2
Child 5–9 kg	0.3–0.45 m^2
Child 10–14 kg	0.45–0.6 m^2
Child 15–19 kg	0.6–0.8 m^2
Child 20–24 kg	0.8–0.9 m^2
Child 25–29 kg	0.9–1.1 m^2
Child 30–39 kg	1.1–1.3 m^2

Footnote:

Example: if the recommended dose is given as 400mg/m^2 twice per day, then for a child in the weight range 15–19 kg the recommended dose will be:

(0.6–0.8) x 400 = 244–316 mg twice per day

	Dosage	Form	Dose according to body weight				
			3–<6 kg	6–<10 kg	10–<15 kg	15–<20 kg	20–29 kg
Abacavir—see separate table for HIV drugs, page 350							
Adrenaline—see Epinephrine							
Aminophylline *For asthma*	Oral: 6 mg/kg	Tablets: 100 mg	1/4	1/2	3/4	1	1 1/2
		Tablets: 200 mg	—	1/4	1/2	1/2	3/4
	IV: *Calculate EXACT dose based on body weight where possible; use these doses only where this is not possible*						
	Loading dose: IV: 5–6 mg/kg (max. 300 mg) slowly over 20–60 minutes	250 mg/10ml vial	1 ml	1.5 ml	2.5 ml	3.5 ml	5 ml
	Maintenance dose: IV: 5 mg/kg up to every 6 hours		1 ml	1.5 ml	2.5 ml	3.5 ml	5 ml
	OR by continuous infusion 0.9 mg/kg/hour		*calculate EXACT dose*				

Give IV loading dose only if the child has not taken aminophylline or theophylline within 24 hours.
For dosage and dosage intervals for apnoea in neonates and premature infants see page 62.

	Dosage	Form	Dose according to body weight 3–<6 kg	6–<10 kg	10–<15 kg	15–<20 kg	20–29 kg
Amodiaquine	Oral: 10 mg/kg daily for 3 days	Tablet 153 mg base	—	—	1	1	1
Amoxicillin	15 mg/kg three times per day	250 mg tablet	1/4	1/2	3/4	1	1 1/2
		Syrup (containing 125 mg/5 ml)	2.5 ml	5 ml	7.5 ml	10 ml	—
For pneumonia	25 mg/kg two times a day	250 mg tablet	1/2	1	1 1/2	2	2 1/2
		Syrup (containing 125 mg/5 ml)	5 ml	10 ml	15 ml	—	—
Amphotericin *For oesophageal candidiasis*	0.25 mg/kg/day increasing to 1 mg/kg/day as tolerated by IV infusion over 6 hours daily for 10–14 days	50 mg vial	—	2–8 mg	3–12 mg	4.5–18 mg	6–24 mg
Ampicillin	Oral: 25 mg/kg four times a day§	250 mg tablet	1/2	1	1	1 1/2	2
	IM/IV: 50 mg/kg every 6 hours	Vial of 500 mg mixed with 2.1 ml sterile water to give 500 mg/2.5 ml	1 ml†	2 ml	3 ml	5 ml	6 ml

§ These oral doses are for mild disease. If oral ampicillin is required after a course of injectable ampicillin for severe disease, the oral dose must be 2–4 times higher than that given here.

† For dosages and dosage intervals in neonates and premature infants, see page 62.

Anti TB antibiotics—see details on page 352

	Dosage	Form	Dose according to body weight 3–<6 kg	6–<10 kg	10–<15 kg	15–<20 kg	20–29 kg
Artemether *For severe malaria*	**Loading dose:** IM: 3.2 mg/kg	40 mg/1 ml ampoule 80 mg/1 ml ampoule	0.4 ml 0.2 ml	0.8 ml 0.4 ml	1.2 ml 0.6 ml	1.6 ml 0.8 ml	2.4 ml 1.2 ml
	Maintenance dose: IM: 1.6 mg/kg	40 mg/1 ml ampoule 80 mg/1 ml ampoule	0.2 ml 0.1 ml	0.4 ml 0.2 ml	0.6 ml 0.3 ml	0.8 ml 0.4 ml	1.2 ml 0.6 ml
Give the maintenance dose daily for a minimum of 3 days until the patient can take oral treatment with an effective anti-malarial.							
Artemether/ lumefantrine *For uncomplicated malaria*	Oral: 1.5/12 mg/kg twice daily for 3 days	Tablet: 20mg artemether/ 120mg lumefantrine	—	1	1	2	2§
§ From 25 kg: 3 tablets/dose							
Artesunate *For severe malaria*	**Loading dose:** IV: 2.4 mg/kg given by IV bolus	60 mg artesunic acid (already dissolved in 0.6 ml of saline/sodium bicarbonate) in 3.4 ml of saline/glucose	0.8 ml	1.6 ml	2.4 ml	3.2 ml	4.6 ml
	Maintenance dose: IV: 1.2 mg/kg		0.4 ml	0.8 ml	1.2 ml	1.6 ml	2.3 ml
For malaria (non severe) In combination therapy	Oral: 2.5 mg once daily for 3 days	Tablet 50 mg	—	—	1	1	1

The IV solution should be prepared just before use. Dilute both the loading and maintenance doses by dissolving 60 mg artesunic acid (which is already dissolved in 0.6 ml of 5% sodium bicarbonate) in 3.4 ml of 5% glucose. Give the maintenance dose at 12 and 24 hours, and then daily for 6 days. If the patient is able to swallow, give the daily dose orally.

	Dosage	Form	Dose according to body weight				
			3–<6 kg	6–<10 kg	10–<15 kg	15–<20 kg	20–29 kg
Aspirin	Oral: 10–20 mg/kg 4–6 hourly	300 mg tablet	—	1/4	1/2	3/4	1
Note: avoid in young children, if possible, because of the risk of Reye's syndrome.							
Benzathine penicillin—see penicillin							
Benzyl penicillin—see penicillin							
Bupivicaine	up to 1mg/kg	0.25% solution					
Caffeine citrate	*For use in neonates, see page 63.*						
Cefotaxime	IM/IV: 50 mg/kg every 6 hours	Vial of 500 mg mixed with 2 ml sterile water OR vial of 1 g mixed with 4 ml sterile water OR vial of 2 g mixed with 8 ml sterile water	0.8 ml§	1.5 ml	2.5 ml	3.5 ml	5 ml

§ For dosage and dosage intervals in neonates and premature infants see page 63.

	Dosage	Form	Dose according to body weight				
			3–<6 kg	6–<10 kg	10–<15 kg	15–<20 kg	20–29 kg
Ceftriaxone	IM/IV: 80 mg/kg/day as a single dose given over 30 min	Vial of 1 g mixed with 9.6 ml sterile water to give 1g/10 ml *OR* vial of 2 g mixed with 19 ml of sterile water to give 2g/20 ml	3 ml§	6 ml	10 ml	14 ml	20 ml
For meningitis	IM/IV: 50 mg/kg every 12 hours (max single dose 4 g)		2 ml	4 ml	6 ml	9 ml	12.5 ml
	OR						
	IM/IV: 100 mg/kg once daily		4 ml	8 ml	12 ml	18 ml	25 ml
For ophthalmia neonatorum	IM: 50 mg/kg single dose max 125 mg		*calculate EXACT dose*				

§ For dosage and dosage intervals in neonates and premature infants, see page 64.

Cefalexin	12.5 mg/kg four times per day	250 mg tablet	1/4	1/2	3/4	1	1 1/4

DRUGS

	Dosage	Form	Dose according to body weight 3–<6 kg	6–<10 kg	10–<15 kg	15–<20 kg	20–29 kg
Chloramphenicol§	*Calculate EXACT dose based on body weight. Only use these doses if this is not possible.*						
For meningitis	IV: 25 mg/kg every 6 hours (maximum 1g per dose)	vial of 1 g mixed with 9.2 ml sterile water to give 1 g/10ml	0.75–1.25 ml†	1.5–2.25 ml	2.5–3.5 ml	3.75–4.75 ml	5–7.25 ml
For cholera	IM: 20 mg/kg every 6 hours for 3 days	vial of 1 g mixed with 3.2 ml sterile water to give 1 g/4ml	0.3–0.5 ml†	0.6–0.9 ml	1–1.4 ml	1.5–1.9 ml	2–2.9 ml
For other conditions	Oral: 25 mg/kg every 8 hours (maximum 1g per dose	125 mg/5ml suspension (palmitate)	3–5 ml	6–9 ml	10–14 ml	15–19 ml	—
		250 mg capsule	—	—	1	1½	2

§ Phenobarbital reduces and phenytonin increases chloramphenicol levels when given together.
† For dosage and dosage intervals in neonates and infants, see page 64.

	Dosage	Form	3–<6 kg	6–<10 kg	10–<15 kg	15–<20 kg	20–29 kg
Oily chloramphenicol (for treatment of meningocccal meningitis during epidemics)	100 mg/kg single dose; maximum of 3 grams	IM: vial of 0.5 gram in 2 ml	1.2–2 ml	2.4–3.6 ml	4–5.6 ml	6–7.6 ml	8–11.6 ml

	Dosage	Form	Dose according to body weight 3–<6 kg	6–<10 kg	10–<15 kg	15–<20 kg	20–29 kg
Chloroquine	Oral: Once a day for 3 days: 10 mg/kg on days 1 and 2 5 mg/kg on day 3	150 mg tablet		Day 1: 1/2 Day 2: 1/2 Day 3: 1/2	Day 1: 1 Day 2: 1 Day 3: 1/2	Day 1: 1 1/2 Day 2: 1 Day 3: 1	Day 1: 1 1/2 Day 2: 1 1/2 Day 3: 1
		100 mg tablet	Day 1: 1/2 Day 2: 1/2 Day 3: 1/2	Day 1: 1 Day 2: 1 Day 3: 1/2	Day 1: 1 1/2 Day 2: 1 1/2 Day 3: 1/2	Day 1: 2 Day 2: 2 Day 3: 1	Day 1: 2 1/2 Day 2: 2 1/2 Day 3: 1
		50 mg base/ 5 ml syrup	Day 1: 5.0 ml Day 2: 5.0 ml Day 3: 2.5 ml	Day 1: 7.5 ml Day 2: 7.5 ml Day 3: 5.0 ml	Day 1: 15 ml Day 2: 15 ml Day 3: 10 ml	— — —	— — —
Chlorphenamine	IM/IV or SC: 0.25 mg/kg once (can be repeated up to 4 times in 24 hours	10 mg in 1 ml IV solution 4 mg tablet	0.1 ml	0.2 ml	0.3 ml	0.5 ml	0.6 ml
	Oral: 2–3 times daily	Tablet: 4 mg	—	—	—	—	1/2
Ciprofloxacin	Oral: 10–15 mg/kg per dose given twice per day for 5 days (max 500 mg per dose)	100 mg tablet 250 mg tablet	1/2 1/4	1 1/2	1 1/2 1/2	2 1	3 1 1/2

Ciprofloxacin in children: use is only warranted if the benefits outweigh the risks of arthropathy.

	Dosage	Form	Dose according to body weight				
			3–<6 kg	6–<10 kg	10–<15 kg	15–<20 kg	20–29 kg
Cloxacillin/ flucloxacillin/ oxacillin§	IV: 25–50 mg/kg every 6 hours (50 mg/kg dose in brackets)	vial of 500 mg mixed with 8 ml sterile water to give 500 mg/10 mls	2–(4) ml§	4–(8) ml	6–(12) ml	8–(16) ml	12–(24) ml
	IM	vial of 250 mg mixed with 1.3 ml sterile water to give 250 mg/1.5 ml	0.6 (1.2) ml§	1 (2) ml	1.8 (3.6) ml	2.5 (5) ml	3.75 (7.5) ml
		250 mg capsule	1/2 (1)§	1 (2)	1 (2)	2 (3)	2 (4)
For treating abscesses	15 mg/kg every 6 hours	250 mg capsule	1/4	1/2	1	1 1/2	2 1/2

§ For dosage and dosage intervals in neonates and premature infants, see page 64.

	Dosage	Form	3–<6 kg	6–<10 kg	10–<15 kg	15–<20 kg	20–29 kg
Codeine *For analgesia*	Oral: 0.5–1 mg/kg every 6–12 hours	15 mg tablet	1/4	1/4	1/2	1/2	1 1/2

	Dosage	Form	Dose according to body weight 3–<6 kg	6–<10 kg	10–<15 kg	15–<20 kg	20–29 kg
Cotrimoxazole§ (trimethoprim-sulfamethoxazole, TMP-SMX)	4 mg trimethoprim/kg and 20 mg sulfa-methoxazole/kg two times per day	Oral: adult tablet (80 mg TMP + 400 mg SMX)	1/4§	1/2	1	1	1
		Oral: paediatric tablet (20 mg TMP + 100 mg SMX)	1	2	3	3	4
		Oral: syrup (40 mg TMP + 200 mg SMX per 5 ml)	2 ml§	3.5 ml	6 ml	8.5 ml	—

Note: For interstitial pneumonia in children with HIV give 8 mg/kg TMP and 40 mg SMX/kg 3 times a day for 3 weeks.
§ If the child is aged <1 month, give cotrimoxazole (1/2 paediatric tablet or 1.25 ml syrup) twice daily. Avoid cotrimoxazole in neonates who are premature or jaundiced.

	Dosage	Form	3–<6 kg	6–<10 kg	10–<15 kg	15–<20 kg	20–29 kg
Deferoxamine *For iron poisoning*	15 mg/kg/hr IV to maximum of 80 mg/kg in 24 hours or 50 mg/kg IM up to a maximum of 1g IM	500 mg ampoule	2	2	2	2	2
Dexamethasone *For severe viral croup*	Oral: 0.6mg/kg single dose	0.5 mg tablets IM: 5 mg/ml	0.5 ml	0.9 ml	1.4 ml	2 ml	3 ml

	Dosage	Form	Dose according to body weight 3–<6 kg	6–<10 kg	10–<15 kg	15–<20 kg	20–29 kg
Diazepam							
For convulsions	Rectal: 0.5 mg/kg	10 mg/2 ml solution	0.4 ml§	0.75 ml	1.2 ml	1.7 ml	2.5 ml
	IV: 0.2–0.3 mg/kg		0.25 ml§	0.4 ml	0.6 ml	0.75 ml	1.25 ml
For sedation before procedures	0.1–0.2 mg/kg IV						

§ Give phenobarbital (20 mg/kg IV or IM) instead of diazepam to neonates. If convulsions continue, give 10 mg/kg IV or IM after 30 minutes. The maintenance dose of oral phenobarbital is 2.5–5 mg/kg.

Didanosine—see separate table for HIV drugs, page 350

	Dosage	Form	3–<6 kg	6–<10 kg	10–<15 kg	15–<20 kg	20–29 kg
Digoxin	*These doses are for oral digoxin. Give as an initial loading dose followed by twice daily maintenance doses, starting 6 hours after the loading dose as set out below:*						
	Loading dose: 15 micrograms per kg, once only	62.5 microgram tablets	$^{3}/_{4}$–1	1$^{1}/_{2}$–2	2$^{1}/_{2}$–3$^{1}/_{2}$	3$^{1}/_{2}$–4$^{1}/_{2}$	—
		125 microgram tablets	—	—	1–1$^{1}/_{2}$	1$^{3}/_{4}$–2	2$^{1}/_{2}$–3
	Maintenance dose: (Start 6 hours after loading dose) 5 micrograms per kg every 12 hours (max 250 micrograms per dose)	62.5 microgram tablets	$^{1}/_{4}$–$^{1}/_{2}$	$^{1}/_{2}$–$^{3}/_{4}$	$^{3}/_{4}$–1	1$^{1}/_{4}$–1$^{1}/_{2}$	1$^{1}/_{2}$–2$^{1}/_{4}$

Efavirenz—see separate table for HIV drugs, page 348

	Dosage	Form	Dose according to body weight				
			3–<6 kg	6–<10 kg	10–<15 kg	15–<20 kg	20–29 kg
Epinephrine (adrenaline)							
For wheeze	*Calculate EXACT dose based on body weight (as rapid-acting bronchodilator)* 0.01 ml/kg (up to a maximum of 0.3 ml) of 1:1000 solution (or 0.1 ml/kg of 1:10 000 solution) given sub-cutaneously with a 1 ml syringe						
For severe viral croup	a trial of 2 ml of 1:1000 nebulized solution		—	2 ml	2 ml	2 ml	2 ml
For anaphylaxis	0.01 ml/kg of 1:1000 solution or 0.1 ml/kg of 1:10 000 solution given subcutaneously with a 1 ml syringe						
Note: Make a 1:10 000 solution by adding 1 ml of 1:1000 solution to 9 ml of normal saline or 5% glucose.							
Erythromycin§ (estolate)	Oral: 12.5 mg/kg 4 times a day for 3 days	250 mg tablet	1/4	1/2	1	1	1 1/2

§ Must NOT be given together with theophylline (aminophylline) due to risk of serious adverse reactions.

	Dosage	Form	Dose according to body weight 3–<6 kg	6–<10 kg	10–<15 kg	15–<20 kg	20–29 kg
Fluconazole	3–6 mg/kg once a day	50 mg/5 ml oral suspension	—	—	5 ml	7.5 ml	12.5 ml
		50 mg capsule	—	—	1	1–2	2–3
Flucloxacillin—see cloxacillin							
Furazolidone	1.25 mg/kg 4 times per day for 3 days	Oral: 100 mg tablet	—	—	1/4	1/4	1/4
Furosemide (frusemide) *For cardiac failure*	Oral or IV: 1–2 mg/kg every 12 hours	20 mg tablets IV 10 mg/ml	1/4–1/2 0.4–0.8 ml	1/2–1 0.8–1.6 ml	1/2–1 1.2–2.4 ml	1–2 1.7–3.4 ml	1 1/4–2 1/2 2.5–5 ml
Gentamicin§	*Calculate EXACT dose based on body weight and only use these doses where this is not possible.*						
	7.5 mg/kg once per day	IM/IV: vial containing 20 mg (2ml at 10 mg/ml) undiluted	2.25–3.75 ml†	4.5–6.75 ml	7.5–10.5 ml	—	—
		IM/IV: vial containing 80 mg (2ml at 40 mg/ml) mixed with 6 ml sterile water	2.25–3.75ml†	4.5–6.75 ml	7.5–10.5 ml	—	—
		IM/IV: vial containing 80 mg (2ml at 40 mg/ml) undiluted	0.5–0.9 ml†	1.1–1.7 ml	1.9–2.6 ml	2.8–3.5 ml	3.75–5.4 ml

§ Beware of the risk of adverse effects with theophylline. In administering an aminoglycoside (gentamicin, kanamycin), it is preferable to avoid use of undiluted 40 mg/ml gentamicin.

† For dosage and dosage intervals in neonates and premature infants, see page 65.

	Dosage	Form	Dose according to body weight 3–<6 kg	6–<10 kg	10–<15 kg	15–<20 kg	20–29 kg
Gentian violet	Topical application to skin						
Ibuprofen	5–10 mg/kg orally 6–8 hourly to a maximum of 500 mg per day	200 mg tablet	—	1/4	1/4	1/2	3/4
		400 mg tablet	—	—	—	1/4	1/2
Iron	Once per day for 14 days	Iron/folate tablet (ferrous sulfate 200 mg + 250 µg folate = 60 mg elemental iron	—	—	1/2	1/2	1
		Iron syrup (ferrous fumarate, 100 mg per 5 ml = 20 mg/ml elemental iron)	1 ml	1.25 ml	2 ml	2.5 ml	4 ml
Kanamycin	Calculate EXACT dose based on body weight. Only use these doses if this is not possible.						
	IM/IV: 20 mg/kg once a day	250 mg vial (2 ml at 125 mg/ml)	0.5–0.8 ml†	1–1.5 ml	1.6–2.2 ml	2.4–3 ml	3.2–4.6 ml

† For dosage and dosage intervals in neonates and premature infants, see page 65.

	Dosage	Form	Dose according to body weight 3–<6 kg	6–<10 kg	10–<15 kg	15–<20 kg	20–29 kg
Ketamine§							
For anaesthesia in major procedures	*Calculate EXACT dose based on surface area (see page 325) or body weight.*						
	IM: **Loading dose:** 5–8 mg/kg		20–35 mg	40–60 mg	60–100 mg	80–140 mg	125–200 mg
	IM: **Further dose:** 1–2 mg/kg (if required)		5–10 mg	8–15 mg	12–25 mg	15–35 mg	25–50 mg
	IV: **Loading dose:** 1–2 mg/kg		5–10 mg	8–15 mg	12–25 mg	15–35 mg	25–50 mg
	IV: **Further dose:** 0.5–1 mg/kg(if required)		2.5–5 mg	4–8 mg	6–12 mg	8–15 mg	12–25 mg
For light anaesthesia in minor procedures	IM: 2–4 mg/kg IV: 0.5–1 mg/kg						
§ Dose details and method of administration are given on page 229–230.							
Lamivudine—see separate table for HIV drugs, page 348							
Lidocaine	Apply topically (see page 222) Local injection 4–5 mg/kg/dose as local anaesthetic						
Mebendazole	100 mg 2 times a day for 3 days	100 mg tablet	—	—	1	1	1
	500 mg once only	100 mg tablet	—	—	5	5	5
Mefloquine	10 mg/kg orally	250 mg tablet	—	1/2	1/2	1	1
Not recommended for children <5 months of age due to limited data.							

	Dosage	Form	Dose according to body weight				
			3–<6 kg	6–<10 kg	10–<15 kg	15–<20 kg	20–29 kg
Metoclopramide *For nausea/ vomiting)*	0.1–0.2 mg/kg every 8 hours as required	10 mg tablets	—	—	1/4	1/4	1/2
		Injection: 5 mg/ml	—	—	0.5 ml	0.7 ml	1 ml
Metronidazole	Oral: 7.5 mg/kg 3 times a day for 7 days§	200 mg tablet	—	1/4	1/2	1/2	1
		400 mg tablet	—	—	1/4	1/4	1/2
§ For the treatment of giardiasis, the dose is 5 mg/kg; for amoebiasis, 10 mg/kg.							
Morphine	*Calculate EXACT dose based on weight of the child.* Oral: 0.2–0.4 mg/kg 4–6 hourly; increase if necessary for severe pain IM: 0.1–0.2 mg/kg 4–6 hourly IV: 0.05–0.1 mg/kg 4–6 hourly or 0.005–0.01 mg/kg/hour by IV infusion						
Nalidixic acid	Oral: 15 mg/kg 4 4 times a day for 5 days	250 mg tablet	1/4	1/2	1	1	1 1/2
Nelfinavir—see separate table for HIV drugs, page 351							
Nevirapine—see separate table for HIV drugs, page 348							
Nystatin	Oral:100 000–200 000 units into the mouth	oral suspension 100,000 units/ml	1–2ml	1–2ml	1–2ml	1–2ml	1–2ml
Oxacillin—see cloxacillin							
Paracetamol	10–15 mg/kg, up to 4 times a day	100 mg tablet	—	1	1	2	3
		500 mg tablet	—	1/4	1/4	1/2	1/2

	Dosage	Form	Dose according to body weight 3–<6 kg	6–<10 kg	10–<15 kg	15–<20 kg	20–29 kg
Paraldehyde	Rectal: 0.3–0.4 ml/kg IM: 0.2 ml/kg	5 ml vial	1.4 ml 0.8 ml	2.4 ml 1.5 ml	4 ml 2.4 ml	5 ml 3.4 ml	7.5 ml 5 ml
PENICILLIN **Benzathine benzylpenicillin**	50 000 units/kg once a day	IM: vial of 1.2 million units mixed with 4 ml sterile water	0.5 ml	1 ml	2 ml	3 ml	4 ml
Benzylpenicillin (penicillin G) *General dosage*	IV: 50 000 units/kg every 6 hours	vial of 600 mg mixed with 9.6 ml sterile water to give 1 000 000 units/10 ml	2 ml§	3.75 ml	6 ml	8.5 ml	12.5 ml
	IM:	vial of 600 mg (1 000 000 units) mixed with 1.6 ml sterile water to give 1,000,000 units/2 ml	0.4 ml§	0.75 ml	1.2 ml	1.7 ml	2.5 ml
For meningitis	100 000 units/kg every 6 hours	IV IM	4 ml§ 0.8 ml§	7.5 ml 1.5 ml	12 ml 2.5 ml	17 ml 3.5 ml	25 ml 5 ml
Procaine benzylpenicillin	IM: 50 000 units/kg once a day	3 g vial (3 000 000 units) mixed with 4 ml sterile water	0.25 ml	0.5 ml	0.8 ml	1.2 ml	1.7 ml

§ For dosage and dosage intervals in neonates and premature infants, see page 66.

	Dosage	Form	Dose according to body weight				
			3–<6 kg	6–<10 kg	10–<15 kg	15–<20 kg	20–29 kg
Phenobarbital	IM: **Loading dose:** 15 mg/kg IM	200 mg/ml solution	0.4 ml§	0.6 ml	1.0 ml	1.5 ml	2.0 ml
	Oral or IM: **Maintenance dose:** 2.5–5 mg/kg	0.1 ml	0.15 ml	0.25 ml	0.35 ml	0.5 ml	
§ Give phenobarbital (20 mg/kg IV or IM) instead of diazepam to neonates. If convulsions continue, give 10 mg/kg IV or IM after 30 minutes.							
Pivmecillinam	Oral: 20 mg/kg 4 4 times a day for 5 days	200 mg tablet	1/2	3/4	1	1 1/2	2
Potassium	2–4 mmol/kg/day						
Prednisolone§	Oral: 1 mg/kg twice a day for 3 days	5 mg tablet	1	1	2	3	5

§ 1 mg prednisolone is equivalent to 5 mg hydrocortisone or 0.15 mg dexamethasone.

	Dosage	Form	Dose according to body weight 3–<6 kg	6–<10 kg	10–<15 kg	15–<20 kg	20–29 kg
Quinine (mg/kg expressed as mg of quinine hydrochloride salt)	IV: **Loading dose:** 20 mg salt/kg given slowly over 4 hours after diluting with 10 ml/kg of IV fluid		*Loading dose is double the maintenance dose given below*				
	IV: **Maintenance dose:** 10 mg salt/kg given slowly over 2 hours after diluting with 10 ml/kg of IV fluid	IV (undiluted): quinine dihydrochloride injection 150 mg/ml (in 2 ml ampoules)	0.3 ml	0.6 ml	1 ml	1.2 ml	2 ml
	If IV infusion is not possible, quinine dihydrochloride can be be given in the same dosages by IM injection.	IV (undiluted): quinine dihydrochloride injection 300 mg/ml (in 2 ml ampoules)	0.2 ml	0.3 ml	0.5 ml	0.6 ml	1 ml
		IM quinine dihydro-chloride (diluted): in normal saline to a concentration of 60 mg salt/ml	1 ml	1.5 ml	2.5 ml	3 ml	5 ml
		Oral: quinine sulfate 200 mg tablet	1/4	1/2	3/4	1	1 1/2
		Oral: quinine sulfate 300 mg tablet	—	—	1/2	1/2	1

	Dosage	Form	Dose according to body weight				
			3–<6 kg	6–<10 kg	10–<15 kg	15–<20 kg	20–29 kg
Quinine *(continued)*							
Note: At 12 hours after the start of the loading dose, give the maintenance dose listed here over 2 hours. Repeat every 12 hours. Switch to oral treatment (10 mg/kg 3 times daily) when the child is able to take it, to complete a 7 days' treatment with quinine tablets or give a single dose of SP (see below).							
Ritonavir—see separate table for HIV drugs, page 352							
Salbutamol	Oral: 1 mg per dose <1 year 2 mg per dose 1–4 years	syrup: 2 mg/5 ml	2.5 ml	2.5 ml	5 ml	5 ml	5 ml
	Acute episode 6–8 hourly	tablets: 2 mg tablets: 4 mg	1/2 1/4	1/2 1/4	1 1/2	1 1/2	1 1/2
	Inhaler with spacer: 2 doses contains 200 µg	metered dose inhaler containing 200 doses					
	Nebulizer: 2.5 mg/dose	5 mg/ml solution 2.5 mg in 2.5 ml single dose units					
Saquinavir—see separate table for HIV drugs, page 352							
Silver sulfadiazine—apply topically to area of affected skin							

	Dosage	Form	Dose according to body weight				
			3–<6 kg	6–<10 kg	10–<15 kg	15–<20 kg	20–29 kg
Spectinomycin *For neonatal ophthalmia*	IM: 25 mg/kg single dose (maximum of 75 mg)	2 gram vial in 5 ml diluent	0.25 ml	—	—	—	—
Sulfadoxine-pyrimethamine (SP)	Oral: 25 mg sulfadoxine and 1.25 mg pyrimethamine/kg single doses only	tablet (500 mg sulfadoxine + 25 mg pyrimethamine)	1/4	1/2	1	1	1 1/2
Topical TAC (tetracaine, adrenaline, cocaine): Apply topically before painful procedures.							
Tetracycline§	12.5 mg/kg 4 times a day for 3 days	250 mg tablet	—	1/2	1/2	1	1
§ Give to children only for treatment of cholera because of permanent staining of teeth.							
Vitamin A	Once per day for 2 days	200 000 IU capsule	—	1/2	1	1	1
		100 000 IU capsule	1/2	1	2	2	2
		50 000 IU capsule	1	2	4	4	4
Zidovudine—see separate table for HIV drugs, page 349							

DRUGS

Anti-retrovirals

	Dosage	Form	Dose according to body weight 3–<6 kg	6–<10 kg	10–<15 kg	15–<20 kg	20–29 kg
Calculate EXACT dose based on surface area (see page 325) or body weight. Note that children with HIV infection are often stunted.							
FIRST LINE DRUGS							
Efavirenz (EFV)	Oral: 15 mg/kg once per day (at night)	syrup 30 mg/ml 50 mg capsules 200 mg capsules					
Note: For children over 10 kg and over 3 years only							
Lamivudine (3TC)	Oral: 4 mg/kg twice per day (maximum of 150 mg per dose)	10 mg/ml suspension 150 mg tablet					
	Oral: in neonates: 2 mg/kg twice per day	10 mg/ml suspension					
Nevirapine (NVP)	Oral: 120–200 mg/m² twice per day (maximum 200 mg per dose)	syrup 10 mg/ml 200 mg tablet					

Experience with ARV dosages in children is limited and due to change. For dosage of individual formulations, refer to national guidelines or www.who.int/hiv

	Dosage	Form	Dose according to body weight				
			3–<6 kg	6–<10 kg	10–<15 kg	15–<20 kg	20–29 kg
Calculate EXACT dose based on surface area (see page 325) or body weight. Note that children with HIV infection are often stunted.							
Stavudine (d4T)	1 mg/kg twice per day	Oral: liquid suspension 1 mg/ml Oral: capsules 15 mg Oral: capsules 20 mg	***Experience with ARV dosages in children is limited and due to change. For dosage of individual formulations, refer to national guidelines or www.who.int/hiv***				
Zidovudine (ZDV; AZT)	4 mg/kg twice per day	Oral: 10 mg/ml liquid Oral: capsules 100 mg Oral: tablets 300 mg					
COMBINATIONS							
Duovir (3TC+ZDV)	Twice daily	Oral: tablets of 150 mg 3TC *plus* 300 mg ZDV *plus*	***Experience with ARV dosages in children is limited and due to change. For dosage of individual formulations, refer to national guidelines or www.who.int/hiv***				
Note: Must be used with either NVP or EFV.							
Triomune (3TC+d4T+NVP)	Twice daily	Oral: tablets of 150 mg 3TC *plus* 200 mg NVP *plus* 30 mg d4T *OR* 150 mg 3TC *plus* 200 mg NVP *plus* 40 mg d4T					

	Dosage	Form	Dose according to body weight				
			3–<6 kg	6–<10 kg	10–<15 kg	15–<20 kg	20–29 kg
Calculate EXACT dose based on surface area (see page 325) or body weight. Note that children with HIV infection are often stunted.							
SECOND LINE DRUGS							
Abacavir (ABC, GW 1592U89, Ziagen)	Oral: 8 mg/kg Twice per day only for children > 3 months (maximum of 300 mg per dose)	liquid suspension 20 mg/ml tablets 300 mg					
Didanosine (ddI, dideoxyinosine)	Oral: Young infants <3 months 50 mg/m² twice per day Children > 3months 120 mg/m² twice per day	enteric coated powder in capsules 30 mg (=25 mg) 60 mg (=50 mg) 115 mg (=100 mg) 170 mg (=150 mg) 230 mg (=200 mg) 285 mg (=250 mg)					
	Combine sachets containing different doses to obtain the required dose.						

Experience with ARV dosages in children is limited and due to change. For dosage of individual formulations, refer to national guidelines or www.who.int/hiv

Note: 75 mg = sachet of 50 mg plus sachet of 25 mg; 125 mg = sachet of 100 mg plus sachet of 25 mg; 150 mg = sachet of 150 mg; 200 mg = sachet of 200 mg. Tablets are poorly tolerated.

	Dosage	Form	Dose according to body weight 3–<6 kg	6–<10 kg	10–<15 kg	15–<20 kg	20–29 kg
Calculate EXACT dose based on surface area (see page 325) or body weight. Note that children with HIV infection are often stunted.							
Lopinavir/ritonavir (LPV/r)	Oral: Child 7–15 kg: 12 mg/kg lopinavir; 3 mg/kg ritonavir Child 15–40 kg: 10 mg/kg lopinavir; 2.5 mg/kg ritonavir Twice per day (children over 6 months only)	suspension 80 mg/ml lopinavir 20 mg/ml ritonavir capsules 133.3 mg lopinavir 33.3 mg ritonavir	***Experience with ARV dosages in children is limited and due to change. For dosage of individual formulations, refer to national guidelines or <u>www.who.int/hiv</u>***				
Nelfinavir (NFV)	Child over 2 years: 45–55 mg/kg (maximum of 2 g per dose) twice per day	250 mg tablet					
Saquinavir	50 mg/kg three times per day	capsule 200 mg soft gel					

Anti-tuberculosis antibiotics

Calculate exact dose based on body weight

Essential anti-TB drug (abbreviation)	Mode of action	Daily dose: mg/kg (range)	Intermittent dose: 3 times/week mg/kg (range)
Ethambutol (E)	Bacteriostatic	20 (15–25)	30 (25–35)
Rifampicin (R)	Bactericidal	10 (8–12)	10 (8–12)
Isoniazid (H)	Bactericidal	5 (4–6)	10 (8–12)
Pyrazinamide (Z)	Bactericidal	25 (20–30)	35 (30–40)
Streptomycin (S)	Bactericidal	15 (12–18)	15 (12–18)
Thioacetazone (T)	Bacteriostatic	3	Not applicable

Note: Avoid thioacetazone in a child who is known to be HIV-infected or when the likelihood of HIV infection is high, because severe (sometimes fatal) skin reactions can occur.

Notes

Notes

DRUGS

APPENDIX 3

Equipment size for children

Appropriate sizes of paediatric equipment according to age (weight) of child

Equipment	0–5 months (3–6 kg)	6–12 months (4–9 kg)	1–3 years (10–15 kg)	4–7 years (16–20 kg)
Airway and breathing				
Laryngoscope	straight blade	straight blade	child macintosh	child macintosh
Uncuffed tracheal tube	2.5–3.5	3.5–4.0	4.0–5.0	5.0–6.0
Stylet	small	small	small/ medium	medium
Suction catheter (FG)	6	8	10/12	14
Circulation				
IV cannula	24/22	22	22/18	20/16
Central venous cannula	20	20	18	18
Other equipment				
Nasogastric tube†	8	10	10–12	12
Urinary catheter†	5 feeding tube	5 feeding tube/F8	Foley 8	Foley 10

† Sizes in French gauge (FG) or Charrière, which are equivalent and indicate the circumference of the tube in millimetres.

Notes

APPENDIX 4

Intravenous fluids

The following table gives the composition of intravenous fluids that are commercially available and commonly used in neonates, infants and children. For consideration on which fluid to use in particular circumstances, see the disease-specific chapters, e.g. for shock (pages 12–13), for neonates (page 51), for severely malnourished children (179), for surgical procedures (232), and for general supportive therapy (273). Please note that none of the fluids contains sufficient calories for the long-term nutritional support of children, but that some fluids contain less than others. Wherever feeding and fluids by mouth or nasogastric tube are possible, this is preferable.

	Composition						
IV fluid	Na^+ mmol/l	K^+ mmol/l	Cl^- mmol/l	Ca^{++} mmol/l	Lactate mmol/l	Glucose g/l	Calories /l
Ringer's lactate (Hartmann's)	130	5.4	112	1.8	27	–	–
Normal saline (0.9% NaCl)	154	–	154	–	–	–	–
5% Glucose	–	–	–	–	–	50	200
10% Glucose	–	–	–	–	–	100	400
0.45 NaCl / 5% glucose	77	–	77	–	–	50	200
0.18% NaCl / 4% glucose	31	–	31	–	–	40	160
Darrow's solution	121	35	103	–	53	–	–
Half-strength Darrow's with 5% glucose*	61	17	52	–	27	50	200
Half-strength Ringer's lactate with 5% glucose	65	2.7	56	1	14	50	200

* Please note that half-strength Darrow's solution often comes without glucose and glucose needs to be added before use.

Notes

APPENDIX 5

Assessing nutritional status

A5.1 Calculating the child's weight-for-age

To calculate a child's weight for age, use the table below or the chart on page 363. For using the table:

- Locate the row containing the child's age in the central column of Table 34.
- Look to the left in that row for boys, and to the right for girls.
- Note where the child's weight lies with respect to the weights recorded in this row.
- Look up the adjacent column to read the weight-for-age of the child.

  Example 1: Boy: age 5 months, weight 5.3 kg; He is between -2 and -3 SD

  Example 2: Girl: age 27 months, weight 6.5 kg; She is less than -4 SD.

The lines in the chart on page 363 correspond to -2 (low weight-for-age) and -3 SD (very low weight-for-age).

Please note that you should use Table 35 on page 365 for weight-for-height to determine whether a child is severely malnourished.

WEIGHT/HEIGHT

Table 34. Weight-for-age

Boys' weight (kg)					Age	Girls' weight (kg)				
-4SD	-3SD	-2SD	-1SD	Median	(months)	Median	-1SD	-2SD	-3SD	-4SD
1.63	2.04	2.45	2.86	3.27	**0**	3.23	2.74	2.24	1.75	1.26
1.55	2.24	2.92	3.61	4.29	**1**	3.98	3.39	2.79	2.19	1.59
1.76	2.62	3.47	4.33	5.19	**2**	4.71	4.03	3.35	2.67	1.99
2.18	3.13	4.08	5.03	5.98	**3**	5.40	4.65	3.91	3.16	2.42
2.73	3.72	4.70	5.69	6.68	**4**	6.05	5.25	4.46	3.66	2.87
3.34	4.33	5.32	6.31	7.30	**5**	6.65	5.82	4.98	4.15	3.31
3.94	4.92	5.89	6.87	7.85	**6**	7.21	6.34	5.47	4.60	3.73
4.47	5.44	6.41	7.37	8.34	**7**	7.71	6.80	5.90	5.00	4.09
4.92	5.89	6.85	7.82	8.78	**8**	8.16	7.22	6.29	5.35	4.42
5.30	6.27	7.24	8.21	9.18	**9**	8.56	7.59	6.63	5.66	4.70
5.62	6.60	7.58	8.56	9.54	**10**	8.92	7.92	6.93	5.93	4.94
5.88	6.88	7.87	8.87	9.86	**11**	9.24	8.22	7.20	6.17	5.15

Boys' weight (kg)					Age	Girls' weight (kg)				
-4SD	-3SD	-2SD	-1SD	Median	(months)	Median	-1SD	-2SD	-3SD	-4SD
6.09	7.11	8.12	9.14	10.15	**12**	9.53	8.48	7.43	6.39	5.34
6.26	7.30	8.34	9.38	10.41	**13**	9.79	8.72	7.65	6.57	5.50
6.40	7.46	8.53	9.59	10.65	**14**	10.03	8.93	7.84	6.74	5.64
6.51	7.60	8.69	9.78	10.87	**15**	10.25	9.13	8.01	6.89	5.78
6.60	7.72	8.84	9.96	11.08	**16**	10.45	9.31	8.17	7.04	5.90
6.68	7.83	8.98	10.13	11.28	**17**	10.64	9.49	8.33	7.18	6.02
6.76	7.93	9.11	10.29	11.47	**18**	10.83	9.65	8.48	7.31	6.14
6.83	8.04	9.25	10.45	11.66	**19**	11.01	9.82	8.64	7.46	6.27
6.91	8.15	9.38	10.61	11.85	**20**	11.19	9.99	8.80	7.60	6.41
7.00	8.26	9.52	10.78	12.04	**21**	11.37	10.16	8.96	7.75	6.54
7.08	8.37	9.65	10.94	12.22	**22**	11.55	10.33	9.12	7.90	6.68
7.17	8.48	9.79	11.10	12.41	**23**	11.73	10.50	9.28	8.05	6.82
7.84	8.97	10.09	11.22	12.34	**24**	11.80	10.62	9.45	8.28	7.10
7.85	9.03	10.20	11.37	12.54	**25**	12.01	10.81	9.61	8.40	7.20
7.87	9.09	10.30	11.52	12.74	**26**	12.23	10.99	9.76	8.53	7.29
7.89	9.15	10.41	11.68	12.94	**27**	12.43	11.17	9.91	8.65	7.39
7.91	9.22	10.52	11.83	13.13	**28**	12.63	11.35	10.06	8.77	7.48
7.94	9.28	10.63	11.98	13.33	**29**	12.83	11.52	10.21	8.89	7.58
7.97	9.36	10.74	12.13	13.52	**30**	13.03	11.69	10.35	9.01	7.67
8.00	9.43	10.85	12.28	13.71	**31**	13.22	11.85	10.49	9.13	7.76
8.04	9.51	10.97	12.43	13.89	**32**	13.40	12.01	10.63	9.24	7.85
8.09	9.58	11.08	12.58	14.08	**33**	13.58	12.17	10.76	9.35	7.94
8.13	9.66	11.20	12.73	14.26	**34**	13.76	12.33	10.90	9.46	8.03
8.18	9.75	11.31	12.88	14.44	**35**	13.93	12.48	11.03	9.57	8.12
8.24	9.83	11.43	13.03	14.62	**36**	14.10	12.63	11.15	9.68	8.21
8.29	9.92	11.55	13.18	14.80	**37**	14.27	12.78	11.28	9.79	8.29
8.35	10.01	11.67	13.32	14.98	**38**	14.44	12.92	11.41	9.89	8.38
8.42	10.10	11.79	13.47	15.16	**39**	14.60	13.06	11.53	9.99	8.46
8.48	10.19	11.91	13.62	15.33	**40**	14.76	13.20	11.65	10.10	8.54
8.55	10.29	12.03	13.77	15.51	**41**	14.91	13.34	11.77	10.20	8.62
8.62	10.39	12.15	13.91	15.68	**42**	15.07	13.48	11.89	10.29	8.70
8.70	10.48	12.27	14.06	15.85	**43**	15.22	13.61	12.00	10.39	8.78
8.77	10.58	12.40	14.21	16.02	**44**	15.37	13.74	12.12	10.49	8.86
8.85	10.68	12.52	14.35	16.19	**45**	15.52	13.88	12.23	10.58	8.94
8.93	10.79	12.64	14.50	16.36	**46**	15.67	14.00	12.34	10.68	9.01
9.01	10.89	12.77	14.65	16.53	**47**	15.81	14.13	12.45	10.77	9.09

Boys' weight (kg)					Age	Girls' weight (kg)				
-4SD	-3SD	-2SD	-1SD	Median	(months)	Median	-1SD	-2SD	-3SD	-4SD
9.10	11.00	12.90	14.79	16.69	**48**	15.96	14.26	12.56	10.86	9.16
9.18	11.10	13.02	14.94	16.86	**49**	16.10	14.39	12.67	10.95	9.23
9.27	11.21	13.15	15.09	17.03	**50**	16.25	14.51	12.77	11.04	9.30
9.36	11.32	13.28	15.23	17.19	**51**	16.39	14.63	12.88	11.13	9.37
9.45	11.43	13.40	15.38	17.36	**52**	16.53	14.76	12.98	11.21	9.44
9.54	11.54	13.53	15.53	17.52	**53**	16.67	14.88	13.09	11.30	9.51
9.64	11.65	13.66	15.67	17.69	**54**	16.81	15.00	13.19	11.38	9.57
9.73	11.76	13.79	15.82	17.85	**55**	16.95	15.12	13.29	11.46	9.64
9.82	11.87	13.92	15.97	18.02	**56**	17.09	15.25	13.40	11.55	9.70
9.92	11.99	14.05	16.12	18.18	**57**	17.24	15.37	13.50	11.63	9.76
10.02	12.10	14.18	16.26	18.34	**58**	17.38	15.49	13.60	11.71	9.82
10.11	12.21	14.31	16.41	18.51	**59**	17.52	15.61	13.70	11.79	9.88
10.21	12.33	14.44	16.56	18.67	**60**	17.66	15.73	13.80	11.87	9.94
10.31	12.44	14.57	16.71	18.84	**61**	17.81	15.85	13.90	11.95	9.99
10.41	12.56	14.70	16.85	19.00	**62**	17.96	15.98	14.00	12.02	10.04
10.50	12.67	14.84	17.00	19.17	**63**	18.10	16.10	14.10	12.10	10.10
10.60	12.78	14.97	17.15	19.33	**64**	18.25	16.23	14.20	12.17	10.15
10.70	12.90	15.10	17.30	19.50	**65**	18.40	16.35	14.30	12.25	10.20
10.79	13.01	15.23	17.45	19.67	**66**	18.56	16.48	14.40	12.32	10.25
10.89	13.13	15.36	17.60	19.84	**67**	18.71	16.61	14.50	12.40	10.29
10.99	13.24	15.49	17.75	20.00	**68**	18.87	16.74	14.60	12.47	10.34
11.08	13.35	15.63	17.90	20.17	**69**	19.03	16.87	14.70	12.54	10.38
11.18	13.47	15.76	18.05	20.34	**70**	19.19	17.00	14.81	12.62	10.42
11.27	13.58	15.89	18.20	20.51	**71**	19.36	17.13	14.91	12.69	10.46
11.36	13.69	16.02	18.35	20.69	**72**	19.52	17.27	15.01	12.76	10.50
11.45	13.80	16.15	18.51	20.86	**73**	19.70	17.41	15.12	12.83	10.54
11.54	13.91	16.29	18.66	21.03	**74**	19.87	17.55	15.22	12.90	10.57
11.63	14.02	16.42	18.81	21.21	**75**	20.05	17.69	15.33	12.97	10.61
11.71	14.13	16.55	18.97	21.38	**76**	20.23	17.83	15.43	13.04	10.64
11.80	14.24	16.68	19.12	21.56	**77**	20.42	17.98	15.54	13.11	10.67
11.88	14.35	16.81	19.28	21.74	**78**	20.61	18.13	15.65	13.18	10.70
11.96	14.45	16.94	19.43	21.92	**79**	20.80	18.28	15.76	13.24	10.72
12.04	14.56	17.07	19.59	22.10	**80**	21.00	18.44	15.87	13.31	10.75
12.12	14.66	17.20	19.75	22.29	**81**	21.20	18.59	15.99	13.38	10.77
12.19	14.76	17.33	19.90	22.47	**82**	21.41	18.76	16.10	13.45	10.79
12.26	14.86	17.46	20.06	22.66	**83**	21.62	18.92	16.22	13.52	10.81

Boys' weight (kg)					Age	Girls' weight (kg)				
-4SD	-3SD	-2SD	-1SD	Median	(months)	Median	-1SD	-2SD	-3SD	-4SD
12.33	14.96	17.59	20.22	22.85	**84**	21.84	19.09	16.34	13.58	10.83
12.39	15.06	17.72	20.38	23.04	**85**	22.06	19.26	16.46	13.65	10.85
12.46	15.15	17.85	20.54	23.24	**86**	22.29	19.43	16.58	13.72	10.86
12.52	15.25	17.97	20.70	23.43	**87**	22.53	19.61	16.70	13.79	10.87
12.57	15.34	18.10	20.87	23.63	**88**	22.76	19.79	16.82	13.85	10.88
12.63	15.43	18.23	21.03	23.83	**89**	23.01	19.98	16.95	13.92	10.89
12.68	15.52	18.35	21.19	24.03	**90**	23.26	20.17	17.08	13.99	10.90
12.72	15.60	18.48	21.36	24.24	**91**	23.51	20.36	17.21	14.06	10.91
12.77	15.69	18.61	21.52	24.44	**92**	23.77	20.55	17.34	14.13	10.92
12.81	15.77	18.73	21.69	24.65	**93**	24.03	20.75	17.48	14.20	10.92
12.84	15.85	18.85	21.86	24.86	**94**	24.30	20.95	17.61	14.27	10.93
12.87	15.92	18.98	22.03	25.08	**95**	24.57	21.16	17.75	14.34	10.93
12.90	16.00	19.10	22.20	25.30	**96**	24.84	21.37	17.89	14.41	10.94
12.92	16.07	19.22	22.37	25.52	**97**	25.12	21.58	18.03	14.49	10.94
12.94	16.14	19.34	22.54	25.74	**98**	25.41	21.79	18.18	14.56	10.94
12.96	16.21	19.46	22.71	25.97	**99**	25.70	22.01	18.32	14.63	10.95
12.97	16.28	19.58	22.89	26.19	**100**	25.99	22.23	18.47	14.71	10.95
12.98	16.34	19.70	23.06	26.43	**101**	26.29	22.45	18.62	14.79	10.96
12.98	16.40	19.82	23.24	26.66	**102**	26.59	22.68	18.77	14.87	10.96
12.99	16.46	19.94	23.42	26.90	**103**	26.89	22.91	18.93	14.95	10.97
12.99	16.52	20.06	23.60	27.14	**104**	27.20	23.14	19.08	15.03	10.97
12.98	16.58	20.18	23.78	27.38	**105**	27.51	23.38	19.24	15.11	10.98
12.98	16.64	20.30	23.97	27.63	**106**	27.82	23.61	19.40	15.20	10.99
12.97	16.70	20.43	24.15	27.88	**107**	28.14	23.85	19.57	15.28	11.00
12.97	16.76	20.55	24.34	28.13	**108**	28.46	24.10	19.73	15.37	11.01
12.96	16.82	20.67	24.53	28.39	**109**	28.79	24.34	19.90	15.46	11.02
12.95	16.87	20.80	24.72	28.65	**110**	29.11	24.59	20.07	15.55	11.03
12.94	16.93	20.93	24.92	28.91	**111**	29.44	24.84	20.24	15.65	11.05
12.93	16.99	21.05	25.12	29.18	**112**	29.78	25.10	20.42	15.74	11.06
12.91	17.05	21.18	25.32	29.45	**113**	30.12	25.36	20.60	15.84	11.08
12.90	17.11	21.31	25.52	29.72	**114**	30.45	25.62	20.78	15.94	11.10
12.89	17.17	21.45	25.72	30.00	**115**	30.80	25.88	20.96	16.04	11.12
12.88	17.23	21.58	25.93	30.28	**116**	31.14	26.14	21.15	16.15	11.15
12.87	17.30	21.72	26.14	30.57	**117**	31.49	26.41	21.33	16.25	11.18
12.86	17.36	21.86	26.36	30.86	**118**	31.84	26.68	21.52	16.36	11.21
12.86	17.43	22.00	26.57	31.15	**119**	32.19	26.95	21.72	16.48	11.24

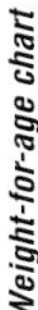

Weight-for-age chart

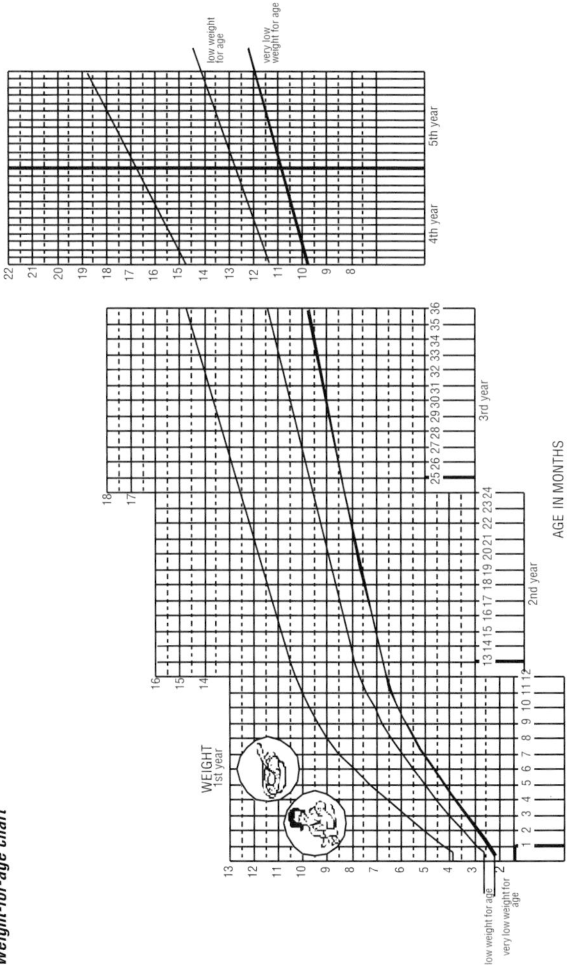

WEIGHT
1st year

2nd year

3rd year

4th year

5th year

AGE IN MONTHS

low weight for age

very low weight for age

A5.2 **Calculating the child's weight-for-length**

Determining child's % weight-for-length or SD weight-for-length

Refer to Table 35 on page 365.

- Locate the row containing the child's length in the central column of Table 35.
- Look to the left in that row for boys, and to the right for girls.
- Note where the child's weight lies with respect to the weights recorded in this row.
- Look up the adjacent column to read the weight-for-length of the child.

Example 1: Boy: length 61 cm, weight 5.3 kg;
this child is -1SD weight-for-length (90% of the median).

Example 2: Girl: length 67 cm, weight 4.3 kg;
this child is less than -4SD weight-for-length (less than 60% of the median).

Table 35. WHO/NCHS normalized reference weight-for-length (49–84 cm) and weight-for-height (85–110 cm), by sex

Boys' weight (kg)						Girls' weight (kg)				
-4SD 60%	-3SD 70%	-2SD 80%	-1SD 90%	Median	Length (cm)	Median	-1SD 90%	-2SD 80%	-3SD 70%	-4SD 60%
1.8	2.1	2.5	2.8	3.1	**49**	3.3	2.9	2.6	2.2	1.8
1.8	2.2	2.5	2.9	3.3	**50**	3.4	3	2.6	2.3	1.9
1.8	2.2	2.6	3.1	3.5	**51**	3.5	3.1	2.7	2.3	1.9
1.9	2.3	2.8	3.2	3.7	**52**	3.7	3.3	2.8	2.4	2
1.9	2.4	2.9	3.4	3.9	**53**	3.9	3.4	3	2.5	2.1
2	2.6	3.1	3.6	4.1	**54**	4.1	3.6	3.1	2.7	2.2
2.2	2.7	3.3	3.8	4.3	**55**	4.3	3.8	3.3	2.8	2.3
2.3	2.9	3.5	4	4.6	**56**	4.5	4	3.5	3	2.4
2.5	3.1	3.7	4.3	4.8	**57**	4.8	4.2	3.7	3.1	2.6
2.7	3.3	3.9	4.5	5.1	**58**	5	4.4	3.9	3.3	2.7
2.9	3.5	4.1	4.8	5.4	**59**	5.3	4.7	4.1	3.5	2.9
3.1	3.7	4.4	5	5.7	**60**	5.5	4.9	4.3	3.7	3.1
3.3	4	4.6	5.3	5.9	**61**	5.8	5.2	4.6	3.9	3.3
3.5	4.2	4.9	5.6	6.2	**62**	6.1	5.4	4.8	4.1	3.5
3.8	4.5	5.2	5.8	6.5	**63**	6.4	5.7	5	4.4	3.7
4	4.7	5.4	6.1	6.8	**64**	6.7	6	5.3	4.6	3.9
4.3	5	5.7	6.4	7.1	**65**	7	6.3	5.5	4.8	4.1
4.5	5.3	6	6.7	7.4	**66**	7.3	6.5	5.8	5.1	4.3
4.8	5.5	6.2	7	7.7	**67**	7.5	6.8	6	5.3	4.5
5.1	5.8	6.5	7.3	8	**68**	7.8	7.1	6.3	5.5	4.8
5.3	6	6.8	7.5	8.3	**69**	8.1	7.3	6.5	5.8	5
5.5	6.3	7	7.8	8.5	**70**	8.4	7.6	6.8	6	5.2
5.8	6.5	7.3	8.1	8.8	**71**	8.6	7.8	7	6.2	5.4
6	6.8	7.5	8.3	9.1	**72**	8.9	8.1	7.2	6.4	5.6
6.2	7	7.8	8.6	9.3	**73**	9.1	8.3	7.5	6.6	5.8
6.4	7.2	8	8.8	9.6	**74**	9.4	8.5	7.7	6.8	6
6.6	7.4	8.2	9	9.8	**75**	9.6	8.7	7.9	7	6.2
6.8	7.6	8.4	9.2	10	**76**	9.8	8.9	8.1	7.2	6.4
7	7.8	8.6	9.4	10.3	**77**	10	9.1	8.3	7.4	6.6
7.1	8	8.8	9.7	10.5	**78**	10.2	9.3	8.5	7.6	6.7
7.3	8.2	9	9.9	10.7	**79**	10.4	9.5	8.7	7.8	6.9
7.5	8.3	9.2	10.1	10.9	**80**	10.6	9.7	8.8	8	7.1

Boys' weight (kg)					Length (cm)	Girls' weight (kg)				
-4SD 60%	-3SD 70%	-2SD 80%	-1SD 90%	Median		Median	-1SD 90%	-2SD 80%	-3SD 70%	-4SD 60%
7.6	8.5	9.4	10.2	11.1	**81**	10.8	9.9	9	8.1	7.2
7.8	8.7	9.6	10.4	11.3	**82**	11	10.1	9.2	8.3	7.4
7.9	8.8	9.7	10.6	11.5	**83**	11.2	10.3	9.4	8.5	7.6
8.1	9	9.9	10.8	11.7	**84**	11.4	10.5	9.6	8.7	7.7
7.8	8.9	9.9	11	12.1	**85**	11.8	10.8	9.7	8.6	7.6
7.9	9	10.1	11.2	12.3	**86**	12	11	9.9	8.8	7.7
8.1	9.2	10.3	11.5	12.6	**87**	12.3	11.2	10.1	9	7.9
8.3	9.4	10.5	11.7	12.8	**88**	12.5	11.4	10.3	9.2	8.1
8.4	9.6	10.7	11.9	13	**89**	12.7	11.6	10.5	9.3	8.2
8.6	9.8	10.9	12.1	13.3	**90**	12.9	11.8	10.7	9.5	8.4
8.8	9.9	11.1	12..3	13.5	**91**	13.2	12	10.8	9.7	8.5
8.9	10.1	11.3	12.5	13.7	**92**	13.4	12.2	11	9.9	8.7
9.1	10.3	11.5	12.8	14	**93**	13.6	12.4	11.2	10	8.8
9.2	10.5	11.7	13	14.2	**94**	13.9	12.6	11.4	10.2	9
9.4	10.7	11.9	13.2	14.5	**95**	14.1	12.9	11.6	10.4	9.1
9.6	10.9	12.1	13.4	14.7	**96**	14.3	13.1	11.8	10.6	9.3
9.7	11	12.4	13.7	15	**97**	14.6	13.3	12	10.7	9.5
9.9	11.2	12.6	13.9	15.2	**98**	14.9	13.5	12.2	10.9	9.6
10.1	11.4	12.8	14.1	15.5	**99**	15.1	13.8	12.4	11.1	9.8
10.3	11.6	13	14.4	15.7	**100**	15.4	14	12.7	11.3	9.9
10.4	11.8	13.2	14.6	16	**101**	15.6	14.3	12.9	11.5	10.1
10.6	12	13.4	14.9	16.3	**102**	15.9	14.5	13.1	11.7	10.3
10.8	12.2	13.7	15.1	16.6	**103**	16.2	14.7	13.3	11.9	10.5
11	12.4	13.9	15.4	16.9	**104**	16.5	15	13.5	12.1	10.6
11.2	12.7	14.2	15.6	17.1	**105**	16.7	15.3	13.8	12.3	10.8
11.4	12.9	14.4	15.9	17.4	**106**	17	15.5	14	12.5	11
11.6	13.1	14.7	16.2	17.7	**107**	17.3	15.8	14.3	12.7	11.2
11.8	13.4	14.9	16.5	18	**108**	17.6	16.1	14.5	13	11.4
12	13.6	15.2	16.8	18.3	**109**	17.9	16.4	14.8	13.2	11.6
12.2	13.8	15.4	17.1	18.7	**110**	18.2	16.6	15	13.4	11.9

SD = standard deviation score or Z-score; although the interpretation of a fixed percent-of-median value varies across age and height, and generally the two scales cannot be compared; the approximate percent-of-the median values for -1 and -2SD are 90% and 80% of median respectively (*Bulletin of the World Health Organization*, 1994, **72**: 273–283).

Length is measured below 85 cm; height is measured 85 cm and above. Recumbent length is on average 0.5 cm greater than standing height, although the difference is of no importance to the individual child. A correction may be made by deducting 0.5 cm from all lengths above 84.9 cm if standing height cannot be measured.

Notes

Notes

APPENDIX 6

Job aids and charts

A pocket book does not allow the reproduction in a size to be readable of job aids and charts which people might find useful for their daily work. Several such job aids can be found in the manual *Management of the child with a serious infection or severe malnutrition.*

In addition, they can be downloaded in PDF format from the website of the WHO Department of Child and Adolescent Health and Development

http://www.who.int/child-adolescent-health/

Charts include:

- Monitoring chart
- Mother's card
- Weight chart
- 24-hour food-intake chart
- Daily ward feed chart

Notes

Index

Notes